Intracerebral Hemorrhage Therapeutics

Bruce Ovbiagele • Adnan I. Qureshi
Editors

Intracerebral Hemorrhage Therapeutics

Concepts and Customs

Springer

Editors
Bruce Ovbiagele
University of California, San Francisco
Medical Center
San Francisco, CA
USA

Adnan I. Qureshi
University of Minnesota
Minneapolis, MN
USA

ISBN 978-3-319-77062-8 ISBN 978-3-319-77063-5 (eBook)
https://doi.org/10.1007/978-3-319-77063-5

Library of Congress Control Number: 2018952921

This Springer imprint is published by the registered company Springer Nature Switzerland AG
The registered company address is: Gewerbestrasse 11, 6330 Cham, Switzerland

Foreword

What a breath of fresh air, this book with 12 deeply researched chapters, focusing on intracerebral hemorrhage therapeutics! It reflects a new mindset, emerging in the past decade, with concepts and practices, indeed new medical care customs, about treating a problem that had long eluded therapy.

For centuries, Galenic admonitions about the poor prognosis of "apoplexy," or the futility of treatment advocated in Avicenna's Canon of Medicine ("*Falej, La'tAalej*" translated as do not treat apoplectic stroke), had taken hold on our collective mindsets. Surely, intracerebral hemorrhage, accounting for a small fraction of strokes, has been recognized to exact disproportionate mortality, case disability, cost of care, and lost productivity. It was best prevented, mostly by chronic blood pressure control. But once blood was spilt in the brain or ventricles, it seemed to be an insurmountable disease. A doctor seemed best able to explain and prognosticate that the more blood spilt, the worse the outlook and provide comfort to patient and family and advice about hospice or long-term nursing care. Many doctors were taught, until recently, that survival may be worse than death, for patient, family, and society, after a bad intracerebral hemorrhage. It seemed that all damage occurs when the brain bleeds, and little could be done thereafter.

Yet new concepts emerged in the past decade, mostly with earlier diagnosis on the coattail of rapid transport of all stroke victims to hospitals, driven by the "time is brain" concepts of acute ischemic stroke management. It became clear that, in many cases of intracerebral hemorrhage, the bleed is still expanding in the early hours after symptom onset, with progressive clinical deterioration. Indeed, this hemorrhagic expansion has a huge impact on outcome and is modifiable, especially in the setting of coagulopathy and intractable blood pressure elevations. Limiting eventual volume of the bleed with rapid reversal of coagulopathy and blood pressure control can in fact improve outcome. Diagnostic studies now identify patients at risk of further hematoma expansion, and rigorous clinical trials have provided new guidelines for blood pressure control in the acute state. Other studies have mandated a new stance on rapid reversal of coagulopathy. These have impacted policies on the rapid transport, urgent diagnosis, and acute resuscitation of patients with intracerebral hemorrhage. Treatment of hydrocephalus and elevated intracranial pressure offers another opportunity to prevent secondary deterioration. Etiologic screening has come into play, as several special pathologies call for individualized management stances (venous thrombosis, arteriovenous malformations, moyamoya disease, cerebral aneurysms).

The concept of thrombotoxicity, modulating clinical decline over days rather than hours after an intracerebral hemorrhage, has reinvigorated questions about the value of evacuating the hematoma, not as much to reverse acute damage, but to prevent secondary sequelae and enhance survival and recovery potential. Yes, clinical trials of early and delayed hematoma evacuation by craniotomy have been disappointing, but we must remember that countless young patients with impending herniation, including expanding supratentorial lobar bleeds and cerebellar hematomas, have always been excluded from such trials and many have benefited from emergent surgery. Decompressive craniectomy has been deployed in many young patients with tight cranial vault, and dramatic gratifying recoveries have been recorded.

More recently, another glimmer of hope has emerged from the use of thrombolysis for enhanced evacuation of hematoma by intraventricular and intracerebral catheters. Feasibility and safety have been demonstrated in randomized clinical trials, protocols have been optimized, and the effectiveness of these therapies is being assessed in ongoing studies. Other minimally invasive surgical tools are being developed, with the same aim of injury-sparing hematoma evacuation. Indeed, perihematoma edema is blunted by such interventions, a critical proof of concept, and mortality is clearly improved. Effect on functional outcome, optimal patient selection and timing of intervention, and comparative techniques are motivating novel hypotheses and a new therapeutic discourse.

Critical care of the brain-injured patient and other multisystem support contribute to the prevention of countless secondary sequelae. Ethical issues have reinvigorated discussions regarding informed consent and the unresponsive patient, family and social dynamics, disparities of care, the implementation of advanced directives, or end of life management. And most exciting are new concepts about biomarkers and medical modifications of secondary injury and potential restorative interventions to enhance recovery.

This book cannot be more timely. It is edited by leaders in the field, with contributions by innovators who helped shape the above "concepts and customs." It tackles all the exciting innovations, and much more, with a mature pragmatic clinical perspective and scientific rigor. Each of the 12 chapters contains pearls of wisdom, likely to benefit actual patients. Students, novices, and experts can benefit from the knowledge and experiences shared herein. Moreover, the book instills the new way of thinking about intracerebral hemorrhage therapeutics in its new age.

Issam A. Awad, MD,MSc,FACS,FAANS,FAHA,MA(hon)
The John Harper Seeley Professor of Neurological Sciences
Professor of Surgery (Neurosurgery) and Neurology
University of Chicago Medicine and Biological Sciences
Chicago, IL, USA

Preface

Intracerebral hemorrhage (ICH) is a serious condition for which early aggressive care is often warranted. This book provides a framework for goal-targeted management of the patient with spontaneous nontraumatic intracerebral hemorrhage, which represents a major cause of morbidity and mortality throughout the world. While ICH has unfortunately trailed behind ischemic stroke with regard to compelling scientific evidence from clinical trials to guide management, over the past several years, advances in brain imaging have resulted in a better understanding of the pathophysiology of ICH, and there has been a welcome rise in the number of clinical trials assessing the impact of various interventions to improve ICH outcomes. With this backdrop, it is an opportune time to summarize current knowledge of ICH and its management from a practical view.

Intracerebral Hemorrhage Therapeutics is a timely and consolidated resource for clinicians, which captures novel strategies and the ever-increasing pace of discovery that is transforming what we know about ICH and its treatment. Topics addressed in a comprehensive yet practical manner in the book include prehospital/emergency department care, early inpatient workup, antithrombotic- and thrombolytic-related strokes, optimal blood pressure management, avoidance of medical complications, surgical interventions, outcome prognostication, recurrence prevention, rehabilitation/recovery, special situations, systems of care, and the design of clinical trials for patients with ICH. Procedures, processes, and helpful decision-making algorithms are presented with the aid of complementary illustrations that facilitate understanding of practical aspects and enable the reader to promptly retrieve relevant information. Prominent academicians with broad clinical practice experience from all over the world present the underlying evidence (or lack thereof) behind prevailing therapeutic strategies for treating ICH. Throughout, the style delivered is both holistic and multidisciplinary. It should however be noted that the book is primarily focused on ICH management in adults, and not necessarily in children and neonates.

As appropriate, each chapter reviews currently available therapies, discusses key controversial or unresolved management issues, and highlights promising future areas of therapeutic focus under investigation. In areas, where evidence is limited or lacking, our expert contributors provide their own management recommendations. Reference lists at the end of each chapter direct readers to important articles for more thorough reading on a particular subject.

Intracerebral Hemorrhage Therapeutics will be of value to primary care physicians, geriatricians, emergency care physicians, hospitalists, general neurologists, neuro-hospitalists, vascular neurologists in training, and vascular neurology board recertification candidates, because it provides a detailed review of the most current evidence-based therapies for routine management of ICH patients and a glimpse of promising future treatment strategies. Moreover, the book allows practitioners in other disciplines to become more familiar with the terminology and techniques that vascular neurologists and neurosurgeons frequently use to aid them in their ICH management practice.

Finally, we are especially grateful to our contributors for lending their time and expertise, our families for providing their moral support, as well as our patients and trainees for teaching us so much.

San Francisco, CA, USA Bruce Ovbiagele
Minneapolis, MN, USA Adnan I. Qureshi

Contents

Contributors

Benjamin A. Abramoff, MD Physical Medicine and Rehabilitation, Emory University Hospital, Atlanta, GA, USA

Rushna Ali, MD Department of Neurosurgery, Vanderbilt University, Nashville, TN, USA

Chirantan Banerjee, MD, MPH Department of Neurology, Medical University of South Carolina, Charleston, SC, USA

Samir R. Belagaje, MD, FAAN Neurology and Rehabiliation Medicine, Emory University, Atlanta, GA, USA

Maria Beran, MD Physical Medicine and Rehabilitation, Emory University Hospital, Atlanta, GA, USA

Saqib Chaudhry, MD Departments of Neurology and Neuro-critical Care, University of Pennsylvania, Philadelphia, PA, USA

Matthew L. Flaherty, MD Department of Neurology and Rehabilitation Medicine, University of Cincinnati Academic Health Center, Cincinnati, OH, USA

Aravind Ganesh, MD Calgary Stroke Program, Department of Clinical Neurosciences, Cumming School of Medicine, University of Calgary, Calgary, Canada

Centre for Prevention of Stroke and Dementia, Nuffield Department of Clinical Neurosciences, University of Oxford, Oxford, UK

Nicole R. Gonzales, MS Department of Neurology, McGovern Medical School, Houston, TX, USA

Nitin Goyal, MD Department of Neurology, University of Tennessee Health Science Center, Memphis, TN, USA

Nabeel A. Herial, MD, MPH Departments of Neurology and Neurosurgery, Sidney Kimmel Medical College, Thomas Jefferson University, Philadelphia, PA, USA

Michael D. Hill, MD, MSc, FRCPC Calgary Stroke Program, Department of Clinical Neurosciences, Cumming School of Medicine, University of Calgary, Calgary, Canada

Department of Radiology, Department of Community Health Sciences, Department of Medicine, Hotchkiss Brain Institute, Cumming School of Medicine, University of Calgary, Calgary, AB, Canada

Muhammad Fawad Ishfaq, MD Department of Neurology, University of Tennessee Health Science Center, Memphis, TN, USA

Odysseas Kargiotis, MD, PhD Stroke Unit, Metropolitan Hospital, Piraeus, Greece

Muhib Khan, MD Spectrum Health Neuroscience Institute, Michigan State University, Grand Rapids, MI, USA

Nicole D. Mahdi, MD Stroke Program, Northwest Hospital, The Sandra and Malcolm Berman Brain and Spine Institute, Baltimore, MD, USA

Shahram Majidi, MD Department of Neurosurgery, Icahn School of Medicine at Mount Sinai, New York, MD, USA

Marc Malkoff, MD Department of Neurology, University of Tennessee Health Science Center, Memphis, TN, USA

Paul Mazaris, MD Spectrum Health Neuroscience Institute, Michigan State University, Grand Rapids, MI, USA

Adeola Olowu, MD Department of Neurology, McGovern Medical School, Houston, TX, USA

Bruce Ovbiagele, MD, MSc, MAS, MBA University of California, San Francisco Medical Center, San Francisco, CA, USA

Abhi Pandhi, MD Department of Neurology, University of Tennessee Health Science Center, Memphis, TN, USA

Jan C. Purrucker, MD Department of Neurology, Heidelberg University Hospital, Heidelberg, Germany

Adnan I. Qureshi, MD University of Minnesota, Minneapolis, MN, USA

Venkatakrishna Rajajee, MBBS Departments of Neurology and Neurosurgery, University of Michigan, Ann Arbor, MI, USA

Gustavo Rodriguez, MD, PhD Department of Neurology, Texas Tech University, El Paso, TX, USA

Magdy Selim, MD, PhD Department of Neurology, Stroke Division, Beth Israel Deaconess Medical Center, Boston, MA, USA

Fazeel Siddiqui, MD Department of Neurology, Southern Illinois University, Springfield, IL, USA

Brian Silver, MD Department of Neurology, University of Massachusetts, Worcester, MA, USA

Justin Singer, MD Spectrum Health Neuroscience Institute, Michigan State University, Grand Rapids, MI, USA

Alejandro M. Spiotta, MD Department of Neurosurgery, Medical University of South Carolina, Charleston, SC, USA

Thorsten Steiner, MD, MME Department of Neurology, Heidelberg University Hospital, Heidelberg, Germany

Department of Neurology, Klinikum Frankfurt Höchst, Frankfurt a.M., Germany

Jose I. Suarez, MD Division of Neurosciences Critical Care, Departments of Anesthesiology and Critical Care Medicine, Neurology, and Neurosurgery, The Johns Hopkins University School of Medicine, Baltimore, MD, USA

Georgios Tsivgoulis, MD, FESO Second Department of Neurology, "Attikon" Hospital, School of Medicine, University of Athens, Athens, Greece

Department of Neurology, The University of Tennessee Health Science Center, Memphis, TN, USA

Raymond D. Turner, MD Department of Neurosurgery, Medical University of South Carolina, Charleston, SC, USA

Jan Vargas, MD Department of Neurosurgery, Medical University of South Carolina, Charleston, SC, USA

Craig A. Williamson, MD Departments of Neurology and Neurosurgery, University of Michigan, Ann Arbor, MI, USA

Chapter 1
Prehospital and Emergency Department Management of Intracerebral Hemorrhage

Muhammad Fawad Ishfaq, Nitin Goyal, Abhi Pandhi, and Marc Malkoff

Background

Stroke is a leading cause of death and disability worldwide and a very common vascular disease prevalent globally spreading like a pandemic [1, 2]. Stroke can be ischemic or hemorrhagic in nature. Intracerebral hemorrhage (ICH) is the second most common subtype of stroke and a critical disease usually leading to severe disability or death [3]. ICH is defined as bleeding in the brain parenchyma. Incidence of ICH is 12–15 cases per 100,000 individual or about 40,000 cases per year in the United States [4]. ICH can be defined as "deep" located within the deep brain parenchyma such as the internal capsule, brain stem, or thalamus, or it can be "lobar" located in cortical–subcortical areas and follows a lobar pattern across one or multiple lobes of the brain. Deep ICH accounts for about two third of spontaneous ICH cases, and lobar ICH accounts for the remaining one third [5].

Hypertension is by far the most common risk factor. Other common risk factors are cerebral amyloid angiopathy, hematological abnormality, anticoagulation use, drug or alcohol abuse, and chronic kidney disease [6].

ICH mortality is about 40% at 30 days, making ICH one of the most deadly acute medical events. At 1 year, the mortality is 50%. Around 50% of the deaths happen in 48–72 h of ictus and are related to neurological complications (i.e., mass effect, increased intracranial pressure, and/or herniation) [7]. Many deaths also occur in the setting of withdrawal of support due to presumed poor prognosis. In the acute setting, predictors of early mortality are hematoma size, hematoma expansion, older age, coma, intraventricular hemorrhage (IVH), and infratentorial location [8].

M. F. Ishfaq · N. Goyal · A. Pandhi · M. Malkoff (✉)
Department of Neurology, University of Tennessee Health Science Center, Memphis, TN, USA
e-mail: mmalkoff@uthsc.edu

B. Ovbiagele, A. I. Qureshi (eds.), *Intracerebral Hemorrhage Therapeutics*,
https://doi.org/10.1007/978-3-319-77063-5_1

ICH is a medical emergency and delays in treatment result in worse outcome. Around 20% of patients will experience a decrease in the Glasgow Coma Scale of two or more points between the prehospital assessment and the initial evaluation in the emergency department [9]. Moreover, around 20% of patients demonstrate continued deterioration within the first hours after hospital arrival [10, 11]. Therefore aggressive prehospital and emergency department treatment is cornerstone for effective management of patients with ICH.

Initial management should focus on urgent stabilization of cardiorespiratory variables and treatment of intracranial complications [12]. Recent advances such as newer laboratory testing and rapid computed tomography for diagnosis, blood pressure reduction to reduce hematoma expansion, and new anticoagulant reversal agents may allow for improved outcomes. In this book chapter, we will discuss about different aspects of prehospital and emergency management of ICH.

Prehospital Stroke Care

Recent technological innovations have opened new perspectives for stroke diagnosis and treatment before the patient arrives at the hospital. These include presumed stroke diagnosis by paramedics, mobile telemedicine for remote clinical examination and imaging, mobile stroke units with integrated CT scanners, and point-of-care laboratories in ambulances [13]. Algorithms for prehospital treatment for either ischemic or hemorrhagic stroke are parallel to each other. In this section of the manuscript, we will discuss several aspects of prehospital care for patients with ICH.

Public Awareness

Time is saved if stroke symptoms are recognized early, and both the family and bystanders play a major role. Early recognition leads to early 911 call and early treatment and thus better outcomes not only for hemorrhagic but ischemic strokes as well. Multiple modalities for increasing awareness have come along including printed materials, audiovisual aids, and billboard advertisements targeting patient population, family members including children and relatives [14–16]. The effects of the campaigning were seen to be effective but for a short span only, and thus repetition and continuous promotion is the key [17]. Despite the continuous campaigning, only 53% of the population is using EMS services. The National Hospital Ambulatory Medical Care Survey (NHAMCS) reported that with use of 911 and EMS services, prehospital delays are less and patient's door to CT or MRI times are shorter as well [18]. Early alarm has been associated with female gender, higher education and socioeconomic status, presence of bystanders, family history of stroke, and acute and severe symptoms [19, 20].

Emergency Medical System Services

Emergency medical system (EMS) personal are involved since 911 activation and dispatch, response to on site, triage and stabilization in field, patient transport ground or air, and prehospital notification. The primary objective is to provide airway management if needed, provide cardiovascular support, and transport the patient to the closest facility prepared to care for patients with acute stroke [21, 22]. The secondary objective for EMS personal is to obtain a focused history regarding the symptom onset time; nature of clinical symptoms; relevant past medical and surgical history, medication, and drug use; and contact information for family. Another important role of EMS providers is the prehospital notification so that critical pathways can be initiated and consulting services alerted. Advance notice by EMS has been shown to significantly shorten time to computed tomography (CT) scanning in the ED [21, 23].

Accuracy of EMS in identifying stroke (ischemic or hemorrhagic) symptoms is highly variable ranging from 30% to 83% [24, 25]. There are various scales available that can be used by EMS personal for identification of suspected stroke patients including Cincinnati prehospital stroke scale [26], Los Angeles prehospital stroke screen [27], or Face Arm Speech Test (FAST) scale assessment [28]. Certain clinical features suggest the diagnosis of ICH over ischemic stroke are vomiting, systolic blood pressure > 220 mmHg at onset, severe headache, coma or decreased level of consciousness, and symptom progression over minutes or hours. However, none of these clinical features are specific [29].

Several prehospital interventions known to influence outcomes, including administration of supplemental oxygen [30, 31], fluid resuscitation preferably with normal saline (avoiding dextrose containing solutions as it can exacerbate cerebral injury), keeping head of bed up for suspected hemorrhagic stroke, identifying hypo- or hyperglycemia with a finger stick glucose testing and treating it promptly, and insertion of angiography compatible IV lines, are routinely provided by EMS personal en route to the hospital in suspected stroke patients.

Mobile Stroke Unit

The concept of taking stroke care to the patient by deployment of mobile stroke units (MSU) is rapidly expanding. Mobile stroke units enable time-sensitive diagnosis and delivery of ultra-early stroke treatment. Walter and colleagues launched the first MSU in 2010 in Saarland, Germany, with a Mercedes-Benz Vario 815D ambulance that included conventional ambulance equipment; a small portable 8-slice CT scan; a telemedicine system for transmission of digital imaging, communication, and real-time video of patient clinical examination; and a point-of-care laboratory system [32].

Then came STEMO in Berlin with CT head and CT angiography capability, but only one CT angiography was done [33–35]. The first MSU in the United States was launched at University of Texas, Houston, followed by Cleveland Clinic MSU and then University of Tennessee, Memphis, MSU [36–38].

The concept of MSU can be very useful for hyper-acute management of ICH. Early detection of ICH on CT head on MSU allows EMS personal to triage patient and to make sure patient is being transported to a tertiary care center with services of neurology, neurosurgery, neurocritical care, and neurointerventional specialist [13]. Hematoma expansion occurs early after ictus in ICH most commonly within 4.5–6 h from onset [21]. Whether very early aggressive reduction systolic blood pressure in the MSU could effectively improve functional outcome in ICH remains unknown, but the MSU provides a unique environment to test this hypothesis. Other than blood pressure lowering, MSUs may serve as a powerful platform for study of hemorrhage control agents as well as neuroprotective drugs in the management of ICH [39]. The BEST-MSU study reported enrolling 4 ICH cases from their first 26 patients, and aggressive BP lowering was provided within the first hour of symptom onset [40]. Use of continuous infusion antihypertensive agents by MSU teams promotes improved blood pressure control of these fragile cases while ensuring provision of close hemodynamic monitoring. Additionally, MSU teams that stock reversal agents for coagulopathic ICH are well suited to rapidly support hemostasis alongside standard management while alerting both neurosurgery and neurocritical care teams of CT/CT angiography findings and pending patient needs [40, 41]. Administration of hyperosmolar agents including mannitol or hypertonic saline, in consultation with neurocritical care team, can be carried out if clinical signs of herniation are present while en route to avoid delay and preventing complete herniation. Detailed prehospital workup with CT angiography allows the determination of vessel leak (so-called spot sign) in ICH patients. However, the cost-effectiveness of MSUs is still a concern.

Role of Mobile Telemedicine

Telemedicine-enabled ambulance-based evaluation reduces time to imaging and treatment. Non-stroke-capable hospitals are also able to get stroke expertise from stroke experts via telemedicine. Telemedicine has been shown to be safe and promotes early triaging and treatment and better clinical outcome. Telemedicine also helps in identifying severe patients which can benefit more by transferring to tertiary stroke centers [42, 43].

Emergency Department Stroke Care

All the major stroke centers are working toward the concept of "Time is brain" which holds true for both ischemic and hemorrhagic strokes [44, 45]. Timely evaluation, diagnosis, and treatment of patients with ICH should be performed expeditiously in emergency department (ED) because clinical deterioration is common in the first few hours. In addition to prehospital notification provided by EMS, there should be an effective and quick communication between EMS transport and ED staff as soon as patient arrives in ED so that rapid clinical evaluation by adequately trained nurses and physicians can be possible [46]. The hospitals without on-site presence of stroke or neurosurgery consultants can also easily be benefited by the telemedicine which allows rapid visualization of clinical and neurological data, providing neurosurgical expertise within minutes to peripheral hospital. Telemedicine can also help to transfer such patients to tertiary care centers when necessary [42, 43].

Primary management of ICH in ED include rapid clinical evaluation, laboratory studies including blood glucose and coagulation defects, diagnostic imaging studies, management of blood pressure and early intracranial complications such as hydrocephalus or impending herniation, and admission to stroke unit or neuroscience intensive care unit (NICU).

Rapid Clinical Evaluation

Rapid clinical evaluation by trained nursing staff and physician is the most vital and earliest part of management of ICH patients in the ED. History can help to evaluate possible vascular risk factors and any triggering agents such as medicine, alcohol, illicit drugs, or other underlying pathologies such as intracranial vascular malformation, cancer, or hematological disorders. Effective physical examination should include vital sign, focused general and cardiovascular exam, and detailed neurological exam including severity scale. Different severity scales are being used for the assessment of ICH, and the most used is ICH score which provides clinical grading scale for outcome after ICH [47]. When the patient arrives to ED, it is difficult to predict that it is ischemic or hemorrhagic stroke; therefore commonly used ischemic stroke scale known as the National Health Institute Stroke Scale may be helpful in ICH as well to assess the severity of deficits. However these scales should be not be used as solo measures to grade prognosis [48, 49].

Laboratory Studies

Laboratory studies include complete blood count, complete metabolic panel, toxicology screen, coagulation profile, urine studies, and other relevant studies deemed significant by history. Early diagnosis and reversal of any triggering factors such as coagulation defects, blood glucose, etc. can play a vital role in better prognosis of patients with ICH.

Neuroimaging Evaluation

In any patients with acute stroke symptoms, it's impossible to know if stroke is ischemic or hemorrhagic based on clinical symptoms alone; therefore rapid neuroimaging evaluation is a must to make the diagnosis and elucidate the etiology of ICH. Neuroimaging usually comprises the combination of any of the following, computerized tomography (CT) head, CT angiography, CT perfusion, magnetic resonance (MR) brain, MR angiography, and MR venography or conventional angiography. CTH without contrast is considered to be the gold standard due to its high sensitivity for diagnosing ICH, rapidity, cost-effectiveness, and easy availability [50, 51]. CT head also gives useful information about location, intraventricular extension, hydrocephalus, presence and degree of edema, and midline shift or brainstem compression secondary to the mass effect from the hematoma [51]. Both CT head and MR brain are equally sensitive to identify ICH, but CT head better visualizes intraventricular and subarachnoid bleed, and MR brain is better at identifying prior hemorrhages, hemorrhagic transformation of ischemic stroke, and underlying structural lesions (i.e., neoplasms and vascular malformations). Given the cost, duration of the examination, and poor tolerability for some patients, MR is less commonly used in the ED for workup of ICH [52].

ICH volume is a strong predictor of ICH outcome as larger hematomas have a poorer prognosis. Intracerebral hematoma volume can be rapidly estimated in the ED with the ABC/2 technique. A is the maximum ICH diameter (in cm) estimated visually; B is the maximum ICH diameter perpendicular to A (in cm), and C is the total number of CT slices with the ICH seen in the vertical plane multiplied by the CT slice thickness (typically 5 mm or 0.5 cm). A, B, and C numbers are then multiplied together and divided by 2 [53, 54]. The location of ICH on CT head, along with the patients' age and medical history, provides important information about the etiology of ICH. In general, deep ICHs are hypertensive, and lobar ICHs are caused by secondary causes, such as cerebral amyloid angiopathy, coagulopathy, vascular malformations, tumors, dural arteriovenous fistulas, and vasculitis, and warrant further investigation such as contrasted MR, CT, or MR angiography or conventional angiogram [55]. A small percentage of lobar ICH can be hypertensive as well [56].

A "spot" sign on post-contrast CT is a small enhancing foci within the hematoma, related to vascular leak at the point of enhancement; the presence of the "spot" sign seems to independently predict hematoma enlargement [53]. The ICH patients with spot sign are at risk of immediate worsening, and several ongoing studies are investigating role of ultra-intensive blood pressure control or hemostatic therapy in this subgroup of patients [53, 57–60].

Computed tomography angiography (CTA) is a useful diagnostic tool in the acute setting of ICH. It is the most widely available noninvasive technique for the detection of vascular abnormalities as secondary cause of ICH [60]. Prompt detection of these lesions is crucial and has a significant impact on patient management. Although CTA is an excellent noninvasive screening tool, digital subtraction angiography remains the gold standard investigation for diagnosis and for possible endovascular treatment of cerebral vascular malformations. The main drawback of CTA is contrast and the additional radiation exposure. Although some clinicians are concerned about the risk of contrast-induced nephropathy, there is a debate in the literature whether this entity exists. In patients with poor kidney function, contrast allergies, or other contraindications to CTA, brain vessel imaging can be achieved through MR angiography [53, 60]. Conventional digital subtraction angiography is often indicated in patients with SAH and ICH with abnormal calcifications or blood in atypical locations or presentation or in young patients with no obvious cause for ICH. MRI is equally sensitive as is CTH to pick up ICH, but ICH evaluation on MRI depends primarily on the age of the hematoma and the type of MR sequence (i.e., T1 or T2 weighted). The signal intensity on MR depends on the specific form of Hb present, hyper-acute >24 h appear isointense on T1 and slightly hyperintense on T2; acute 1–3 days appear slightly hypointense on T1 and very hypointense on T2; early subacute >3 days appear very hyperintense on T1 and very hypointense on T2; late subacute >7 days appear very hyperintense on T1 and very hyperintense on T2; chronic center >14 days appear isointense on T1 and slightly hyperintense on T2; and chronic rim >14 days appear slightly hypointense on T1 and very hypointense on T2 [61].

After diagnosis, emergency providers should arrange for rapid admission to a stroke unit or neuroscience intensive care unit (at their own hospital if available or via transfer) and initiate early management, while the patient is awaiting this bed. The following management procedures should be initiated in the ED rather than waiting until after transfer to an intensive care unit, stroke unit, or other hospital.

Airway Protection

Generalized endotracheal intubation is indicated in patients with reduced consciousness to protect airway, bulbar dysfunctional leading to inability to handle secretions, or concomitant respiratory or cardiac problems leading to respiratory distress. In these clinical situations, induction of GETA should be done as in a rapid sequence technique with careful attention to minimize large hemodynamic fluctuations or fluctuations in intracranial pressure if monitoring is being done [62].

Blood Pressure Management

The underlying reason for high blood pressure in stroke patients is not absolutely clear. Most of patients with ICH have chronically uncontrolled hypertension and elevation of blood pressure at time of presentation to hospital is merely a reflection of the poorly controlled blood pressure. Cushing–Kocher response resulting from compression from brain stem may also play a vital role for elevated blood pressure to maintain cerebral perfusion. Acute stress response leading to abnormal neurohumoral mechanism may also cause acute high blood pressure during ICH. Blood pressure increase is associated with higher risk of hematoma expansion, neurological deterioration, poor outcome, and death. The pathophysiology behind hematoma expansion is not well understood. It is not clear whether it reflects leakage, rebleeding, or both. After vessel rupture, an initial hematoma forms, causing secondary vessel rupture due to mass effect, and also triggers an avalanche of further vessel ruptures, but the real mechanism leading to final hematoma volume remains unclear. Hematoma expansion occurs early in the course of ICH, and early CT scan repetition is warranted to detect it [63, 64].

ATACH-I trial failed to find any significant relationship between SBP reduction and hematoma expansion, perihematomal edema, and 3-month outcome among patients with ICH [65]. INTERACT1 (intensive blood pressure reduction in acute cerebral hemorrhage trial-1) showed that patients within 6 h of ICH with rapid reduction of SBP to <140 mmHg to be safe [66]; but INTERACT 2 (intensive blood pressure reduction in acute cerebral hemorrhage trial-2) failed to meet its primary end point, and did not definitively show improved outcome with intensive BP treatment (SBP target <140 mmHg) [67–69]. The most robust and latest data on BP management come from the ATACH-2 trial (antihypertensive treatment of acute cerebral hemorrhage II), a large clinical trial randomizing patients to one of two different systolic blood pressure (SBP) control strategies, SBP 110–139 mmHg vs SBP 140–179 mmHg, which showed that patients with ICH and tight SBP control of 110–139 mmHg did not result in a lower rate of death or disability than standard reduction to a target of 140–179 mmHg [70]. The main limitation in ATACH-2 trial is that patient randomized to have intensive treatment had ultra-intensive control of blood pressure, i.e., the mean minimum systolic blood pressure during the first 2 h was 128.9 ± 16 mmHg versus 141.1 ± 14.8 mmHg in the standard-treatment group. Such intense systolic blood pressure control led to higher percentage of patients with any serious adverse events (25.6% vs. 20.0%).

The current American Heart Association guidelines suggest that the early lowering of BP to 140 mmHg is safe and can be effective for patients with ICH presenting with a 150–220 mmHg systolic blood pressure [21].

To avoid hypotension, short half-life antihypertensive, such as labetalol or nicardipine, is recommended to control blood pressure in patients with ICH [21, 64]. Clevidipine monotherapy has recently shown promising effects in terms of safe rapid blood pressure reduction in ICH patients leading to decreased hematoma expansion [71].

Thromboprophylaxis in ICH Patients

Deep vein thrombosis (DVT) prophylaxis is tricky in patients with ICH as they have tendency to bleed more with conventional medications used for DVT prophylaxis; therefore intermittent pneumatic sequential compression devices (SCDs) are indicated in such patients beginning the day of hospital admission. DVT prophylaxis can be started with conventional low-dose molecular weight heparin or unfractionated heparin once intracranial bleed has been stopped after 3–4 days of onset of the ICH [72–74]. ICH patients with symptomatic DVT or PE can be given one of the following two options, systemic anticoagulation or IVC filter placement, depending on various factors such as comorbidities including prothrombotic conditions, cause of hemorrhage, time from hemorrhage onset, and hematoma stability.

Hemostatic Treatment

(a) Platelet function

Limited data is available to support the reversal strategy to improve platelet function in patients with ICH who are taking antiplatelet medications. PATCH trial failed to show beneficial effect of platelet transfusion over standard care for people taking antiplatelet therapy before intracerebral hemorrhage [75]. However, patients with severe thrombocytopenia, 50,000–100,000, should receive replacement therapy with platelet transfusion [72].

(b) Anticoagulant-Associated Coagulopathy

Anticoagulants and coagulation defect may lead to intracranial hematoma expansion and subsequently clinical deterioration and death. In case of warfarin coagulopathy, recommendations are to discontinue warfarin, administer intravenous vitamin K, and factor repletion [72–74]. INCH trial [76] showed that in patients with vitamin K antagonist-related intracranial hemorrhage, prothrombin complex concentrates (PCC) may be preferred over fresh frozen plasma (FFP) due to rapid action causing INR normalization in short period of time and leading to smaller hematoma expansion [67, 68]. The optimal INR target is still debated, and proposed target value range less than 1.5. rFVIIa is not recommended for reversal in ICH [77]. FAST trial failed to prove the beneficial effects of hemostatic therapy with rFVIIa in terms of survival or functional outcome after ICH, but it significantly reduced growth of the hematoma [78].

Protamine sulfate may be considered to reverse heparin in patients with acute ICH at the dose of 1 mg per 100 units of heparin (maximum dose up to 50 mg).

Novel oral anticoagulants (NOACs) or direct oral anticoagulants (DOACs) are increasingly being used as an alternative to warfarin. The most commonly used are the factor Xa inhibitors apixaban, rivaroxaban, and edoxaban and the direct thrombin inhibitor dabigatran. Functions of these agents do not need to be monitored by laboratory studies such as INR. Limited data is available on reversal of these newer agents by antagonists. Administration of vit K for reversal of these newer agents is futile; however charcoal (<2 h intake of NOACs) PCC, FEIBA, and rFVIIa have showed some promising effects which needed to be further investigated [79, 80]. Idarucizumab has been recently licensed and proved effective for reversal of dabigatran [81]. Andexanet alfa has also shown promising effect in reversal of rivaroxaban, apixaban, and edoxaban and is likely to be soon licensed for use in patients with ICH [82–84].

(c) Recombinant tissue plasminogen activator (rtPA)-associated coagulopathy may lead to hemorrhagic conversion of ischemic stroke, symptomatic ICH being the most dangerous complication. To prevent the hemorrhagic conversion of ischemic stroke, it is recommended to strictly control blood pressure and avoid antithrombotic medication in the first 24 h following the infusion of rtPA. Limited data is available to standardize the treatment of post rtPA ICH. It is recommended to immediately discontinue rtPA and administer any of the following compounds: cryoprecipitate, antifibrinolytic, aminocaproic acid, vitamin K, FFP, PCC, platelet transfusion, or recombinant activated factor VII A [85].

Intracranial Pressure Management

Current AHA/ASA guidelines suggest ICP monitoring with parenchymal or ventricular devices in patients with coma, significant IVH with hydrocephalus, and evidence of transtentorial herniation, with a cerebral perfusion pressure target of 50–70 mmHg. ICP increase can be avoided or treated by elevation of the head to 30, adequate sedation, or avoidance of hyponatremia [21]. ICH who are at risk of transtentorial herniation may also benefit from hyperosmolar therapy with mannitol or hypertonic saline.

Surgical Management of ICH

Surgery in patients with neurologically asymptomatic ICH is not clearly beneficial. Supratentorial hematoma evacuation in deteriorating patients might be considered as a life-saving measure. STICH and STICH II were undertaken to determine whether early surgery reduces mortality and improve neurological outcome compared with conservative management for supratentorial ICH [86, 87]. Both STICH and STICH II failed to clearly identify the beneficial role of surgery in patients supratentorial hemorrhages, but subgroup analysis of STICH [86] suggested that patients with lobar hemorrhages within 1 cm of the cortical surface might benefit from surgery which led to STICH II trial that specifically included the ICH patients with superficial lobar hemorrhage.

Supratentorial ICH patients who are in a coma, have large hematomas with midline shift, or have elevated ICP refractory to medical management may also have mortality benefit from decompressive craniectomy with or without hematoma evacuation [86, 87].

The role of minimally invasive clot also is uncertain [88, 89]. The Minimally Invasive Surgery Plus Recombinant Tissue-Type Plasminogen Activator for ICH Evacuation Trial II (MISTIE II) showed a significant reduction in perihematomal edema in the hematoma evacuation group. Such a promising effect in MISTIE II led researchers to continue a randomized phase 3 clinical trial of minimally invasive hematoma evacuation (MISTIE III) which is currently in progress [90]. Apollo devices have also been studied for minimally invasive evacuation of ICH and intraventricular hemorrhage, but further studies are required to prove benefit from this promising technology [91].

Emergent surgical removal of the hemorrhage is also recommended in patient with cerebellar hemorrhage who have neurological deterioration, brain stem compression, or neurologically or hydrocephalus from ventricular obstruction [88, 89].

Intraventricular administrations of thrombolytics or any other endoscopic treatment of IVH are clinically unproven in terms of efficacy [92].

Blood Glucose Management

No specific blood glucose target level is recommended, but tight glycemic control has been shown to be associated with better outcome [93]. The AHA/ASA guidelines suggest to avoid both hyperglycemia and hypoglycemia [21].

Temperature Management

Optimal temperature management is still unclear, but it is recommended to treat fever as it has been associated with poor outcome. The presence of fever is a common finding in patients with ICH, especially in those with extensive IVH [93]. More studies are needed to investigate the role of normothermia or hypothermia and their effect on outcome in patients with ICH.

Seizures and Antiseizure Drugs

The prophylactic administration of antiseizure drug therapy is not recommended, and even some data suggest that phenytoin may worsen outcomes in patients with ICH. Antiseizure medications are administered in the patients with clinical or electroencephalography (EEG) evidence of seizures [94]. The patients with ICH who have impaired mental status that is disproportionate to the degree of brain damage should be considered for continuous EEG monitoring to rule out nonconvulsive seizures.

Transfer to an Intensive Care Unit, Stroke Unit, or Other Hospital

There should be no delay in transfer of patients with ICH to a facility which is better equipped to manage this devastating condition. Furthermore, studies have shown better morbidity and mortality rates in patients who are admitted to dedicated stroke unit.

References

1. Wang H, Naghavi M, Allen C, et al. Global, regional, and national life expectancy, all-cause mortality, and cause-specific mortality for 249 causes of death, 1980-2015: a systematic analysis for the Global Burden of Disease Study 2015. Lancet. 2016;388(10053):1459–544.
2. Portegies ML, Koudstaal PJ, Ikram MA. Cerebrovascular disease. Handb Clin Neurol. 2016;138:239–61.
3. An SJ, Kim TJ, Yoon BW. Epidemiology, risk factors, and clinical features of intracerebral hemorrhage: an update. J Stroke. 2017;19(1):3–10.

4. Gebel JM, Broderick JP. Intracerebral hemorrhage. Neurol Clin. 2000;18(2):419–38.
5. Grysiewicz RA, Thomas K, Pandey DK. Epidemiology of ischemic and hemorrhagic stroke: incidence, prevalence, mortality, and risk factors. Neurol Clin. 2008;26(4):871–95. vii
6. Qureshi AI, Tuhrim S, Broderick JP, Batjer HH, Hondo H, Hanley DF. Spontaneous intracerebral hemorrhage. N Engl J Med. 2001;344(19):1450–60.
7. Vermeer SE, Algra A, Franke CL, Koudstaal PJ, Rinkel GJ. Long-term prognosis after recovery from primary intracerebral hemorrhage. Neurology. 2002;59(2):205–9.
8. Broderick JP, Brott TG, Duldner JE, Tomsick T, Huster G. Volume of intracerebral hemorrhage. A powerful and easy-to-use predictor of 30-day mortality. Stroke. 1993;24(7):987–93.
9. Moon JS, Janjua N, Ahmed S, et al. Prehospital neurologic deterioration in patients with intracerebral hemorrhage. Crit Care Med. 2008;36(1):172–5.
10. Brott T, Broderick J, Kothari R, et al. Early hemorrhage growth in patients with intracerebral hemorrhage. Stroke. 1997;28:1–5.
11. Fan JS, Huang HH, Chen YC, et al. Emergency department neurologic deterioration in patients with spontaneous intracerebral hemorrhage: incidence, predictors, and prognostic significance. Acad Emerg Med. 2012;19:133–8.
12. Elliott J, Smith M. The acute management of intracerebral hemorrhage: a clinical review. Anesth Analg. 2010;110(5):1419–27.
13. Audebert HJ, Saver JL, Starkman S, Lees KR, Endres M. Prehospital stroke care: new prospects for treatment and clinical research. Neurology. 2013;81(5):501–8.
14. Morgenstern LB, Staub L, Chan W, et al. Improving delivery of acute stroke therapy: the TLL temple foundation stroke project. Stroke. 2002;33(1):160–6.
15. Williams O, Noble JM. 'Hip-hop' stroke: a stroke educational program for elementary school children living in a high-risk community. Stroke. 2008;39(10):2809–16.
16. Morgenstern LB, Gonzales NR, Maddox KE, et al. A randomized, controlled trial to teach middle school children to recognize stroke and call 911: the kids identifying and defeating stroke project. Stroke. 2007;38(11):2972–8. Epub 2007 Sep 20
17. Hodgson C, Lindsay P, Rubini F. Can mass media influence emergency department visits for stroke? Stroke. 2007;38(7):2115–22. Epub 2007 May 31
18. Mohammad YM. Mode of arrival to the emergency department of stroke patients in the United States. J Vasc Interv Neurol. 2008;1(3):83–6.
19. Wester P, Rådberg J, Lundgren B, et al. Factors associated with delayed admission to hospital and in-hospital delays in acute stroke and TIA: a prospective, multicenter study.Seek- medical-attention-in-time study group. Stroke. 1999;30(1):40–8.
20. Rosamond WD, Gorton RA, Hinn AR, et al. Rapid response to stroke symptoms: the delay in accessing stroke healthcare (DASH) study. Acad Emerg Med. 1998;5(1):45–51.
21. Hemphill JC 3rd, Greenberg SM, Anderson CS, et al. Guidelines for the Management of Spontaneous Intracerebral Hemorrhage: a guideline for healthcare professionals from the American Heart Association/American Stroke Association. Stroke. 2015;46(7):2032–60.
22. Acker JE 3rd, Pancioli AM, Crocco TJ, et al. Implementation strategies for emergency medical services within stroke systems of care: a policy statement from the American Heart Association/American Stroke Association expert panel on emergency medical services systems and the stroke council. Stroke. 2007;38(11):3097–115.
23. Abdullah AR, Smith EE, Biddinger PD, et al. Advance hospital notification by EMS in acute stroke is associated with shorter door-to-computed tomography time and increased likelihood of administration of tissue-plasminogen activator. Prehosp Emerg Care. 2008;12(4):426–31.
24. Buck BH, Starkman S, Eckstein M, et al. Dispatcher recognition of stroke using the National Academy Medical Priority Dispatch System. Stroke. 2009;40(6):2027–30.
25. Reginella RL, Crocco T, Tadros A, et al. Predictors of stroke during 9-1-1 calls: opportunities for improving EMS response. Prehosp Emerg Care. 2006;10(3):369–73.
26. Kothari RU, Pancioli A, Liu T, et al. Cincinnati prehospital stroke scale: reproducibility and validity. Ann Emerg Med. 1999;33(4):373–8.
27. Kidwell CS, Starkman S, Eckstein M, et al. Identifying stroke in the field. Prospective validation of the Los Angeles prehospital stroke screen (LAPSS). Stroke. 2000;31(1):71–6.

28. Harbison J, Massey A, Barnett L, et al. Rapid ambulance protocol for acute stroke. Lancet. 1999;353(9168):1935.
29. Goldstein LB. Simel DL. Is this patient having a stroke? JAMA. 2005;293:2391–402.
30. Jauch EC, Cucchiara B, Adeoye O, et al. Part 11: adult stroke: 2010 American Heart Association guidelines for cardiopulmonary resuscitation and emergency cardiovascular care. Circulation. 2010;122(18 Suppl 3):S818–28.
31. Peberdy MA, Callaway CW, Neumar RW, et al. Part 9: post-cardiac arrest care: 2010 American Heart Association guidelines for cardiopulmonary resuscitation and emergency cardiovascular care. Circulation. 2010;122(18 Suppl 3):S768–86.
32. Walter S, Kostpopoulos P, Haass A, et al. Bringing the hospital to the patient: first treatment of stroke patients at the emergency site. PLoS One. 2010;5(10):e13758.
33. Hiyama N, Yoshimura S, Shirakawa M, et al. Safety and effectiveness of drip, ship, and retrieve paradigm for acute ischemic stroke: a single center experience. Neurol Med Chir (Tokyo). 2016;56(12):731–6. Epub 2016 Jul 14
34. Kageji T, Obata F, Oka H, et al. Drip-and-ship thrombolytic therapy supported by the Telestroke system for acute ischemic stroke patients living in medically under-served areas. Neurol Med Chir (Tokyo). 2016;56(12):753–8. Epub 2016 Jun 22
35. Walter S, Kostopoulos P, Haass A, et al. Diagnosis and treatment of patients with stroke in a mobile stroke unit versus in hospital: a randomised controlled trial. Lancet Neurol. 2012;11(5):397–404.
36. Weber JE, Ebinger M, Rozanski M, et al. Prehospital thrombolysis in acute stroke: results of the PHANTOM-S pilot study. Neurology. 2013;80(2):163–8.
37. Ebinger M, Kunz A, Wendt M, et al. Effects of golden hour thrombolysis: a prehospital acute neurological treatment and optimization of medical Care in Stroke (PHANTOM-S) substudy. JAMA Neurol. 2015;72(1):25–30.
38. Gierhake D, Weber JE, Villringer K, et al. [Mobile CT: technical aspects of prehospital stroke imaging before intravenous thrombolysis]. [Article in German]. Rofo. 2013;185(1):55–9.
39. Frontera JA, Lewin JJ, Rabinstein AA, et al. Guideline for reversal of antithrombotics in intracranial hemorrhage: executive summary, a statement for healthcare professionals from the Neurocritical care society and Society of Critical Care Medicine. Crit Care Med. 2016;44:2251–7.
40. Gomes JA, Ahrens CL, Hussain MS, et al. Prehospital reversal of warfarin-related coagulopathy in intracerebral hemorrhage in a mobile stroke treatment unit. Stroke. 2015;46(5):e118–20.
41. Bowry R, Parker S, Rajan SS, et al. Benefits of stroke treatment using a mobile stroke unit compared with standard management: the BEST-MSU study run-in phase. Stroke. 2015;46(12):3370–4.
42. Al Kasab S, Adams RJ, Debenham E, et al. Medical University of South Carolina Telestroke: a telemedicine facilitated network for stroke treatment in South Carolina-a progress report. Telemed J E Health. 2017;23:674.
43. Wechsler LR, Demaerschalk BM, Schwamm LH, et al. Telemedicine quality and outcomes in stroke: a scientific statement for healthcare professionals from the American Heart Association/American Stroke Association. Stroke. 2017;48(1):e3–e25.
44. Kim J-T, Fonarow GC, Smith EE, et al. Treatment with tissue plasminogen activator in the golden hour and the shape of the 4.5-hour time-benefit curve in the national United States Get With The Guidelines–Stroke population. Circulation. 2017;135:128–39.
45. Prabhakaran S, O'Neill K, Stein-Spencer L, Walter J, Alberts MJ. Prehospital triage to primary stroke centers and rate of stroke thrombolysis. JAMA Neurol. 2013;70:1126–32.
46. Ikram MA, Wieberdink RG, Koudstaal PJ. International epidemiology of intracerebral hemorrhage. Curr Atheroscler Rep. 2012;14(4):300–6.
47. Qureshi AI, Mendelow AD, Hanley DF. Intracerebral haemorrhage. Lancet. 2009;373(9675):1632–44.
48. Hwang BY, Appelboom G, Kellner CP, et al. Clinical grading scales in intracerebral hemorrhage. Neurocrit Care. 2010;13:141–51.

49. Wang W, Lu J, Wang C, et al. Prognostic value of ICH score and ICH-GS score in Chinese intracerebral hemorrhage patients: analysis from the China National Stroke Registry (CNSR). PLoS One. 2013;8(10):e77421.
50. Macellari F, Paciaroni M, Agnelli G, et al. Neuroimaging in intracerebral hemorrhage. Stroke. 2014;45(3):903–8.
51. Halpin SF, Britton JA, Byrne JV, et al. Prospective evaluation of cerebral angiography and computed tomography in cerebral haematoma. J Neurol Neurosurg Psychiatry. 1994;57(10):1180–6.
52. Wijman CA, Venkatasubramanian C, Bruins S, et al. Utility of early MRI in the diagnosis and management of acute spontaneous intracerebral hemorrhage. Cerebrovasc Dis. 2010;30(5):456–63.
53. Demchuk AM, Dowlatshahi D, Rodriguez-Luna D, et al. Prediction of haematoma growth and outcome in patients with intracerebral haemorrhage using the CT-angiography spot sign (PREDICT): a prospective observational study. Lancet Neurol. 2012;11(4):307–14.
54. Brouwers HB, Chang Y, Falcone GJ, et al. Predicting hematoma expansion after primary intracerebral hemorrhage. JAMA Neurol. 2014;71(2):158–64.
55. Earnest F 4th, Baker HL Jr, Kispert DB, Laws ER Jr. Magnetic resonance imaging vs. computed tomography: advantages and disadvantages. Clin Neurosurg. 1985;32:540–73.
56. Ohtani R, Kazui S, Tomimoto H, et al. Clinical and radiographic features of lobar cerebral hemorrhage: hypertensive versus non-hypertensive cases. Intern Med. 2003;42(7):576–80.
57. Meretoja A, Churilov L, Campbell BC, et al. The spot sign and tranexamic acid on preventing ICH growth--AUStralasia trial (STOP-AUST): protocol of a phase II randomized, placebo-controlled, double-blind, multicenter trial. Int J Stroke. 2014;9(4):519–24.
58. Liu L, Wang Y, Meng X, et al. Tranexamic acid for acute intracerebral hemorrhage growth predicted by spot sign trial: rationale and design. Int J Stroke. 2017;12(3):326–31.
59. Rehmani R, Han A, Hassan J, et al. Role of prothrombin complex concentrate (PCC) in acute intracerebral hemorrhage with positive CTA spot sign: an institutional experience at a regional and state designated stroke center. Emerg Radiol. 2016;24(3):241.
60. Morotti A, Romero JM, Jessel MJ, et al. Effect of CTA tube current on spot sign detection and accuracy for prediction of intracerebral hemorrhage expansion. AJNR Am J Neuroradiol. 2016;37:1781.
61. Boulouis G, van Etten ES, Charidimou A, et al. Association of key Magnetic Resonance Imaging Markers of cerebral small vessel disease with hematoma volume and expansion in patients with lobar and deep intracerebral hemorrhage. JAMA Neurol. 2016;73(12):1440–7.
62. Salhi B, Stettner E. In defense of the use of lidocaine in rapid sequence intubation. Ann Emerg Med. 2007;49(1):84–6.
63. Zheng H, Chen C, Zhang J, et al. Mechanism and therapy of brain edema after intracerebral hemorrhage. Cerebrovasc Dis. 2016;42(3–4):155–69.
64. Manning LS, Robinson TG. New insights into blood pressure control for intracerebral Haemorrhage. Front Neurol Neurosci. 2015;37:35–50.
65. Qureshi AI, Palesch YY, Martin R, et al. Effect of systolic blood pressure reduction on hematoma expansion, perihematomal edema, and 3-month outcome among patients with intracerebral hemorrhage: results from the antihypertensive treatment of acute cerebral hemorrhage study. Arch Neurol. 2010;67(5):570–6.
66. Anderson CS, Huang Y, Wang JG, et al. Intensive blood pressure reduction in acute cerebral haemorrhage trial (INTERACT): a randomised pilot trial. Lancet Neurol. 2008;7:391–9.
67. Delcourt C, Huang Y, Wang J, et al. The second (main) phase of an open, randomised, multicentre study to investigate the effectiveness of an intensive blood pressure reduction in acute cerebral haemorrhage trial (INTERACT2). Int J Stroke. 2010;5:110–6.
68. Anderson CS, Heeley E, Huang Y, et al. Rapid blood-pressure lowering in patients with acute intracerebral hemorrhage. N Engl J Med. 2013;368:2355–65.
69. Anderson C, Heeley E, Heritier S, et al. Statistical analysis plan for the second INTEnsive blood pressure reduction in acute cerebral hemorrhage trial (INTERACT2): a large-scale

investigation to solve longstanding controversy over the most appropriate management of elevated blood pressure in the hyperacute phase of intracerebral hemorrhage. Int J Stroke. 2013;8:327–8.
70. Qureshi AI, Palesch YY, Barsan WG, et al. Intensive blood-pressure lowering in patients with acute cerebral hemorrhage. N Engl J Med. 2016;375(11):1033–43.
71. Graffagnino C, Bergese S, Love J, et al. Clevidipine rapidly and safely reduces blood pressure in acute intracerebral hemorrhage: the ACCELERATE trial. Cerebrovasc Dis. 2013;36(3):173–80.
72. Hunt BJ. Bleeding and coagulopathies in critical care. N Engl J Med. 2014;370(9):847–59.
73. Aguilar MI, Freeman WD. Treatment of coagulopathy in intracranial hemorrhage. Curr Treat Options Neurol. 2010;12(2):113–28.
74. Milling TJ, Refaai MA, Goldstein JN, et al. Thromboembolic events after vitamin K antagonist reversal with 4-factor prothrombin complex concentrate: exploratory analyses of two randomized, plasma-controlled studies. Ann Emerg Med. 2016;67(1):96–105.e5.
75. Baharoglu MI, Cordonnier C, Al-Shahi Salman R, et al. Platelet transfusion versus standard care after acute stroke due to spontaneous cerebral haemorrhage associated with antiplatelet therapy (PATCH): a randomised, open-label, phase 3 trial. Lancet. 2016;387(10038):2605–13.
76. Steiner T, Poli S, Griebe M, et al. Fresh frozen plasma versus prothrombin complex concentrate in patients with intracranial haemorrhage related to vitamin K antagonists (INCH): a randomised trial. Lancet Neurol. 2016;15(6):566–73.
77. Goldstein JN, Refaai MA, Milling TJ Jr, et al. Four-factor prothrombin complex concentrate versus plasma for rapid vitamin K antagonist reversal in patients needing urgent surgical or invasive interventions: a phase 3b, open-label, noninferiority, randomised trial. Lancet. 2015;6736(14):1–11.
78. Mayer SA, Brun NC, Begtrup K, et al. Efficacy and safety of recombinant activated factor VII for acute intracerebral hemorrhage. N Engl J Med. 2008;358(20):2127–37.
79. Kaatz S, Kouides PA, Garcia DA, et al. Guidance on the emergent reversal of oral thrombin and factor Xa inhibitors. Am J Hematol. 2012;87(Suppl 1):141–5.
80. Steiner T, Bo¨hm M, Dichgans M, et al. Recommendations for the emergency management of complications associated with the new direct oral anticoagulants (DOACs), apixaban, dabigatran and rivaroxaban. Clin Res Cardiol. 2013;102(6):399–412.
81. Held V, Eisele P, Eschenfelder CC, et al. Idarucizumab as antidote to intracerebral hemorrhage under treatment with dabigatran. Case Rep Neurol. 2016;8(3):224–8.
82. Nafee T, Aslam A, Chi G, et al. Andexanet alfa for the reversal of anticoagulant activity in patients treated with direct and indirect factor Xa inhibitors. Expert Rev Cardiovasc Ther. 2017;15(4):237–45.
83. da Luz LT, Marchand M, Nascimento B, et al. Efficacy and safety of the drugs used to reverse direct oral anticoagulants: a systematic review and meta-analysis. Transfusion. 2017;57:1834. https://doi.org/10.1111/trf.14096.
84. Hunt BJ, Levi M. Andexanet alfa for factor Xa inhibitor reversal. N Engl J Med. 2016;375(25):2500.
85. Yaghi S, Eisenberger A, Willey JZ. Symptomatic intracerebral hemorrhage in acute ischemic stroke after thrombolysis with intravenous recombinant tissue plasminogen activator: a review of natural history and treatment. JAMA Neurol. 2014;71(9):1181–5.
86. Mendelow AD, Gregson BA, Fernandes HM, et al. Early surgery versus initial conservative treatment in patients with spontaneous supratentorial intracerebral haematomas in the International Surgical Trial in Intracerebral Haemorrhage (STICH): a randomised trial. Lancet. 2005;365:387–97.
87. Mendelow AD, Gregson BA, Mitchell PM, et al. Surgical trial in lobar intracerebral Haemorrhage (STICH II) protocol. Trials. 2011;12:124. https://doi.org/10.1186/1745-6215-12-124.
88. Fung C, Murek M, Z'Graggen WJ, et al. Decompressive hemicraniectomy in patients with supratentorial intracerebral hemorrhage. Stroke. 2012;43:3207–11. https://doi.org/10.1161/STROKEAHA.112.666537.

89. Takeuchi S, Wada K, Nagatani K, Otani N, Mori K. Decompressive hemicraniectomy for spontaneous intracerebral hemorrhage. Neurosurg Focus. 2013;34:E5. https://doi.org/10.3171/2013.2.FOCUS12424.
90. Morgan T, Zuccarello M, Narayan R, Keyl P, Lane K, Hanley D. Preliminary findings of the minimally-invasive surgery plus rtPA for intracerebral hemorrhage evacuation (MISTIE) clinical trial. Acta Neurochir Suppl. 2008;105:147–51.
91. Spiotta AM, Fiorella D, Vargas J, et al. Initial multicenter technical experience with the Apollo device for minimally invasive intracerebral hematoma evacuation. Neurosurgery. 2015;11(Suppl 2):243–51.; discussion 251. https://doi.org/10.1227/NEU.0000000000000698.
92. Yadav YR, Mukerji G, Shenoy R, Basoor A, Jain G, Nelson A. Endoscopic management of hypertensive intraventricular haemorrhage with obstructive hydrocephalus. BMC Neurol. 2007;7:1. https://doi.org/10.1186/1471-2377-7-1.
93. Middleton S, McElduff P, Ward J, et al. Implementation of evidence-based treatment protocols to manage fever, hyperglycaemia, and swallowing dysfunction in acute stroke (QASC): a cluster randomised controlled trial. Lancet. 2011;378(9804):1699–706.
94. De Herdt V, Dumont F, He'non H, et al. Early seizures in intracerebral hemorrhage: incidence, associated factors and outcome. Neurology. 2011;77(20):1794–800.

Chapter 2
Early Inpatient Workup for Intracerebral Hemorrhage

Muhib Khan, Rushna Ali, Justin Singer, Paul Mazaris, and Brian Silver

Spontaneous non-traumatic intracerebral hemorrhage (ICH) is a leading cause of morbidity and mortality around the world. The mortality related to ICH has not changed in the past three decades emphasizing the need for further improvement in care of these patients [1]. In this chapter we will focus on the diagnostic workup of ICH to determine the etiology. It is important to understand the various etiologies of ICH to tailor the investigation accordingly. We have attempted to provide an evidence-based approach using the available data at this time.

Clinical Evaluation

The initial evaluation is focused in the emergency department. However, this clinical evaluation should continue onto the neuro-critical care unit and/or stroke unit [2, 3]. Since intracerebral hemorrhage can be a devastating condition, a baseline severity score should be performed as part of the initial evaluation of patients with ICH. Various severity scales have been developed, but the most widely used scale is ICH score [3–11] and should be used as a standardized severity score for communication between providers [10]. It should not be used as a singular indicator of prognosis and decision for withdrawal of care. The National Institutes of Health Stroke

M. Khan (✉) · J. Singer · P. Mazaris
Spectrum Health Neuroscience Institute, Michigan State University, Grand Rapids, MI, USA

R. Ali
Department of Neurosurgery, Vanderbilt University, Nashville, TN, USA

B. Silver
Department of Neurology, University of Massachussetts, Worcester, MA, USA

B. Ovbiagele, A. I. Qureshi (eds.), *Intracerebral Hemorrhage Therapeutics*,
https://doi.org/10.1007/978-3-319-77063-5_2

Scale (NIHSS) score, which is used for ischemic stroke, may also be useful for continued bedside monitoring in ICH [12, 13].

A complete history is imperative in determining the need for further evaluation. This includes time of symptom onset (or time the patient was last normal) and progression of symptoms over time. Patient and/or family members should be asked about history of prior ischemic stroke or ICH, seizures, liver disease, cancer and hematological disorders, hypertension, diabetes mellitus, and smoking. Current and prior prescribed and over-the-counter medications should be documented specially anticoagulants, antiplatelets, antihypertensives, stimulants (including diet pills), and sympathomimetic drugs. It is important to know about the recent trauma or surgery especially carotid endarterectomy or carotid stenting as these can lead to ICH through hyperperfusion. An assessment of prior cognitive function or dementia is helpful. A history of alcohol or illicit drug use such as cocaine and other sympathomimetic drugs also needs to be evaluated, given that a significant number of these patients with ICH have a past or current history of drug abuse [14, 15].

Laboratory Tests

Laboratory investigation is important in both the evaluation of etiology of ICH and continued care. Complete blood count, electrolytes, blood urea nitrogen, creatinine, glucose, prothrombin time (with INR), activated partial thromboplastin time, cardiac-specific troponin, electrocardiogram (ECG), urinalysis, urine culture, pregnancy test in a woman of childbearing age, and urine toxicology screening [3].

Classification of ICH

In order to efficiently investigate the etiology, it is important to characterize the ICH into different classes. As mentioned earlier, a good system of classification is not available, but some guidance can be sought from published literature.

Intracerebral hemorrhages can be classified according to location into deep, lobar, supratentorial, and infratentorial. This location-based classification helps in determining the severity and prognosis [16]. However, this location-based approach alone is not helpful in determining the etiology and guide diagnostic workup. Therefore, it needs to be combined with further demographic and clinical information. A simple classification is provided by Meretoja et al. designated as SMASH-U (structural vascular lesions, medication, cerebral amyloid angiopathy, systemic disease, hypertension, or undetermined) [17]. This classification provides a stepwise approach to etiological assessment of ICH incorporating demographic, clinical, and imaging context.

This approach provides a simple and practical means by which to classify the pathogenesis of ICH as well as provide prognosis. However, like every other classification system, SMASH-U is not accurate at all times and may misclassify ICH especially when there are more than one possible etiologies [18]. Determining the etiology of ICH is dependent on neuroimaging evaluation which we discuss below.

Neuroimaging

Initial evaluation of ICH in the emergency department should include at least computed tomography (CT). Although certain clinical features can point toward an ICH, neuroimaging is the only definitive way to make a diagnosis [19].

Computed Tomography (CT)

CT is a sensitive and effective modality for identifying acute hemorrhage. It is considered the "gold standard" for initial evaluation of ICH [3]. CT is commonly used in the emergency department due to its convenience and availability. As mentioned earlier, hematoma volume plays a major role in ICH severity, and the ICH score relies on volume calculation. CT is the main modality implied in quantifying the hematoma volume and monitoring expansion [20]. Hemorrhage volume is calculated by the ABC/2 method, where A is the greatest hemorrhage diameter; B, the diameter at 90° to A; and C, the approximate number of CT slices with hemorrhage multiplied by slice thicknesses [21]. Recent studies question the reliability of the ABC/2 method showing that it produces a larger percentage of error compared with planimetry, particularly for irregular-shaped objects [22, 23]. However, ABC/2 method is easy to use assessment tool in the acute situation.

CT scan has the ability to approximate the age of hematomas based on the density measured in Hounsfield units. Hyperacute ICH is seen as a uniform and smooth hyper-intense signal. Evolving hematomas start showing fluid levels as hypodense bloody serum layered above hyperdense settled blood [24]. Further evolution leads to a hypodense region around the hematoma, as a result of the edema that surrounds the brain tissue. Consequently mass effect can be detected at this time. Subacutely, the hematoma shrinks in about 20 days after onset becoming less intense. This process can take up to 2 months and eventually a confined region of modest hypodensity can be seen [25].

Magnetic Resonance Imaging

CT scan is highly sensitive in identifying intracerebral hemorrhage as mentioned earlier. Multimodal magnetic resonance imaging (MRI) has excellent ability to delineate hyperacute ischemia [26]. Stroke MRI protocols which include T1, T2, gradient echo (GE), fluid-attenuated inversion recovery, and diffusion-weighted images are widely used nowadays [27]. T1- and T2-weighted MRI sequences are able to detect subacute and chronic blood. However, with technological advancement, gradient recalled echo (GRE) is sensitive in detecting hyperacute ICH [28–32]. MRI is able to identify ICH from the blood degradation product deoxyhemoglobin which has paramagnetic properties. GRE shows areas of hyperintensity in the ICH core usually surrounded by hypointense boundaries. Hyperintense signals are found bordering the central ICH on T2 images, whereas a hypointense signal is seen on T1 indicating vasogenic edema [27, 29–31]. MRI has shown comparable accuracy to CT in detecting ICH in hyperacute phase.

MRI brain has its limitations as well. Patient factors such as critical illness, presence of a pacemaker, metallic implants, and claustrophobia preclude some patients from getting an MRI. Easy availability is another issue which is a factor in the acute situation [33, 34]. MRI is superior to CT in detecting underlying causes of ICH, including vascular malformations, tumors, and cerebral vein thrombosis [35]. MRI is highly sensitive for detecting cavernomas which can lead to ICH [36]. Contrast-enhanced MR venography shows the thrombosed segment of the venous sinus and correlates well with conventional angiogram [37, 38]. Cerebral microhemorrhages (CMB) have been shown to increase the risk of ICH [39] and point toward a diagnosis cerebral amyloid angiopathy (CAA) [40]. MRI is superior to CT in detecting these silent lesions and helps in etiological assessment. CMB have been shown to increase the risk of recurrent ICH, and detecting these may be helpful in further management of these patients with regard to antiplatelet and anticoagulation treatment [41]. Moreover, MRI helps in quantifying the burden the small vessel disease in patients with ICH [42].

For the abovementioned reasons, it is important to carefully select patients with ICH who should have evaluation by MRI. Although no established protocols are available, a logical approach is suggested by Kamal et al. utilizing the Hong Kong criteria which were originally developed for catheter angiography [35]. Kamal et al. recommend an MRI brain for patients with ICH with age less than 45 years and no history of hypertension or who present with lobar hemorrhage [35, 43].

Computed Tomographic Angiography

Computed tomographic angiography (CTA) in the initial phase can reveal a spot sign, which is extravasation of contrast within the hematoma [44]. The spot sign is predictive of hematoma enlargement with high sensitivity (63%) and specificity (90%) [45]. The spot sign is associated with a poor prognosis; however its impact on clinical decision-making still needs further evaluation [46]. CTA performed in the initial 3–4 days from symptom onset has a high accuracy for detecting vascular lesions. Its easy availability and noninvasive nature make it a promising modality in the initial workup of ICH [47, 48]. However, it comes with its own risk of exposure to radiation, contrast-induced nephropathy (CIN), and allergic reaction [49]. Cost is another issue related to diagnostic studies and should be factored in. Therefore, it should be reserved for patients in whom the suspicion for underlying vascular lesion is high.

Magnetic Resonance Angiography

Magnetic resonance angiography (MRA) is a noninvasive modality used to identify vascular lesions responsible for ICH. MRA is useful in avoiding radiation and iodinated-contrast. The sensitivity (0.98) and specificity (0.99) is comparable to CTA [50]. Limitations are similar to MRI such as accessibility and patient-related factors. It is a good alternative for patients who cannot undergo CTA.

Digital Subtraction Angiography (DSA)

Patients who have subarachnoid hemorrhage (SAH) in addition to ICH, noncircular hematoma, edema out of proportion to the hemorrhagic mass seen on CT at admission, lobar ICH, and young age might point toward an underlying vascular lesion [3]. DSA should be considered in these cases. It can reveal underlying conditions such as arteriovenous malformations, aneurysms, moyamoya disease, vasculitis, reversible cerebral vasoconstriction syndrome, and cerebral vein thromboses. Factors such as young age, absence of history of hypertension, and lobar hemorrhage can increase the yield of angiogram [51]. Timing of DSA is important in improving yield as well as diagnosing vascular lesions promptly to treat them. Repeat angiogram can improve the yield in certain patients. DSA is associated with the risks of transient and permanent neurological deficits and should be kept in mind. Therefore, careful selection of patients for repeat angiogram is warranted [52, 53].

CTA vs MRA vs DSA

It is difficult to compare these modalities due to variation in studies evaluating each modality [50]. Combining CTA with DSA or MRA with DSA improves the diagnostic yield. Patient selection should be based on demographics, known risk factors, ICH location, and imaging features. A simplified approach to the diagnostic workup is provided by Macellari et al. [54] They propose a stepwise approach to diagnostic evaluation incorporating CT, CTA, MRI, and DSA. The choice of each modality is guided by clinical and imaging findings [54].

Other Causes of ICH

Hematological disorders account for about 8% of all spontaneous ICH. Most of these are attributed to coagulopathy caused by anticoagulant and antiplatelet use [55]. However a significant number is due to clotting factor deficiencies, thrombocytopenia and lymphoproliferative disorders.

Thrombocytopenia has multiple causes with some general mechanism: (1) decreased platelet production due to congenital disorders and bone marrow damage, (2) increased platelet destruction as seen in idiopathic thrombocytopenic purpura (ITP) and disseminated intravascular coagulation (DIC), (3) abnormal sequestration in the spleen as seen in cirrhosis, and (4) toxins such as alcohol, drugs, and uremia [56]. Idiopathic thrombocytopenic purpura (ITP) can lead to ICH in about 1% of the patients with ITP. The risk is high with very low platelet counts of less than 20,000/mm [3].

Cytotoxic drugs, antimalarial agents, antiepileptic medications, furosemide, digoxin, and estrogens have been shown to cause thrombocytopenia [57]. Uremia causes both a decrease in the number of platelets and dysfunction leading to ICH [58]. Alcohol causes thrombocytopenia through folate deficiency, splenic sequestration, and direct toxic effects of alcohol on the bone marrow [59]. It also causes platelet dysfunction. Therefore, a platelet count should always be tested in patients with ICH. In addition, a select number of patients should have their platelet function tested.

Coagulation factor deficiencies are rare conditions causing ICH in young patients [56]. Hemophilia A and B are rare conditions caused by a deficiency of coagulation factors VIII (hemophilia A) and IX (hemophilia B). Intracerebral hemorrhage is a serious complication of hemophilia leading to mortality [60]. The incidence is between 2.2% and 7.8% in hemophiliacs [61]. Most of these patients are young, and the mean age of hemophiliacs presenting with ICH is 15 years [62]. Other congenital coagulation factor deficiencies such as vWF deficiency, congenital afibrinogenemia, and factors V, VII, and XIII can lead to ICH [63–67].

Hypercoagulable states such as antiphospholipid syndrome, prothrombin mutation, and factor V Leiden deficiency can lead to ICH through mechanism cerebral venous thrombosis [68–70]. Patients with leukemia have a high (15%) incidence ICH. Of the subtypes, acute myeloid leukemia (AML) has a higher incidence of 22%. ICH is mediated through DIC, thrombocytopenia, and leukostasis [71]. Therefore, it is important to test for these coagulation factors both quantitative and qualitatively specially in young patients with ICH.

Intracranial Vasculopathy

Approximately 12% of patients with Primary CNS Vasculitis (PCNSV) patients can present with ICH [72]. The mean age of presentation is 50 years with a range between 30 and 68 years. Headache, cognitive deficits, and systemic vasculitis manifestations are presenting features. Therefore, when suspected diagnostic workup should include MRI brain with contrast, lumbar puncture, cerebral angiogram, and brain biopsy. Prompt diagnosis leads to a proper treatment with steroids and immunosuppressive medications [72].

Reversible cerebral vasoconstriction syndrome (RCVS) can lead to ICH in 12% of patients at presentation. Mean age of presentation is 43.5 years with a female predominance. Sudden maximum intensity headache is a common presenting symptom. Diagnostic evaluation should include extensive medication history including over-the-counter medications, MRI brain, cerebral angiogram, and transcranial Doppler ultrasound. A trial of magnesium and calcium channel blockers is warranted to relieve headache [73].

Brain tumors have the potential to cause ICH with an overall incidence between 2% and 4%. Most of these brain tumors causing ICH are metastases of extracranial origin (36%), followed by glioblastoma multiforme (30%) and benign primary intracranial neoplasms (18%). A high number of these patients (58%) have ICH as a presenting feature of neoplastic disease [74]. Therefore, patients with no risk factors of spontaneous ICH should undergo MRI brain with contrast and potential CT chest, abdomen, and pelvis to look for neoplastic lesions. In some cases, a biopsy might help with diagnosis [74].

Conclusion

ICH is a devastating disease with high morbidity and mortality. Proper diagnostic workup is essential to effective management and should be guided by demographics, history, clinical features, imaging, and laboratory findings.

References

1. van Asch CJ, Luitse MJ, Rinkel GJ, van der Tweel I, Algra A, Klijn CJ. Incidence, case fatality, and functional outcome of intracerebral haemorrhage over time, according to age, sex, and ethnic origin: a systematic review and meta-analysis. Lancet Neurol. 2010;9:167–76.
2. Hafeez S, Behrouz R. The safety and feasibility of admitting patients with Intracerebral hemorrhage to the step-down unit. J Intensive Care Med. 2016;31:409–11.
3. Hemphill JC 3rd, Greenberg SM, Anderson CS, et al. Guidelines for the management of spontaneous intracerebral hemorrhage: a guideline for healthcare professionals from the American Heart Association/American Stroke Association. Stroke. 2015;46:2032–60.
4. Bernstein RA, Hemphill JC. Critical care of acute ischemic stroke. Curr Neurol Neurosci Rep. 2001;1:587–92.
5. Bruce SS, Appelboom G, Piazza M, et al. A comparative evaluation of existing grading scales in intracerebral hemorrhage. Neurocrit Care. 2011;15:498–505.
6. Ji R, Shen H, Pan Y, et al. A novel risk score to predict 1-year functional outcome after intracerebral hemorrhage and comparison with existing scores. Crit Care. 2013;17:R275.
7. Rost NS, Smith EE, Chang Y, et al. Prediction of functional outcome in patients with primary intracerebral hemorrhage: the FUNC score. Stroke. 2008;39:2304–9.
8. Wei JW, Heeley EL, Wang JG, et al. Comparison of recovery patterns and prognostic indicators for ischemic and hemorrhagic stroke in China: the ChinaQUEST (qUality evaluation of stroke care and treatment) registry study. Stroke. 2010;41:1877–83.
9. Weimar C, Benemann J, Diener HC, German Stroke Study C. Development and validation of the Essen Intracerebral Haemorrhage score. J Neurol Neurosurg Psychiatry. 2006;77:601–5.
10. Morgenstern LB, Zahuranec DB, Sanchez BN, et al. Full medical support for intracerebral hemorrhage. Neurology. 2015;84:1739–44.

11. Hemphill JC 3rd, Farrant M, Neill TA Jr. Prospective validation of the ICH score for 12-month functional outcome. Neurology. 2009;73:1088–94.
12. Fonarow GC, Pan W, Saver JL, et al. Comparison of 30-day mortality models for profiling hospital performance in acute ischemic stroke with vs without adjustment for stroke severity. JAMA. 2012;308:257–64.
13. Smith EE, Shobha N, Dai D, et al. A risk score for in-hospital death in patients admitted with ischemic or hemorrhagic stroke. J Am Heart Assoc. 2013;2:e005207.
14. Kalani R, Liotta EM, Prabhakaran S. Diagnostic yield of universal urine toxicology screening in an unselected cohort of stroke patients. PLoS One. 2015;10:e0144772.
15. Shoamanesh A, Catanese L, Romero JR, et al. High prevalence of cerebral microbleeds in inner city young stroke patients. J Stroke Cerebrovascular Diseases: Off J National Stroke Assoc. 2016;25:733–8.
16. Hwang DY, Dell CA, Sparks MJ, et al. Clinician judgment vs formal scales for predicting intracerebral hemorrhage outcomes. Neurology. 2016;86:126–33.
17. Meretoja A, Strbian D, Putaala J, et al. SMASH-U: a proposal for etiologic classification of intracerebral hemorrhage. Stroke. 2012;43:2592–7.
18. Yeh SJ, Tang SC, Tsai LK, Jeng JS. Pathogenetical subtypes of recurrent intracerebral hemorrhage: designations by SMASH-U classification system. Stroke. 2014;45:2636–42.
19. Goldstein LB, Simel DL. Is this patient having a stroke? JAMA. 2005;293:2391–402.
20. Zimmerman RD, Maldjian JA, Brun NC, Horvath B, Skolnick BE. Radiologic estimation of hematoma volume in intracerebral hemorrhage trial by CT scan. AJNR Am J Neuroradiol. 2006;27:666–70.
21. Kothari RU, Brott T, Broderick JP, et al. The ABCs of measuring intracerebral hemorrhage volumes. Stroke. 1996;27:1304–5.
22. Divani AA, Majidi S, Luo X, et al. The ABCs of accurate volumetric measurement of cerebral hematoma. Stroke. 2011;42:1569–74.
23. Khan M, Baird GL, Elias R, et al. Comparison of intracerebral hemorrhage volume calculation methods and their impact on scoring tools. J Neuroimag: Off J Am Soc Neuroimag. 2017;27:144–8.
24. Zilkha A. Intraparenchymal fluid-blood level: a CT sign of recent intracerebral hemorrhage. J Comput Assist Tomogr. 1983;7:301–5.
25. Herold S, von Kummer R, Jaeger C. Follow-up of spontaneous intracerebral haemorrhage by computed tomography. J Neurol. 1982;228:267–76.
26. Baird AE, Warach S. Magnetic resonance imaging of acute stroke. J Cerebral Blood Flow Metabolism: Off J Int Soc Cerebral Blood Flow Metab. 1998;18:583–609.
27. Wintermark M, Fiebach J. Imaging of brain parenchyma in stroke. Handb Clin Neurol. 2009;94:1011–9.
28. Edelman RR, Johnson K, Buxton R, et al. MR of hemorrhage: a new approach. AJNR Am J Neuroradiol. 1986;7:751–6.
29. Patel MR, Edelman RR, Warach S. Detection of hyperacute primary intraparenchymal hemorrhage by magnetic resonance imaging. Stroke. 1996;27:2321–4.
30. Linfante I, Llinas RH, Caplan LR, Warach S. MRI features of intracerebral hemorrhage within 2 hours from symptom onset. Stroke. 1999;30:2263–7.
31. Schellinger PD, Jansen O, Fiebach JB, Hacke W, Sartor K. A standardized MRI stroke protocol: comparison with CT in hyperacute intracerebral hemorrhage. Stroke. 1999;30:765–8.
32. Kidwell CS, Saver JL, Mattiello J, et al. Diffusion-perfusion MR evaluation of perihematomal injury in hyperacute intracerebral hemorrhage. Neurology. 2001;57:1611–7.
33. Singer OC, Sitzer M, du Mesnil de Rochemont R, Neumann-Haefelin T. Practical limitations of acute stroke MRI due to patient-related problems. Neurology. 2004;62:1848–9.
34. Barber PA, Hill MD, Eliasziw M, et al. Imaging of the brain in acute ischaemic stroke: comparison of computed tomography and magnetic resonance diffusion-weighted imaging. J Neurol Neurosurg Psychiatry. 2005;76:1528–33.
35. Kamel H, Navi BB, Hemphill JC 3rd. A rule to identify patients who require magnetic resonance imaging after intracerebral hemorrhage. Neurocrit Care. 2013;18:59–63.

36. Kazim SF, Bhatti ESA. Intracranial cavernous angiomas. J Coll Physicians Surg Pak. : JCPSP. 2010;20:738–43.
37. Bousser MG, Ferro JM. Cerebral venous thrombosis: an update. Lancet Neurol. 2007;6: 162–70.
38. Ihn YK, Jung WS, Hwang SS. The value of T2*-weighted gradient-echo MRI for the diagnosis of cerebral venous sinus thrombosis. Clin Imaging. 2013;37:446–50.
39. Fan YH, Zhang L, Lam WW, Mok VC, Wong KS. Cerebral microbleeds as a risk factor for subsequent intracerebral hemorrhages among patients with acute ischemic stroke. Stroke. 2003;34:2459–62.
40. van Etten ES, Auriel E, Haley KE, et al. Incidence of symptomatic hemorrhage in patients with lobar microbleeds. Stroke. 2014;45:2280–5.
41. Greenberg SM, Eng JA, Ning M, Smith EE, Rosand J. Hemorrhage burden predicts recurrent intracerebral hemorrhage after lobar hemorrhage. Stroke. 2004;35:1415–20.
42. Charidimou A, Martinez-Ramirez S, Reijmer YD, et al. Total magnetic resonance imaging burden of small vessel disease in cerebral amyloid angiopathy: an imaging-pathologic study of concept validation. JAMA Neurol. 2016;73:994–1001.
43. Zhu XL, Chan MS, Poon WS. Spontaneous intracranial hemorrhage: which patients need diagnostic cerebral angiography? A prospective study of 206 cases and review of the literature. Stroke. 1997;28:1406–9.
44. Murai Y, Ikeda Y, Teramoto A, et al. Contrast extravasation on CT angiography predicts hematoma expansion in intracerebral hemorrhage. Neurology. 2007;69:617. author reply
45. Demchuk AM, Dowlatshahi D, Rodriguez-Luna D, et al. Prediction of haematoma growth and outcome in patients with intracerebral haemorrhage using the CT-angiography spot sign (PREDICT): a prospective observational study. Lancet Neurol. 2012;11:307–14.
46. Romero JM, Brouwers HB, Lu J, et al. Prospective validation of the computed tomographic angiography spot sign score for intracerebral hemorrhage. Stroke. 2013;44:3097–102.
47. Yoon DY, Chang SK, Choi CS, Kim WK, Lee JH. Multidetector row CT angiography in spontaneous lobar intracerebral hemorrhage: a prospective comparison with conventional angiography. AJNR Am J Neuroradiol. 2009;30:962–7.
48. Wong GK, Siu DY, Abrigo JM, et al. Computed tomographic angiography and venography for young or nonhypertensive patients with acute spontaneous intracerebral hemorrhage. Stroke. 2011;42:211–3.
49. Hotta K, Sorimachi T, Osada T, et al. Risks and benefits of CT angiography in spontaneous intracerebral hemorrhage. Acta Neurochir. 2014;156:911–7.
50. Josephson CB, White PM, Krishan A, Al-Shahi Salman R. Computed tomography angiography or magnetic resonance angiography for detection of intracranial vascular malformations in patients with intracerebral haemorrhage. Cochrane Database Syst Rev. 2014:CD009372.
51. Cordonnier C, Klijn CJ, van Beijnum J, Al-Shahi Salman R. Radiological investigation of spontaneous intracerebral hemorrhage: systematic review and trinational survey. Stroke. 2010;41:685–90.
52. Hino A, Fujimoto M, Yamaki T, Iwamoto Y, Katsumori T. Value of repeat angiography in patients with spontaneous subcortical hemorrhage. Stroke. 1998;29:2517–21.
53. Willinsky RA, Taylor SM, TerBrugge K, Farb RI, Tomlinson G, Montanera W. Neurologic complications of cerebral angiography: prospective analysis of 2,899 procedures and review of the literature. Radiology. 2003;227:522–8.
54. Macellari F, Paciaroni M, Agnelli G, Caso V. Neuroimaging in intracerebral hemorrhage. Stroke. 2014;45:903–8.
55. del Zoppo GJ, Mori E. Hematologic causes of intracerebral hemorrhage and their treatment. Neurosurg Clin N Am. 1992;3:637–58.
56. Quinones-Hinojosa A, Gulati M, Singh V, Lawton MT. Spontaneous intracerebral hemorrhage due to coagulation disorders. Neurosurg Focus. 2003;15:E3.
57. Burstein SA. Cytokines, platelet production and hemostasis. Platelets. 1997;8:93–104.
58. Carvalho AC. Bleeding in a uremia--a clinical challenge. N Engl J Med. 1983;308:38–9.
59. Cowan DH. Effect of alcoholism on hemostasis. Semin Hematol. 1980;17:137–47.

60. Kerr CB. Intracranial Haemorrhage in Haemophilia. J Neurol Neurosurg Psychiatry. 1964;27:166–73.
61. Silverstein A. Intracranial bleeding in hemophilia. Arch Neurol. 1960;3:141–57.
62. de Tezanos Pinto M, Fernandez J, Perez Bianco PR. Update of 156 episodes of central nervous system bleeding in hemophiliacs. Haemostasis. 1992;22:259–67.
63. Almaani WS, Awidi AS. Spontaneous intracranial hemorrhage secondary to von Willebrand's disease. Surg Neurol. 1986;26:457–60.
64. Ariffin H, Lin HP. Neonatal intracranial hemorrhage secondary to congenital factor VII deficiency: two case reports. Am J Hematol. 1997;54:263.
65. Gerlach R, Raabe A, Zimmermann M, Siegemund A, Seifert V. Factor XIII deficiency and postoperative hemorrhage after neurosurgical procedures. Surg Neurol. 2000;54:260–4. discussion 4–5
66. Mizoi K, Onuma T, Mori K. Intracranial hemorrhage secondary to von Willebrand's disease and trauma. Surg Neurol. 1984;22:495–8.
67. Parameswaran R, Dickinson JP, de Lord S, Keeling DM, Colvin BT. Spontaneous intracranial bleeding in two patients with congenital afibrinogenaemia and the role of replacement therapy. Haemophilia: Off J World Federat Hemophilia. 2000;6:705–8.
68. Nagai S, Horie Y, Akai T, Takeda S, Takaku A. Superior sagittal sinus thrombosis associated with primary antiphospholipid syndrome--case report. Neurol Med Chir. 1998;38:34–9.
69. Provenzale JM, Loganbill HA. Dural sinus thrombosis and venous infarction associated with antiphospholipid antibodies: MR findings. J Comput Assist Tomogr. 1994;18:719–23.
70. Provenzale JM, Ortel TL. Anatomic distribution of venous thrombosis in patients with antiphospholipid antibody: imaging findings. AJR Am J Roentgenol. 1995;165:365–8.
71. Graus F, Rogers LR, Posner JB. Cerebrovascular complications in patients with cancer. Medicine. 1985;64:16–35.
72. Salvarani C, Brown RD Jr, Calamia KT, et al. Primary central nervous system vasculitis presenting with intracranial hemorrhage. Arthritis Rheum. 2011;63:3598–606.
73. Topcuoglu MA, Singhal AB. Hemorrhagic reversible cerebral vasoconstriction syndrome: features and mechanisms. Stroke. 2016;47:1742–7.
74. Schrader B, Barth H, Lang EW, et al. Spontaneous intracranial haematomas caused by neoplasms. Acta Neurochir. 2000;142:979–85.

Chapter 3
Antithrombotic- and Thrombolytic-Related Intracerebral Hemorrhage

Jan C. Purrucker, Matthew L. Flaherty, Gustavo Rodriguez, Saqib Chaudhry, Fazeel Siddiqui, and Thorsten Steiner

Antithrombotic- and Thrombolytic-Related ICH

Case Vignette

Only minutes after dining with her husband, a 77-year-old woman was found by him vomiting and with reduced level of consciousness. She was immediately transported to the closest hospital, a tertiary care center. On admission, her Glasgow Coma Scale score was 8, with no clear lateralizing signs of paresis, but bilateral positive Babinski signs. Emergency medical services personnel reported use of rivaroxaban due to atrial fibrillation, but the last time of intake and dose were unknown. CT scan revealed a small left-sided thalamic intracerebral hemorrhage (ICH) with

J. C. Purrucker
Department of Neurology, Heidelberg University Hospital, Heidelberg, Germany

M. L. Flaherty
Department of Neurology and Rehabilitation Medicine, University of Cincinnati, Academic Health Center, Cincinnati, OH, USA

G. Rodriguez
Department of Neurology, Texas Tech University, El Paso, TX, USA

S. Chaudhry
Departments of Neurology and Neuro-critical Care, University of Pennsylvania, Philadelphia, PA, USA

F. Siddiqui
Department of Neurology, Southern Illinois University, Springfield, IL, USA

T. Steiner (✉)
Department of Neurology, Heidelberg University Hospital, Heidelberg, Germany

Department of Neurology, Klinikum Frankfurt Höchst, Frankfurt a.M., Germany
e-mail: thorsten_steiner@med.uni-heidelberg.de

B. Ovbiagele, A. I. Qureshi (eds.), *Intracerebral Hemorrhage Therapeutics*,
https://doi.org/10.1007/978-3-319-77063-5_3

intraventricular extension (Fig. 3.1). The third and fourth ventricles were nearly occluded, but hydrocephalus had not developed. CT angiography revealed no vascular pathology. Aware of rivaroxaban use, the attending neurologist and neurosurgeon were immediately informed of the necessity of intubation of the patient, preparation of a reversal treatment, and placement of an external ventricular drainage (EVD). However, both responded with several questions, "In the absence of a definite time-window of 'last intake of rivaroxaban,' should one wait for laboratory parameters confirming the effective intake before administration of a reversal treatment?" and "Which dose of the reversal treatment should be administered?", and the neurosurgeon questioned "after reversal treatment, how can I be sure no anticoagulant effect is present before placing an EVD?"

In the following chapter, knowledge about the clinical course and emergency management of ICH related to vitamin K antagonists (VKA), non-vitamin K antagonist oral anticoagulants (NOAC), heparin, thrombolytic agents, and antiplatelet treatment will be provided in order to offer sufficient background knowledge for daily clinical practice.

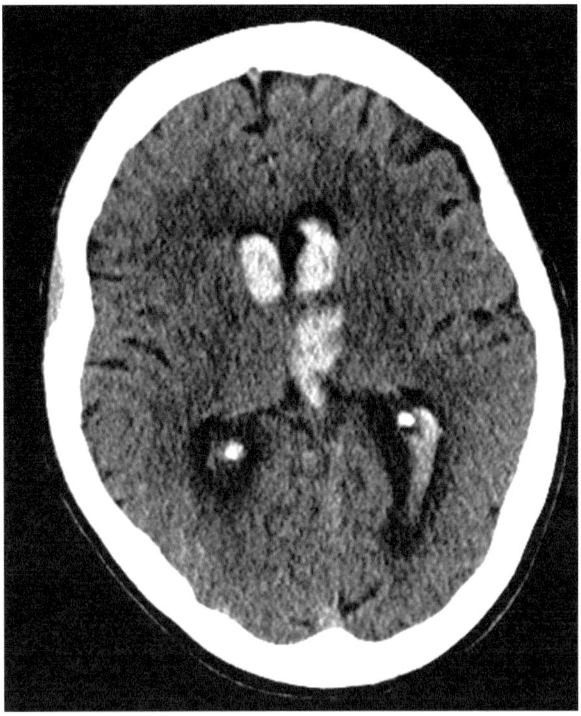

Fig. 3.1 Illustrative CT scan showing left-sided thalamic intracerebral hemorrhage with intraventricular extension (By courtesy of the Department of Neuroradiology, Heidelberg University Hospital)

Pathophysiology of OAC-Related ICH

Small vessel disorders account for approximately 85% of all ICH cases. Chronic disorders such as hypertension can lead to fibrinoid necrosis (lipohyalinosis), characterized by vessel wall thickening, endothelial dysfunction, and local inflammatory processes [1]. Accumulation of beta-amyloid in basement membranes of arterioles and capillaries in cases of cerebral amyloid angiopathy (CAA) causes blood-brain barrier disruptions and microaneurysm formation [2, 3]. While ICH in patients with hypertensive angiopathy occurs mainly in deep cerebral locations, bleedings in CAA are mostly lobar. In contrast, primary ICH related to large vessel disease including arterial aneurysms, arteriovenous malformations, dural fistulas, and venous malformations may be deep or lobar.

Although the exact pathophysiology of ICH in orally anticoagulated patients is not fully understood, it is currently assumed that spontaneous bleedings occur due to mechanisms previously described. In non-anticoagulated patients, rapid coagulation and thus cessation of bleeding lead to (asymptomatic) cerebral microbleed formation in the vast majority of cases. However, in patients treated with antithrombotic agents, bleeding continues, and symptomatic macrobleeds are more likely to form. Therefore, anticoagulation presents a hemorrhagic diathesis (facilitates symptomatic ICH), but may not cause the bleeding itself. Notably, there are indirect hints that formation of micro- and macrobleeds do comprise distinct pathophysiological processes in the context of CAA [4]. Similarly, neuropathological observations question a direct relation between microbleeds and CAA burden [5].

If the initial bleeding is not fatal, hematoma expansion may worsen outcome. In anticoagulated patients, hematoma expansion is frequent and occurs during a longer period compared to non-anticoagulated patients [6, 7]. Hematoma expansion is influenced by at least two phenomena: 1 the pressure gradient between arterial blood extravasating from an injured vessel and the pressure in surrounding tissue and 2 shear forces which may injure adjacent vessels and produce further, secondary sources of bleeding [8]. Immediately after vessel rupture, the vessel-tissue-pressure gradient is highest, but decreases with increasing hematoma volume. However, if adjacent vessels or microaneurysms rupture due to shear forces, hematoma expansion may continue [9]. The two processes build the rational for stringent blood pressure management and immediate reversal of anticoagulation in order to prevent or stem hematoma expansion.

Vitamin K Antagonist-Related ICH

In the pre-NOAC era, vitamin K antagonist-related ICH (VKA-ICH) accounted for 10–25% of all ICH [10, 11], with a rising annual incidence of >4/100,000 persons in 1999 [12]. Although a decline in the incidence of VKA-ICH is expected due to the increasing use of NOACs, VKAs are still widely used and therefore account for a substantial number of ICH cases [13]. Baseline hematoma size is likely larger in VKA-ICH compared to other cases of ICH; however in one study this effect was only seen with supratherapeutic INR (>3) [14]. In contrast, hematoma expansion occurs more frequently in VKA-ICH even when INR levels are within the therapeutic range [6]. In a large retrospective observational study, hematoma expansion was as frequent as 36% in VKA-ICH (Table 3.1) [7]. [Note: While in the latter study hematoma expansion was defined as a relative increase of 33% compared to baseline, the lack of a common agreed definition hampers direct comparison with other studies [15].] In warfarin-related ICH, the period of hematoma growth is prolonged, even beyond the initial 24 h [6] especially if anticoagulation is not reversed.

Intraventricular extension of ICH during anticoagulation with warfarin is also more frequent compared to non-anticoagulated patients, and the risk of IVH is INR dependent, with higher INR levels being associated with a greater risk [16].

Another potential prognostic factor is lobar location of ICH (defined as ICH related to the cortex and cerebellar hemorrhage in the MUCH-Italy study) that was recently found to occur more frequently in VKA-ICH compared to ICH in non-anticoagulated patients [17]. Anticoagulant-related ICH was previously found to preferentially affect the cerebellum, but supratentorial lobar ICH was not associated with anticoagulant use [18]. In a large observational study including only VKA-ICH, there was no relevant difference between patients with deep and lobar hemorrhage (according to the definition by Pezzini; $n = 433$ vs. $n = 422$). However, distribution of hemorrhage was only available for patients with follow-up imaging; thus patients with large lobar hemorrhage with early decision to palliate might not have been included.

The potentially larger baseline hematoma volume and more frequent hematoma expansion including ventricular extension contribute to a less favorable prognosis compared to patients without anticoagulation [19]. VKA-ICH is associated with a high in-hospital mortality (~ 31%) and an unfavorable long-term prognosis with the majority of all patients (56%) being dead at 1-year follow-up [7]. Once discharged with an unfavorable functional status (modified Rankin scale score of 4–5), the chance of significant improvement at 1 year was only 6.3% [7].

Anticoagulation Reversal Treatment (VKA)

In VKA-anticoagulated patients, determination of anticoagulant status is performed by measuring the INR [20]. Point-of-care devices allow for rapid bedside measurements [21]. In contrast to the easy assessment of the anticoagulant activity, until recently there was uncertainty about the best method of anticoagulant reversal. The time-dependent nature of hematoma expansion makes the rapid correction of coagulopathy intuitively attractive. Additionally, observational data suggests that the rapid correction of INR to ≤1.3, coupled with reduction of systolic blood pressure control to <160 mmHg, reduces hematoma expansion (see also Chap. 4) [5]. However, the associations were drawn from retrospective data and therefore might be subject to bias.

Table 3.1 Summary of selected studies on intracerebral hemorrhage related to non-OAC and OAC

	Non-OAC				Mixed					OAC				
Reference	Kazui et al.	Brott et al.	Davis et al.	Mayer et al.	Flibotte et al.	Flaherty et al.	Cucchiara et al.	Huhtakangas et al.	Horstmann et al.	Kuramatsu et al.	Purrucker et al.	Steiner et al.	Connolly et al.	Wilson et al.
#	[49]	[50]	[51]	[52]	[6]	[14]	[53]	[54]	[10]	[7]	[31]	[13]	[42]	[32]
Year	1996	1997	2006	2008	2004	2008	2008	2011	2013	2015	2016	2016	2016	2017
Study type	Retrospective analysis	Prospective observational	Pooled meta-analysis	RCT	Prospective cohort study	Retrospective cohort study	RCT substudy	Retrospective observational	Prospective observational	Retrospective cohort study (VKA)	Prospective observational (NOAC)	RCT (VKA)	Prospective observational (factor Xa antagonists incl. enoxaparin)	Pooled analysis
N	204	103	218	268 (placebo arm)	183 (70 expansion analysis)	258	303 (285 expansion analysis)	982	206 (152 expansion analysis)	853	61	50	14 (ICH only)	91 (NOAC), 403 (VKA)
Age, mean, years	64	63	66	65	76	69	NR (OAC: 75)	69	74[b]	74	76	76	NR	Median: 80
Women, %	37.7%	36.0%	41.7%	37.0%	NR	54.3%	33.9%	46.2%	47.6%	37.9%	41%	38%	NR	45% (NOAC), 51% (VKA)
Oral anticoagulation, No. (%)[c]	0 (0)	0 (0)	0 (0)	0 (0)	42 (23.0)	51 (19.8)	21 (6.9)	182 (18.5)	51 (24.8)	853 (100)	61 (100)	50 (100)	NR	500 (100)

(continued)

Table 3.1 (continued)

	Non-OAC				Mixed					OAC				
Reversal therapy	–	–	(Placebo arms)	(Placebo arm)	VK + FFP	–	Not speci-fied	Partly: VK + PCC	VK + PCC or FFP	VK+/– PCC +-FFP	Partly: PCC	PCC vs. FFP	Andexanet alfa	Partly PCC
Hematoma volume (mL)														
Median (IQR)	NR	NR	NR	NR	NR	NR	Non-OAC: 14.4 (7.9–30.9) OAC: 30.6 (7.4–70.1)	NR	Non-OAC 14.3 (4.9–35.7) OAC: 20.0 (8.3–48.8)	19.3 (6.9–52.8)	10.8 (4.0–30.0)	FFP: 13.2 (0.2–43.9) PCC: 13.0 (0.6–78.1)	NR	NOAC 14.4 (3.6–38.4); VKA 10.6 (4.0–27.9)
Mean (SD)	20.1 (18.0)	26 (29)	25.3 (NR)	22 (24)	NR	d	NR	Non-OAC: 29.6 (37.0) OAC: 47.8 (58.0)	Non-OAC: 26.4 (31.7) OAC: 31.5 (30.2)	NR	23.7 (31.3)	NR	NR (8/14 ≤ 10 ml; 6/14 11–60 mL)	NR
Hematoma expansion														
Predefined time frame analyzed	0–120 h	0–20 h	24 h	21–48 h	0–7 day	–	0–72 h	NR	24–48 h	NR	3–72 h	3 h, 24 h, 72 h	1 h, 12 h	<72 h

Definition of significant expansion	>12.5 ml or > 40%	≥33%	>33%	–	≥33%	NR	≥33%	NR	≥6 ml or ≥ 33%	≥33%	≥6 ml or ≥ 33%	≥33% or death	"effective hemostasis: ≤20%; good hemostasis: >20% ≤35%"	≥6 ml or ≥ 33%
Proportion of patients with significant expansion	19.6%	38.0%	31.6%	NR[e]	Non-OAC 23% OAC: 54%	NR	Non-OAC: 26% OAC: 56%	NR	Non-OAC: 11.7% OAC: 12.5%	36%	38%	24 h: FFP: 60% PCC: 30%	NR (intracranial hemor-rhage, effective/ good hemostasis: 80% (56–94%)	NOAC 40%, VKA 34%

Modified and updated from Purrucker et al. [31]
Abbreviations: *NR* not reported, *RCT* randomized clinical trial, *OAC* oral anticoagulation
[a]References within the main document
[b]Median
[c]Oral anticoagulation = treatment with vitamin K antagonists
[d]Non-OAC (international normalized ratio (INR) < 1.2) 13.4 ml, OAC INR 2.1–3.0 14.0 ml, OAC INR > 3.0 33.2 ml
[e]Estimated mean volume increase 26%
[f]Further secondary imaging endpoints included hematoma expansion ≥15% and/or death

Because VKA block a subunit of the vitamin K epoxide reductase and consequently the synthesis of the vitamin K-dependent coagulation factors (II, VII, IX, and X) [22], administration of vitamin K counteracts this mechanism. Nevertheless, administration of vitamin K does not immediately reverse anticoagulation. Thus, it should be used in order to avoid a rebound after administration of more rapid-acting reversal agents.

Three agents are capable of INR normalization: activated factor VII (aFVII), fresh frozen plasma (FFP), and prothrombin complex concentrate (PCC). According to an international survey [23], all agents are currently in use in various combinations depending on local standards and recommendations, which until recently were not supported by prospective, multicenter, randomized data. PCC contains all vitamin K-dependent coagulation factors, with variable amounts of factor VII. PCCs with no or only little amounts of VII are classified as three-factor PCCs and PCCs including factor VII, as four-factor PCCs. As the latter formulations provide a better correlation with INR reversal, it should be preferentially used, if available [24]. In 2015, a pooled multicenter observational study found that the combination of FFP and PCC was associated with the lowest case fatality and concluded that FFP might be equivalent to PCC. However, in 2016 data from the randomized INCH trial (fresh frozen plasma versus prothrombin complex concentrate in patients with intracranial hemorrhage related to vitamin K antagonists) showed that (four-factor) PCC was more efficient in normalizing the INR (≤1.2 at 3 h) and hematoma expansion seems to occur less frequently in the PCC group [13]. However, due to safety concerns (more hematoma expansion in the FFP group), the trial was halted early, and no effect on clinical outcome was found. Importantly, in the INCH trial, 83% of the patients initially treated with FFP had subsequently received PCC because INR was not below 1.3 after 3 h. Potentially due to this delay, hematoma volumes were larger in the FFP than in the PCC group, supporting an immediate start of reversal treatment once the diagnosis is made by CT or MRI scan. In view of the low efficacy and high doses (translating into high fluid volumes administered in a short time period) necessary in attempting INR reversal with FFP, PCC should be used whenever available. Due to scarce data supporting the use of recombinant factor VIIa and its known risk of inducing thrombotic events, it is only recommended for exceptional circumstances (e.g., Jehovah's witness not accepting blood products) [25]. Although rare, adverse thrombotic events might also occur with PCC. In patients with VKA-ICH, 4.4% of adverse thrombotic events were rated as "possibly" or "probably related" to PCC infusion in a retrospective observational study, but no event was rated as "clearly related." [26] In that study, high doses of PCC (>2000 IU) were associated with occurrence of thrombotic events. Thus, titration of PCC to achieve an INR below a certain threshold seems reasonable. However, the optimal INR target following VKA reversal is unknown. In the INCH trial, 1.2 was chosen [13], while other prospective studies used a target INR value of 1.3 [27, 28].

Recommendations In cases of VKA-ICH, immediate reversal of INR to ≤1.3 should be targeted by administration of a PCC and intravenous vitamin K. For patients in whom the INR is not corrected by the first dose of PCC, it is unknown whether the benefit of repeat dosing outweighs potential risks. General treatment recommendations, especially strict blood pressure control (<160 mmHg systolic), are the same as for ICH not associated with anticoagulants. Future prospective studies will have to show whether a bundle of these measures will indeed help to improve the dismal prognosis of VKA-ICH. Prevention of VKA-ICH by careful selection of patients with an indication for VKA therapy and stringent INR controls to optimize the time within the therapeutic range is necessary.

Non-vitamin K Antagonist Oral Anticoagulant-Related ICH

All NOACs have been shown to significantly reduce the relative risk of ICH compared to warfarin [29]. However a greater acceptance of oral anticoagulation, along with an increasing number of patients with indications for oral anticoagulation caused by increasing numbers of patients with atrial fibrillation and a potential extension of indications (e.g., embolic stroke of undetermined source), may ultimately result in a greater absolute number of NOAC-related hemorrhages. Eighteen to 25% of ICH patients are anticoagulated [10, 30], and according to recent German registry data, 40% of anticoagulant-associated ICHs are now attributable to NOACs [30]. In contrast to the long experience with VKA-related complications, less evidence exists regarding the clinical and radiological course and optimal management of NOAC-associated ICH (NOAC-ICH). The first prospective observational data show a similar rate of hematoma expansion (38%) in NOAC-ICH and VKA-ICH, and prognosis of NOAC-ICH seems unfavorable as well (Table 3.1) [31, 32].

In contrast to VKA-ICH, where INR measurements rapidly allow assessment of the anticoagulation status, coagulation testing in NOAC-treated patients is less straightforward. Sensitivity of routine global coagulation tests, such as INR or activated partial thromboplastin time (aPTT) for detection of relevant anticoagulant activity of NOACs, largely depends on the reagent used, and thus results should be interpreted with caution if the locally used reagent is not known [20, 33]. Thrombin time (TT) – highly sensitive for dabigatran – can be used to rule out any dabigatran effect if normal, but cannot provide a reliable estimate of the effective anticoagulant activity [20]. NOAC-specific coagulation tests (e.g., drug-specific calibrated anti-Xa tests for factor Xa inhibitors or diluted TT/hemoclot assay for dabigatran) should thus be obtained directly at admission if available. Assessment of initial coagulation status is important to clarify the etiology of the bleeding, to guide management of reversal agents, and to provide a baseline for sequential measurements after administration of reversal agents.

Anticoagulation Reversal Treatment (NOAC)

The lack of specific antidotes to the NOACs has been perceived as a major disadvantage relative to VKAs and has limited their adoption by some clinicians. Data from experimental settings suggest that PCC and FFP and activated factor VII are effective in preventing hematoma expansion with rivaroxaban as well as dabigatran [34–36]. In contrast, while a phase I clinical study involving 12 healthy male volunteers showed efficacy in reversal of rivaroxaban after PCC administration, no such effect was observed with dabigatran [37]. According to the first prospective registry data, no effect of PCC on hematoma expansion and functional outcome was observed, but these data are clearly preliminary [31]. In 2015 however, the first specific antidote for a NOAC, idarucizumab for reversal of dabigatran, gained approval from the FDA. Idarucizumab is a humanized monoclonal antibody fragment, which specifically reverses dabigatran, and it was shown effective in a phase III case series replicating positive phase I data [38–40]. More recently the publication of the RE-VERSE AD study results confirmed the reversal of dabigatran in patients with an uncontrolled hemorrhage or those requiring an urgent procedure after the administration of intravenous idarucizumab 5 g. The primary endpoint was the reversal of the anticoagulation effect of dabigatran within 4 h using thrombin time or ecarin clotting time. In a total of 503 patients, the median maximum percentage reversal was 100% (95% CI, 100–100). Only 10 patients experienced recurrent or ongoing hemorrhage out of 114 that were found to have recurrent elevations in the unbound-dabigatran levels between the 12 and 24 h. While only three of these patients required an additional dose of idarucizumab, the explanation suggested for the recurrent elevation in clotting time was redistribution of unbound dabigatran from the extravascular to the intravascular compartment [41]. Another antidote exists for reversal of the oral Xa inhibitors (apixaban, rivaroxaban, and edoxaban) and low-molecular-weight heparin, termed andexanet alfa (a recombinant truncated factor Xa). According to phase I data, it is capable of reversing the anti-factor Xa activity within minutes. In contrast to idarucizumab, in which a single bolus infusion showed long during activity, a rapid rebound after cessation of andexanet alfa infusion is observed, resulting in equal activity levels of the drug vs. placebo group after 1 h. Consequently, a continuous infusion may be needed as long as pharmacologically relevant activity can be expected. The latter depends on individual factors, such as dose, renal function, and concomitant medication, but usually after 24 h, a concentration below 33 ng/ml, currently seen as the lower threshold of clinically relevant activity [20], should be reached. An interim analysis of the prospective multicenter open-label single-arm study ANNEXA-4 (clinicaltrials.gov NCT02329327) evaluated the efficacy and safety of andexanet alfa in patients presenting with major bleeding within 18 h of the last administration of a factor Xa inhibitor (rivaroxaban, apixaban, edoxaban, or enoxaparin) [42]. Forty-seven patients with baseline anti-factor Xa activity over 75 ng/mL were included in the efficacy analysis. In 89% of rivaroxaban (95% CI, 58–94%) and 93% (95% CI, 87–94%) of apixaban-treated patients, anti-factor Xa activity was effectively reduced by bolus administration of andexanet alfa, and levels remained stable during a 2-h continuous infusion. Four hours after cessation of the andexanet alfa infusion, a relevant rebound of the anti-factor Xa activity occurred, such that reductions of 39% (rivaroxaban) and 30% (apixaban) were observed, compared to baseline. Due to the interim nature of the report, patient numbers were small, with only 20 patients with intracranial hemorrhage included in the efficacy analysis (12 ICH, 7 subdural hematoma, 1 subarachnoid hemorrhage). Furthermore, patients with a suspected unfavorable profile (GCS < 7 or estimated ICH volume > 60 mL) were excluded. ICH volume increase after 12 h was ≤30% in 10 of the 12 patients (80%), comparable to the larger study population, where effective hemostasis was reached in 79%. As of October, 2017, andexanet alfa was not yet approved for clinical use by regulatory authorities.

Further antidotes are in development, among them the "universal antidote" aripazine (Ciraparantag or PER977), which may enable reversal of the oral factor Xa inhibitors, the thrombin inhibitor dabigatran, unfractionated heparin, low-molecular-weight heparin, and fondaparinux [43].

Recommendations In view of the similar rate of hematoma expansions in NOAC-ICH compared to VKA-ICH, immediate reversal of anticoagulation in acute NOAC-ICH is prudent. After admission, standard procedures such as strict management of blood pressure should be undertaken. When available, indicators of coagulation status including thrombin time or ecarin clotting time (in the case of dabigatran) and drug-specific concentrations can be obtained. For dabigatran-related ICH, intravenous bolus administration of 5 g of idarucizumab is recommended. If idarucizumab is not available, PCC might be administered, and/or the patient might undergo immediate hemodialysis as dabigatran is dialyzable. In case of the factor Xa inhibitors, in the absence of a specific antidote, PCC may be administered. If specific reversal agents were used, drug-specific concentrations might be remeasured before starting neurosurgical procedures (in case a short postponement is possible). However, nonspecific reversal agents such as PCC do not reliably influence the drug concentration measurements, and thus measurement of the efficacy of the reversal treatment is not possible with standard coagulation tests.

Heparin-Related ICH

Data regarding the natural course of ICH during heparin therapy with either unfractionated heparin (UFH) or low-molecular-weight heparin (LMWH) is scarce. Among patients receiving heparin for non-neurological indications, ICH occurs in <0.1% of the patients [25]. Interestingly, a recent study examining the common practice of "bridging" (i.e., in case of discontinuation of warfarin therapy due to elective surgery, periprocedural use of LMWH until warfarin resumption) found a higher incidence of bleedings among the bridging group compared to those with full discontinuation of anticoagulation: Major bleeding (including ICH) occurred in 3.2% of bridged patients compared to 1.3% in the no-bridging group. In case of UFH-induced ICH, continuous infusion should be stopped immediately, and protamine sulfate (1 mg for every 100 units of heparin administered in the past 2–3 h) should be administered (maximum single dose, 50 mg). If repeated aPTT measurements indicate prolongation, a further 0.5 mg per 100 units heparin should be administered [25]. Recommendations for reversal of subcutaneous LMWH depend on the substance used and dosing: in patients not receiving therapeutic doses, reversal is not generally recommended [25]. In case of enoxaparin, protamine at a dose of 1 mg per mg enoxaparin should be administered (if the last dose of enoxaparin was >8–12 h, 0.5 mg protamine per mg enoxaparin; max. Single dose, 50 mg). In cases of dalteparin, nadroparin, and tinzaparin, 1 mg protamine per 100 IU should be administered (if time from last administration of LMWH is <25 h (~3–5 half-lives)). If protamine is contraindicated or not available, factor VIIa can be considered, although evidence is poor [25]. Full therapeutic doses of fondaparinux might be reversed by administration of PCC or recombinant factor VIIa. The availability of a "universal antidote" might dramatically change recommendations in the near future.

Thrombolytic-Related ICH

Intracerebral hemorrhage is the most feared complication of thrombolytic therapy. Various definitions of (symptomatic) hemorrhage in relation to thrombolytic therapy exist [44]. Recently, an updated anatomical classification set of secondary hemorrhage after ischemic stroke was proposed (the Heidelberg Bleeding Classification, Table 3.2) [45].

A large meta-analysis of randomized trials comparing alteplase vs. placebo found that parenchymal hemorrhage type 2 (Table 3.2) occurred in 6.8% of the patients who received alteplase compared to 1.3% in patients who were not treated (odds ratio (OR), 5.6) [46]. Fatal ICH occurred in 2.7% vs. 0.4% (OR 7.1) [46]. More severe stroke, but not age, increased the absolute risk of ICH [46]. Importantly, rates of ICH are significantly lower in patients receiving thrombolytics in situations other than ischemic stroke [25]. Thrombolytic therapy by plasminogen activators

Table 3.2 Description of secondary hemorrhage after ischemic stroke

Class	Type	Description
1		Hemorrhagic transformation of infarcted brain tissue
1a	HI 1	Scattered small petechiae, no mass effect
1b	HI 2	Confluent petechiae, no mass effect
1c	PH 1	Hematoma within infarcted tissue, occupying <30%, no substantive mass effect
2		Intracerebral hemorrhage within and beyond infarcted brain tissue
	PH 2	Hematoma occupying 30% or more of the infarcted tissue, with obvious mass effect
3		Parenchymal hematoma remote from infarcted brain tissue
3 a		Parenchymal hematoma remote from infarcted brain tissue
3 b		Intraventricular hemorrhage
3 c		Subarachnoid hemorrhage
3 d		Subdural hemorrhage

HI indicates hemorrhagic infarction and PH, parenchymatous hematoma (According to the Heidelberg Bleeding Classification; modified from Rüdiger von Kummer et al. [[45]], Table 3.1 with permission from Wolters Kluwer Health, Inc.

disturbs coagulation for several hours (fibrinogen levels may not be recovered to normal even after 24 h). Low fibrinogen levels (<150 mg/dL) were associated with hematoma expansion in a retrospective analysis [47].

In every case of early neurologic deterioration, thrombolytic therapy should be halted immediately, and follow-up brain imaging (CT scan) must be obtained. If ICH is confirmed, guidelines recommend administration of cryoprecipitate (initial dose, 10 IU). Cryoprecipitate is obtained from thawed and centrifuged FFPs and contains factor VIII, fibronectin, factor XIII, and von Willebrand factor [25]. Target fibrinogen levels are >150 mg/dL (although others still recommend >100 mg/dL). Transfusion of 10 units of cryoprecipitate contains 2 g of fibrinogen, which may raise fibrinogen levels by 70 mg/dL in a 70 kg patient [25]. However, cryoprecipitates are not available at every site. If cryoprecipitate is unavailable, tranexamic acid (10–15 mg/kg body weight) or ε-aminocaproic acid may be administered [25]. Fibrinogen levels should be measured after administration of a reversal agent. Platelet infusions have been advocated in the past but are not recommended in the recent guidelines from the Neurocritical Care Society and Society of Critical Care Medicine [25].

Antiplatelet Medication-Related ICH

Conflicting data exists over the relevance of baseline antiplatelet therapy and risk of hematoma expansion or poor functional outcome following ICH [25]. Nevertheless, as a potential effect on hematoma expansion cannot be excluded by the data available today, discontinuation of antiplatelet therapy in cases of ICH is recommended. After discontinuation of antiplatelet therapy, prolonged effects on thrombocyte function can be observed. In agents producing a "nonreversible" platelet inhibition (such as aspirin, clopidogrel, prasugrel, ticlopidine, or abciximab), effects last up to several days until a relevant number of new thrombocytes are produced. For agents acting as reversible inhibitors (such as ibuprofen, ticagrelor, tirofiban, or eptifibatide), function is restored after 3–5 half-lives [25]. While platelet transfusion may seem a logical treatment for ICH associated with antiplatelet drugs, the best available data does not support this routine practice. The PATCH trial randomized patients with spontaneous acute ICH taking antiplatelet therapy (aspirin, clopidogrel, and/or dipyridamole) to platelet transfusion therapy vs. standard therapy [48]. Platelet transfusion increased the likelihood of death or an unfavorable outcome (OR, 2.05) [48]. While platelet transfusion cannot be recommended in acute spontaneous ICH with prior antiplatelet therapy, it should be noted that patients who were likely to undergo surgical procedures were excluded from the PATCH trial. It remains possible that platelet transfusion may provide a benefit if acute neurosurgical procedures are necessary. In patients requiring immediate surgery, administration of desmopressin can be considered, although higher-class evidence is lacking. Desmopressin releases multimers of factor VIII/von Willebrand factor, supporting platelet adhesion to the endothelium. Desmopressin should be administered as a single dose (0.4 μg/kg body weight) [25].

Conclusion

ICH related to anticoagulant therapy represents a medical emergency and is associated with a high case fatality and unfavorable outcome. Prothrombin concentrate can effectively reverse VKA therapy and should be immediately administered in acute VKA-ICH. For NOAC-associated ICH, specific antidotes are either available (idarucizumab for reversal of dabigatran) or in development (for factor Xa inhibitors)). In cases of ICH associated with antiplatelet therapy, cessation of antiplatelet therapy seems sufficient in most cases, and platelet infusions should not be given.

Literature

1. Fisher CM. Hypertensive cerebral hemorrhage. Demonstration of the source of bleeding. J Neuropathol Exp Neurol. 2003;62(1):104–7.
2. Biffi A, Greenberg SM. Cerebral amyloid angiopathy: a systematic review. J Clin Neurol. 2011;7(1):1–9.
3. Charidimou A, Gang Q, Werring DJ. Sporadic cerebral amyloid angiopathy revisited: recent insights into pathophysiology and clinical spectrum. J Neurol Neurosurg Psychiatry. 2012;83(2):124–37.
4. Greenberg SM, Nandigam RN, Delgado P, Betensky RA, Rosand J, Viswanathan A, et al. Microbleeds versus macrobleeds: evidence for distinct entities. Stroke. 2009;40(7):2382–6.
5. Kovari E, Charidimou A, Herrmann FR, Giannakopoulos P, Bouras C, Gold G. No neuropathological evidence for a direct topographical relation between microbleeds and cerebral amyloid angiopathy. Acta Neuropathol Commun. 2015;3:49.
6. Flibotte JJ, Hagan N, O'Donnell J, Greenberg SM, Rosand J. Warfarin, hematoma expansion, and outcome of intracerebral hemorrhage. Neurology. 2004;63(6):1059–64.
7. Kuramatsu JB, Gerner ST, Schellinger PD, Glahn J, Endres M, Sobesky J, et al. Anticoagulant reversal, blood pressure levels, and anticoagulant resumption in patients with anticoagulation-related intracerebral hemorrhage. JAMA. 2015;313(8):824–36.
8. Schlunk F, Greenberg SM. The pathophysiology of intracerebral hemorrhage formation and expansion. Transl Stroke Res. 2015;6(4):257–63.
9. Greenberg CH, Frosch MP, Goldstein JN, Rosand J, Greenberg SM. Modeling intracerebral hemorrhage growth and response to anticoagulation. PLoS One. 2012;7(10):e48458.
10. Horstmann S, Rizos T, Lauseker M, Mohlenbruch M, Jenetzky E, Hacke W, et al. Intracerebral hemorrhage during anticoagulation with vitamin K antagonists: a consecutive observational study. J Neurol. 2013;260(8):2046–51.
11. Bejot Y, Cordonnier C, Durier J, Aboa-Eboule C, Rouaud O, Giroud M. Intracerebral haemorrhage profiles are changing: results from the Dijon population-based study. Brain. 2013;136(Pt 2):658–64.
12. Flaherty ML, Kissela B, Woo D, Kleindorfer D, Alwell K, Sekar P, et al. The increasing incidence of anticoagulant-associated intracerebral hemorrhage. Neurology. 2007;68(2):116–21.
13. Steiner T, Poli S, Griebe M, Husing J, Hajda J, Freiberger A, et al. Fresh frozen plasma versus prothrombin complex concentrate in patients with intracranial haemorrhage related to vitamin K antagonists (INCH): a randomised trial. Lancet Neurol. 2016;15(6):566–73.
14. Flaherty ML, Tao H, Haverbusch M, Sekar P, Kleindorfer D, Kissela B, et al. Warfarin use leads to larger intracerebral hematomas. Neurology. 2008;71(14):1084–9.
15. Dowlatshahi D, Demchuk AM, Flaherty ML, Ali M, Lyden PL, Smith EE, et al. Defining hematoma expansion in intracerebral hemorrhage: relationship with patient outcomes. Neurology. 2011;76(14):1238–44.

16. Biffi A, Battey TW, Ayres AM, Cortellini L, Schwab K, Gilson AJ, et al. Warfarin-related intraventricular hemorrhage: imaging and outcome. Neurology. 2011;77(20):1840–6.
17. Pezzini A, Grassi M, Paciaroni M, Zini A, Silvestrelli G, Del Zotto E, et al. Antithrombotic medications and the etiology of intracerebral hemorrhage: MUCH-Italy. Neurology. 2014;82(6):529–35.
18. Flaherty ML, Haverbusch M, Sekar P, Kissela BM, Kleindorfer D, Moomaw CJ, et al. Location and outcome of anticoagulant-associated intracerebral hemorrhage. Neurocrit Care. 2006;5(3):197–201.
19. Hanger HC, Fletcher VJ, Wilkinson TJ, Brown AJ, Frampton CM, Sainsbury R. Effect of aspirin and warfarin on early survival after intracerebral haemorrhage. J Neurol. 2008;255(3):347–52.
20. Drouet L, Bal Dit Sollier C, Steiner T, Purrucker J. Measuring non-vitamin K antagonist oral anticoagulant levels: when is it appropriate and which methods should be used? Int J Stroke. 2016;11(7):748–58.
21. Rizos T, Jenetzky E, Herweh C, Hug A, Hacke W, Steiner T, et al. Point-of-care reversal treatment in phenprocoumon-related intracerebral hemorrhage. Ann Neurol [Clinical Trial]. 2010;67(6):788–93.
22. Ansell J, Hirsh J, Poller L, Bussey H, Jacobson A, Hylek E. The pharmacology and management of the vitamin K antagonists: the seventh ACCP conference on antithrombotic and thrombolytic therapy. Chest. 2004;126(3 Suppl):204S–33S.
23. Neal M, Crowther M, Douketis J, Verhovsek M, Stidley C, Garcia D. Reversal of vitamin K antagonist-associated coagulopathy: a survey of current practice. Thromb Res. 2008;122(6):864–6.
24. Voils SA, Baird B. Systematic review: 3-factor versus 4-factor prothrombin complex concentrate for warfarin reversal: does it matter? Thromb Res. 2012;130(6):833–40.
25. Frontera JA, Lewin JJ 3rd, Rabinstein AA, Aisiku IP, Alexandrov AW, Cook AM, et al. Guideline for reversal of Antithrombotics in intracranial hemorrhage: a statement for healthcare professionals from the Neurocritical care society and Society of Critical Care Medicine. Neurocrit Care. 2016;24(1):6–46.
26. Laible M, Jenetzky E, Beynon C, Muller OJ, Sander P, Schuler S, et al. Adverse events following international normalized ratio reversal in intracerebral hemorrhage. Cerebrovasc Dis. 2016;42(5–6):446–54.
27. Goldstein JN, Refaai MA, Milling TJ Jr, Lewis B, Goldberg-Alberts R, Hug BA, et al. Four-factor prothrombin complex concentrate versus plasma for rapid vitamin K antagonist reversal in patients needing urgent surgical or invasive interventions: a phase 3b, open-label, non-inferiority, randomised trial. Lancet. 2015;385(9982):2077–87.
28. Sarode R, Milling TJ Jr, Refaai MA, Mangione A, Schneider A, Durn BL, et al. Efficacy and safety of a 4-factor prothrombin complex concentrate in patients on vitamin K antagonists presenting with major bleeding: a randomized, plasma-controlled, phase IIIb study. Circulation. 2013;128(11):1234–43.
29. Ruff CT, Giugliano RP, Braunwald E, Hoffman EB, Deenadayalu N, Ezekowitz MD, et al. Comparison of the efficacy and safety of new oral anticoagulants with warfarin in patients with atrial fibrillation: a meta-analysis of randomised trials. Lancet. 2014;383(9921):955–62.
30. Pfeilschifter W, Farahmand D, Niemann D, Ikenberg B, Hohmann C, Abruscato M, et al. Estimating the quantitative demand of NOAC antidote doses on stroke units. Cerebrovasc Dis. 2016;42(5–6):415–20.
31. Purrucker JC, Haas K, Rizos T, Khan S, Wolf M, Hennerici MG, et al. Early clinical and radiological course, management, and outcome of intracerebral hemorrhage related to new oral anticoagulants. JAMA Neurol. 2016;73(2):169–77.
32. Wilson D, Seiffge DJ, Traenka C, Basir G, Purrucker JC, Rizos T, et al. Outcome of intracerebral hemorrhage associated with different oral anticoagulants. Neurology. 2017;88(18):1693–700.
33. Purrucker JC, Rizos T, Haas K, Wolf M, Khan S, Heuschmann PU, et al. Coagulation testing in intracerebral hemorrhage related to non-vitamin K antagonist oral anticoagulants. Neurocrit Care. 2017;27:208.

34. Zhou W, Schwarting S, Illanes S, Liesz A, Middelhoff M, Zorn M, et al. Hemostatic therapy in experimental intracerebral hemorrhage associated with the direct thrombin inhibitor dabigatran. Stroke. 2011;42(12):3594–9.
35. Zhou W, Zorn M, Nawroth P, Butehorn U, Perzborn E, Heitmeier S, et al. Hemostatic therapy in experimental intracerebral hemorrhage associated with rivaroxaban. Stroke. 2013;44(3):771–8.
36. Grottke O, Aisenberg J, Bernstein R, Goldstein P, Huisman MV, Jamieson DG, et al. Efficacy of prothrombin complex concentrates for the emergency reversal of dabigatran-induced anticoagulation. Crit Care. 2016;20(1):115.
37. Eerenberg ES, Kamphuisen PW, Sijpkens MK, Meijers JC, Buller HR, Levi M. Reversal of rivaroxaban and dabigatran by prothrombin complex concentrate: a randomized, placebo-controlled, crossover study in healthy subjects. Circulation [Comparative Study]. 2011;124(14):1573–9.
38. Glund S, Stangier J, Schmohl M, Gansser D, Norris S, van Ryn J, et al. Safety, tolerability, and efficacy of idarucizumab for the reversal of the anticoagulant effect of dabigatran in healthy male volunteers: a randomised, placebo-controlled, double-blind phase 1 trial. Lancet. 2015;386(9994):680–90.
39. Reilly PA, van Ryn J, Grottke O, Glund S, Stangier J. Idarucizumab, a specific reversal agent for dabigatran: mode of action, pharmacokinetics and pharmacodynamics, and safety and efficacy in phase 1 subjects. Am J Med. 2016;129(11S):S64–72.
40. Pollack CV Jr, Reilly PA, Eikelboom J, Glund S, Verhamme P, Bernstein RA, et al. Idarucizumab for Dabigatran Reversal. N Engl J Med. 2015;373(6):511–20.
41. Pollack CV Jr, Reilly PA, van Ryn J, Eikelboom JW, Glund S, Bernstein RA, et al. Idarucizumab for dabigatran reversal - full cohort analysis. N Engl J Med. 2017;377(5):431–41.
42. Connolly SJ, Milling TJ Jr, Eikelboom JW, Gibson CM, Curnutte JT, Gold A, et al. Andexanet alfa for acute major bleeding associated with factor Xa inhibitors. N Engl J Med. 2016;375(12):1131–41.
43. Gomez-Outes A, Suarez-Gea ML, Lecumberri R, Terleira-Fernandez AI, Vargas-Castrillon E. Specific antidotes in development for reversal of novel anticoagulants: a review. Recent Pat Cardiovasc Drug Discov. 2014;9(1):2–10.
44. Gumbinger C, Gruschka P, Bottinger M, Heerlein K, Barrows R, Hacke W, et al. Improved prediction of poor outcome after thrombolysis using conservative definitions of symptomatic hemorrhage. Stroke. 2012;43(1):240–2.
45. von Kummer R, Broderick JP, Campbell BC, Demchuk A, Goyal M, Hill MD, et al. The Heidelberg bleeding classification: classification of bleeding events after ischemic stroke and reperfusion therapy. Stroke. 2015;46(10):2981–6.
46. Whiteley WN, Emberson J, Lees KR, Blackwell L, Albers G, Bluhmki E, et al. Risk of intracerebral haemorrhage with alteplase after acute ischaemic stroke: a secondary analysis of an individual patient data meta-analysis. Lancet Neurol. 2016;15(9):925–33.
47. Yaghi S, Boehme AK, Dibu J, Leon Guerrero CR, Ali S, Martin-Schild S, et al. Treatment and outcome of thrombolysis-related hemorrhage: a multicenter retrospective study. JAMA Neurol. 2015;72(12):1451–7.
48. Baharoglu MI, Cordonnier C, Al-Shahi Salman R, de Gans K, Koopman MM, Brand A, et al. Platelet transfusion versus standard care after acute stroke due to spontaneous cerebral haemorrhage associated with antiplatelet therapy (PATCH): a randomised, open-label, phase 3 trial. Lancet. 2016;387(10038):2605–13.
49. Kazui S, Naritomi H, Yamamoto H, Sawada T, Yamaguchi T. Enlargement of spontaneous intracerebral hemorrhage. Incidence and time course. Stroke. 1996;27(10):1783–7.
50. Brott T, Broderick J, Kothari R, Barsan W, Tomsick T, Sauerbeck L, et al. Early hemorrhage growth in patients with intracerebral hemorrhage. Stroke. 1997;28(1):1–5.
51. Davis SM, Broderick J, Hennerici M, Brun NC, Diringer MN, Mayer SA, et al. Hematoma growth is a determinant of mortality and poor outcome after intracerebral hemorrhage. Neurology. 2006;66(8):1175–81.

52. Mayer SA, Brun NC, Begtrup K, Broderick J, Davis S, Diringer MN, et al. Efficacy and safety of recombinant activated factor VII for acute intracerebral hemorrhage. N Engl J Med. 2008;358(20):2127–37.
53. Cucchiara B, Messe S, Sansing L, Kasner S, Lyden P, Investigators C. Hematoma growth in oral anticoagulant related intracerebral hemorrhage. Stroke. 2008;39(11):2993–6.
54. Huhtakangas J, Tetri S, Juvela S, Saloheimo P, Bode MK, Hillbom M. Effect of increased warfarin use on warfarin-related cerebral hemorrhage: a longitudinal population-based study. Stroke. 2011;42(9):2431–5.

Chapter 4
Blood Pressure Management in ICH

Shahram Majidi and Adnan I. Qureshi

Blood Pressure Management in ICH

Elevated blood pressure is a strong and independent risk factor for occurrence of intracerebral hemorrhage (ICH) [1]. Elevated blood pressure (greater than 140/90 mmHg) in the first 24 h from symptom onset has been observed in approximately 80% of patients with primary ICH [2–4]. This high blood pressure in acute phase following ICH, known as acute hypertensive response, is shown to be transient with spontaneous reduction even without antihypertensive therapy [5, 6]. The mechanism of acute hypertensive response following ICH is not fully understood; however, the high prevalence and self-limiting nature of this phenomenon suggest possible hemorrhage specific etiology such as damage to the areas of the brain involved in blood pressure regulation (for example the insula, cingulate cortex, amygdala, prefrontal area, or brainstem compression and increased intracranial pressure) with subsequent functional recovery [7–9].

The management of elevated systolic blood pressure (SBP) in patients with primary ICH has been subject of a long-lasting debate and controversy during the past few decades. Approximately three decades ago, the standard approach was to not treat elevated blood pressure in acute phase in order to avoid subsequent ischemic changes in perihematoma areas. However, during the subsequent years, an alternative hypothesis gained attention which was advocating for aggressive acute blood pressure management to improve patients' outcome by reducing the magnitude of hematoma expansion. Figure 4.1 shows the evolution of our understanding on blood pressure management in patients with ICH.

S. Majidi (✉)
Department of Neurosurgery, Icahn School of Medicine at Mount Sinai, New York, NY, USA

A. I. Qureshi
University of Minnesota, Minneapolis, MN, USA

B. Ovbiagele, A. I. Qureshi (eds.), *Intracerebral Hemorrhage Therapeutics*,
https://doi.org/10.1007/978-3-319-77063-5_4

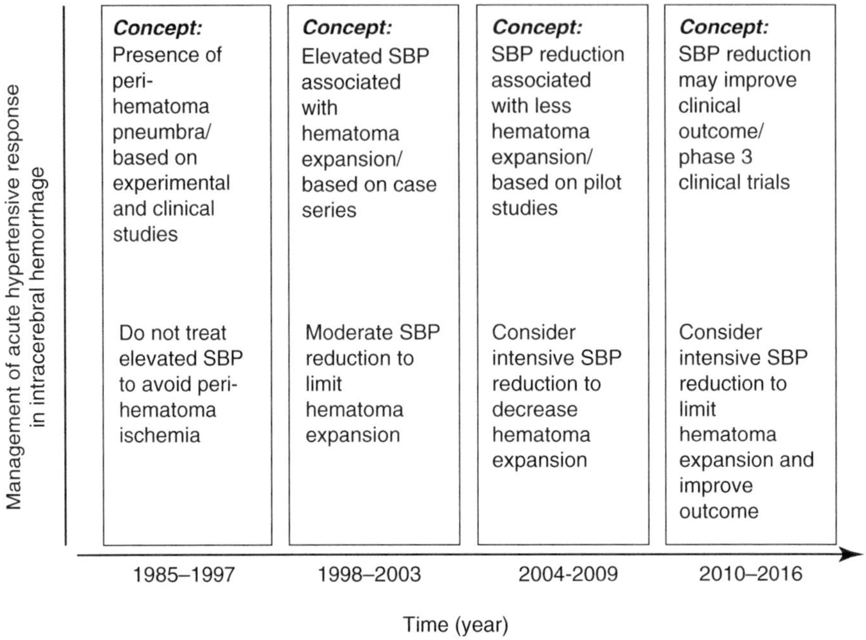

Fig. 4.1 Evolution in the management of elevated blood pressure in acute ICH during the past three decades. (From Majidi et al. [41] with permission of Springer)

Blood Pressure and Outcome in Patients with Intracerebral Hemorrhage

Previous observational studies have identified SBP ≥ 200 mmHg as a predictor of poor outcome and higher mortality rate, early hematoma expansion, and perihematoma edema in patients with primary ICH [10, 11]. In a retrospective analysis of 87 patients with hypertensive ICH, Dandapani et al. [12] found higher rate of mortality and severe morbidity among patients with admission mean arterial pressure (MAP) of >145 mmHg compared to those patient with MAP ≤ 145 mmHg. The Stroke Acute Management with Urgent Risk-factor Assessment and Improvement (SAMURAI)-ICH study [13] was a prospective multicenter observational study to determine the safety and feasibility of early SBP reduction in patients with primary ICH. They recruited 211 patients with primary ICH within 3 h from symptom onset and initial SBP > 180 mmHg. All patients were treated with intravenous nicardipine within 3 h from symptom onset and continued on treatment for 24 h with the SBP goal of <160 mmHg and > 120 mmHg. Blood pressures were measured every 15 min during the initial 2 h and then every 1 h in the following 22 h. The mean SBP during the first 24 h was calculated for each patient. The study demonstrated that the higher mean SBP was independently associated with hematoma expansion (defined as >33% increase in hematoma volume), neurological deterioration (defined as ≥4 points increase in National Institutes of Health Stroke Scale (NIHSS) score or ≥ 2 points decrease in Glasgow Coma Score (GCS) score), and unfavorable outcome (defined as 90-day modified Rankin Scale (mRS) score of 4–6). Essentially, every 10 mmHg increment of mean SBP was associated with a 4.5-fold increase in neurological deterioration, 2-fold increase in unfavorable outcome, and 1.8-fold increase in hematoma expansion. The study also demonstrated that the relative reduction of SBP in first 24 h was inversely associated with higher rate of hematoma expansion, neurological deterioration, and unfavorable outcome [14]. In a retrospective analysis of 76 consecutive patients with hypertensive ICH, Ohwaki et al. [15] found direct association between maximum SBP levels and the rate of hematoma expansion. Only 9% hematoma expansion was observed in patients with SBP goal of less than 150 mmHg whereas 30% hematoma expansion in those patients with SBP goal of less than 160 mmHg. Analysis from secondary analysis from Factor Seven for Acute Hemorrhagic Stroke Trial (FAST) revealed independent association between higher mean arterial pressure (MAP) and presence of intraventricular hemorrhage which is an independent predictor of poor outcome [16].

The primary target of blood pressure reduction in hypertensive ICH is to prevent hematoma expansion and subsequently improve the patient's outcome. Therefore, the time window for blood pressure management in these patients is short and limited as majority of hematoma growth occur in the first few hours after symptom onset. In a pooled analysis using placebo arms of three clinical trials studying dosing, safety, and efficacy of recombinant factor VIIa (rFVIIa) [17–19] and also Cincinnati ICH cohort [20], hematoma expansion reported in 73% of 218 patients within 3 h from symptom onset [21]. In a retrospective analysis of 204 patients with primary ICH, the highest rate of hematoma expansion observed within 3 h from symptom onset which was 36% compared to 16% within 3–6 h and 15% within 6–12 h. Notably, none of the patients with first CT scan obtained within 24–48 h had hematoma expansion (suggesting that hematoma expansion had preceded the first scan) [22]. FAST trial was a randomized, double-blind, placebo-controlled study of 821 patients treated within 4 h of symptom onset with placebo, 20, or 80 μg/kg of rFVIIa [23]. The study demonstrated significant reduction in hematoma expansion in patients who received 80 μg/kg of rFVIIa; however, no improvement in 90-day functional outcome or survival was noted. Pertinent to our current discussion is the subgroup analysis from this study which showed that the reduction in hematoma expansion rate in comparison to placebo group doubled when limiting symptom onset to treatment to 2.5 h [24]. Finally, it should be noted that although the rate of hematoma expansion is highest in the first 3 h, it may still occur in 12–30% of patients between 3 and 24 h from symptom onset; therefore, it is reasonable to maintain adequate blood pressure control during first 24 h [25, 26].

Safety of Early Intensive Blood Pressure Lowering Treatment

The safety of acute SBP reduction in patients with ICH has been confirmed in numerous independent studies. The safety has been assessed by radiological biomarkers or clinical outcomes. In an observational study of 19 patients with primary supratentorial ICH who underwent positron emission tomography (PET) 5–22 h from symptom onset, no evidence of ischemia in the perihematoma region was detected [27]. In a prospective study, perihematoma edema and blood flow were studied in 21 patients with primary ICH. All patients underwent perfusion-weighted MRI and diffusion-weighted MRI study at baseline, 3–5 and 30 days after symptoms onset and relative mean transit time (rMTT), relative cerebral blood flow (rCBF), and relative cerebral blood volume (rCBV) were calculated in each perfusion study. The study found perihematoma oligemia (rMTT>2 s) in patients with ICH volume > 15 ml. This phenomenon was self-limited with spontaneous resolution within 3–5 days after symptom onset, and there was no MRI marker of cerebral ischemia [28]. In a randomized, multicenter, open-label clinical trial (ICH-ADAPT), Butcher et al. studied the effect of blood pressure reduction on perihematoma CBF. They recruited 75 patients with primary ICH with baseline SBP >150 mmHg and within 24 h from symptom onset and assigned the patients to intensive SBP reduction of <150 mmHg or standard SBP reduction of <180 mmHg using intravenous antihypertensive medication with SBP goal to be achieved in 1 h. All patients underwent CT perfusion imaging 2 h after randomization. They found no significant change in CBF in the perihematoma region related to acute blood pressure reduction [29].

In a prospective observational multicenter study, Qureshi et al. [30] studied the feasibility and safety of intravenous antihypertensive treatment for acute hypertension in patients with primary ICH. Elevated blood pressure was defined as SBP ≥ 160 mmHg and/or diastolic blood pressure (DBP) ≥ 110 mmHg documented by at least two measurements 5 min apart. The treatment goal was to maintain SBP <160 mmHg and DBP <100 mmHg for 24 h from onset of symptoms. The study included total of 35 patients, 27 patients required antihypertensive treatment, and 8 other patients were used as control group. They demonstrated lower rate of neurological deterioration (defined as a decrease in initial GCS score ≥ 2) among patients who required antihypertensive treatment (7% versus 26%). The study also found lower rate of hematoma expansion among patients who required antihypertensive treatment (9% versus 13%) and higher chance of functional independence (mRS 0–2) at 30 days among patients who were treated within 6 h from symptom onset compared to those within 6–24 h. Antihypertensive Treatment of Acute Cerebral Hemorrhage (ATACH)-I [31] was a National Institute of Neurological Disorders and Stroke (NINDS)-funded open-labeled pilot trial which was conducted to determine the safety and tolerability of reducing SBP in the acute phase of ICH. A total of 60 patients within 6 h of symptom onset and initial hematoma volume of less than 60 ml were recruited in three different SBP goals. The escalating SBP goals (achieved using intravenous nicardipine) were as follows (1): 170–200 mmHg (2), 140–170 mmHg, and (3) 110–140 mmHg. The SBP goal was maintained for 24 h from symptom onset, and the primary outcome of the study was first to assess the feasibility of achieving and maintaining SBP goals for 18–24 h and to determine the rate of neurological deterioration (defined as decline in the GCS score ≥2 or increase in NIHSS score ≥4 points) within 24 h and serious adverse events within 72 h. The SBP goals were achieved in 90% of the patient by 2 h. The observed proportions of neurological deterioration and serious adverse events were below the pre-specified safety thresholds, and the 3-month mortality rate was lower than expected among all SBP tiers. The post hoc analysis of ATACH I study showed a trend toward lower rates of hematoma expansion, perihematoma edema, and also poor outcome in 90 days among patients with more intensive SBP reduction; however the differences were not statistically significant [32]. Intensive blood pressure reduction in acute cerebral hemorrhage (INTERACT)-I [33] trial was another randomized clinical trial that assessed the safety and efficacy of intensive SBP reduction in patients with acute ICH. The study included patients ≥ 18 years old of age with primary ICH within 6 h from symptom onset and elevated SBP which was defined as at least two measurements of 150–220 mmHg recorded ≥ 2 min apart. A total of 404 subjects were recruited and randomly assigned to either standard SBP reduction (with SBP goal <180 mmHg) or intensive SBP reduction (with SBP goal <140 mmHg). The SBP goal was to achieve within 1 h and maintained for 7 days or until discharge from hospital. The primary efficacy outcome of study was proportional change in hematoma volume at 24 h. There was no evidence of increased rate of adverse events or worse outcome at 90 days among intensive SBP reduction group. They also found 8% absolute risk reduction in the rate of hematoma expansion (defined as an increase in volume > 33% or > 12.5 ml in the first 24 h) in intensive SBP reduction group (15% versus 23%, $p = 0.05$). Notably, substantial reduction in the rate of hematoma growth was observed among intensive SBP reduction group recruited within 4 h from symptom onset (15 vs 30% in guideline group, relative risk reduction 54%, 95% CI: 30–88%) and also among subjects with initial SBP greater than 180 mmHg (17 vs 32% with relative risk reduction 47%, 95% CI: 6–70%).

Efficacy of Early Intensive Blood Pressure Lowering Treatment

Following promising observations from ATACH I and INTERACT I studies and also other studies such as ICH-ADAPT and SAMURAI-ICH, two phase 3, randomized, double-blind, multicenter international clinical trials were launched to independently determine the efficacy of intensive SBP reduction in patients with acute primary ICH.

In the second intensive blood pressure reduction in acute cerebral hemorrhage trial (INTERACT II) [34], a total of 2839 patients from 144 hospitals in 21 countries with ICH within 6 h of symptom onset were randomized to either intensive SBP reduction which was defined as target of <140 mmHg within 1 h or standard SBP reduction which was target of <180 mmHg. Patients with primary hypertensive ICH were required to have at least two SBP measurements between 150 and 220 mmHg recorded at least 2 min apart to be eligible for enrollment. The target SBP goal in each group was maintained for 7 days. The study did not show any significant difference in the rate of 90-day major disability and death (mRS: 3–6) between the two treatment groups. Also, there was no significant reduction in the rate of hematoma expansion among the intensive SBP reduction group. However, in the ordinal analysis of 90 day mRS, higher rate of functional recovery was observed among intensive SBP reduction group. Patients in the intensive SBP reduction group reported better physical and mental health-related quality of life in the European Quality of Life 5 Dimension (EQ-5D) health utility score obtained at 90 days. The post hoc analysis of INTERACT II study showed lowest rate of death and major disability at 90 days (mRS 3–5) among patients who had larger SBP reduction (≥20 mmHg) which was achieved within 1 h of randomization and maintained for 7 days [35]. As further evidence on importance of faster and greater SBP reduction, sub-analysis of INTERACT II study revealed the lowest mean absolute hematoma expansion in patients who achieved SBP < 140 mmHg within 1 h compared to those who required over 6 h (2.6 ml versus 5.4 ml) [36]. There are some issues and limitations which need to be considered for the interpretation of INTERACT II study results including 1) patients with large hematoma volume and midline shift and low GCS score were not included in the study. Indeed, 70% of the patients had baseline hematoma volume of <15 ml; therefore, the safety and efficacy of intensive SBP reduction in large ICH and patients with unfavorable characteristics were not tested in this study. 2) Substantial percentage (34%) of patients in the intensive SBP reduction group did not achieve SBP goal, and only one third of the patients in the intensive SBP reduction group achieved SBP goal within 1 h. The benefit of intensive SBP reduction might have been different if intensive SBP reduction goal had been achieved in a larger proportion of the patients and in a faster time period.

Based on INTERACT II results, several organizations including European Stroke Organization and American Heart Association/American Stroke Association (AHA/ASA) updated their guideline for ICH management. In the updated 2015 AHA/ASA guideline for management ICH, acute SBP reduction to <140 mmHg in ICH patients presenting with SBP between 150 and 220 mmHg and without contraindication to acute BP treatment is mentioned as safe and feasible which can be effective in improving clinical outcome. However, it is highlighted that data pertaining to the safety and efficacy of intensive SBP reduction in patients with higher SBP (>220 mmHg) and larger hematoma volume and those who require decompressive craniotomy is limited [37].

Antihypertensive Treatment of Acute Cerebral Hemorrhage (ATACH) II trial was a NINDS-funded randomized double-blind controlled clinical trial which recruited patients with primary supratentorial ICH from 2010 to 2015 in the United States, Europe, and Asia [38]. ATACH II study was highly anticipated to solidify the evidence for efficacy of intensive SBP reduction in acute ICH following promising trends seen in INTERACT II study. However, ATACH II study was prematurely terminated by Data Safety and Monitoring Board (DSMB) before reaching target 1280 subjects recruitment for futility after interim analysis revealed no significant difference in outcome between the intensive SBP reduction group and standard SBP reduction group. Briefly, ATACH II clinical trial recruited patients with primary ICH within 4.5 h from symptom onset with initial SBP ≥180 mmHg. The patients were randomly assigned to SBP target of 110–139 mmHg (intensive treatment) or a target of 140–179 mmHg (standard treatment). The SBP goals were maintained for

24 h in both groups because the primary therapeutic target of SBP reduction mainly occurs within this time frame. Nicardipine infusion was used for blood pressure reduction in both groups, and the primary outcome of the study was defined as death or major disability (mRS >3) at 90-day follow-up. A total of 1000 subjects were recruited in the study, 500 patients in each group with mean admission SBP of 200 ± 27 and 201 ± 27 mmHg in intensive treatment group and standard treatment group, respectively. There was no significant difference between the two groups in regard to the rate of 90-day death or major disability (38.7% versus 37.7%), the quality of life assessment via EQ-5D, or the rate of hematoma expansion. Moreover, the rate of renal adverse events within 7 days after enrollment was significantly higher among intensive SBP reduction group (9.0% versus 4.0%, $p = 0.002$). There are several issues that need to be taken into consideration for proper interpretation of ATACH II results: 1) only 10% of all subjects had initial hematoma volume greater than 30 ml, and more than half of the patients had admission GCS score of 15; therefore, similar to INTERACT II, the result of ATACH II cannot be generalized to patients with unfavorable characteristics including larger hemorrhage and low GCS score on admission. 2) primary treatment failure occurred in 12% of patients in intensive SBP reduction group versus less than 1% of patients in standard SBP reduction group. It can be argued that if higher proportion of the patients had met the treatment goal, the outcome benefit could have been different. 3) considering the high rate of favorable outcome among both arms of ATACH II study in comparison to previously published studies, it is also possible that standardized intensity of medical care and monitoring provided throughout the study sites and blunting of blood pressure fluctuations may have provided therapeutic benefits independent of the magnitude of SBP reduction. Table 4.1. summarizes all clinical trials addressing SBP management in patients with primary ICH.

In summary, ATACH II and INTERACT II, as two largest clinical trials addressing acute blood pressure treatment in patients with ICH, both failed to demonstrate improved functional outcome with intensive SBP reduction to <140 mmHg in comparison to standard SBP goal of <180 mmHg in acute primary ICH. Figure 4.2 demonstrates the blood pressure profile within the first 24 h among study arms in both studies. As evident in this figure, the SBP profile of intensive SBP reduction group in INTERACT II study is similar to standard SBP reduction group of ATACH II study. The results of these two studies suggest that perhaps SBP reduction to 140–150 mmHg in patients with acute ICH provides the maximum outcome benefit as further reduction to less than 140 mmHg was associated with higher rate of adverse events without further improvement of clinical outcome. However, the safety and possible outcome benefits of intensive SBP reduction in certain groups of ICH patients including patients with large hematoma volume, midline shift, increased ICP, and lower admission GCS score remain unclear. Further sub-analysis from ATACH II study and pooled analysis from these two trials might answer some of these questions. Future studies should focus on utilization of MRI and MR perfusion in acute ICH for better delineation of the pathophysiology, magnitude, and natural history of secondary brain injury and its association with patient's SBP profile during the acute phase after ICH ictus. Prior studies of MRI in patients with

Table 4.1. Summary of completed prospective clinical trials that studied acute hypertensive response treatment in ICH patient

Study	Design	Patient included	Mean initial ICH volume (ml) median (range)	Intervention	Primary outcome	No. of subjects	Results
Intracerebral Hemorrhage Acutely Decreasing Arterial Pressure Trial (ICH-ADAPT) [29]	Multicenter, open-label, randomized, blinded-point trial	ICH within 24 h of symptom onset and SBP ≥150 mmHg	23.25 (±24.82)[a]	IV labetalol to reduce SBP to <150 mmHg, control group based on AHA guideline	Pre-hematomal rCBF measured with CT perfusion 2 h after treatment	82	Perihematomal rCBF was not lower among patients randomized to SBP <150 mmHg ($p = 0.18$)
Antihypertensive Treatment in Acute Cerebral Hemorrhage (ATACH-1) [31]	Prospective, multicenter, open-label, safety, and tolerability study	ICH within 6 h of symptom onset and SBP ≥200 mmHg	13.74 (±14.21)[a]	Stepwise BP control to test three tiers of SBP reduction: 170–200 mmHg 140–170 mmHg and 110–140 mmHg using IV nicardipine	[1] Neurological deterioration within 24 h [2]. Serious adverse events within 72 h from treatment initiation	60	Low rate of serious adverse events and neurological deterioration among all three tiers. No difference in average SBP change between patients with and those without neurological deterioration ($p = 0.47$)
Intensive Blood Pressure Reduction in Acute Cerebral Hemorrhage – (INTERACT I) Pilot Study [33]	Randomized, open-label, active-control, parallel-assignment, safety/efficacy study	ICH within 6 h of symptom onset and SBP >150 and ≤ 200 mmHg	13.45 (±13.05)[a]	Intensive SBP lowering to <140 mmHg within 1 h; control group with SBP goal of <180 mmHg	Proportional change in hematoma volume in 24 h and mortality and poor outcome (defined as mRS 3–6) at 90 days	400	Early intensive BP reduction feasible, safe and reduces the rate of hematoma expansion by 8% ($p = 0.05$)

Intensive Blood Pressure Reduction in Acute Cerebral Hemorrhage – INTERACT II [35]	Randomized, open-treatment, blinded end-point clinical trial	ICH within 6 h from symptom onset with at least two SBP reads between 150 and 220 mmHg	11 (6–20)	Intensive SBP lowering to <140 mmHg within 1 h; control group with SBP goal of <180 mmHg	Death or major disability (defined as mRS > 2) at 90 days	2794	No significant change in the rate of death or major disability. However, ordinal analysis of mRS suggested improved outcome (OR: 0.87; 95% CI: 0.77–1.00; $p = 0.04$)
Antihypertensive Treatment in Acute Cerebral Hemorrhage – ATACH II [38]	Randomized multicenter, two-arm, open-label clinical trial	ICH patients within 4.5 h from symptom onset with at least one SBP record of ≥180 mmHg	10 (1–79)	Intensive SBP control with goal of 110–139 mmHg, control group with SBP goal of 140–179 mmHg	Death or severe disability (defined as mRS 4–6) at 90 days	1000	No difference in the rate of death or severe disability ($p = 0.72$). Higher rate of renal complications in 7 day among intensive SBP group ($p = 0.002$)

Abbreviations used: *ICH* intracerebral hemorrhage, *rCBF* relative cerebral blood flow, *SBP* systolic blood pressure, *mRS* modified Rankin Scale

[a]Mean (±SD)

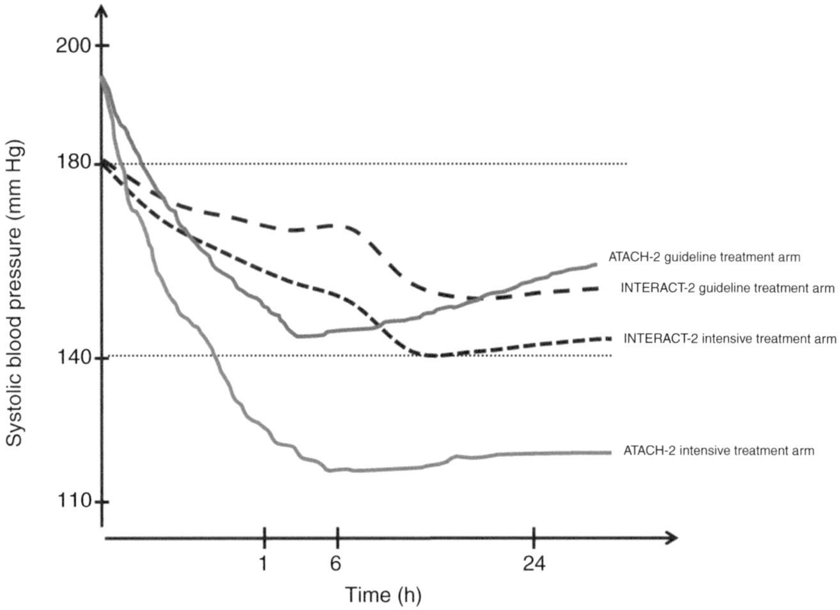

Fig. 4.2 Comparison of mean SBP profile in the first 24 h after randomization in standard SBP reduction and intensive SBP reduction group in INTERACT II (black dash lines) with mean minimum SBP profile for same groups in ATACH II (gray lines). (From Majidi et al. [41] with permission of Springer)

acute ICH have shown remote areas of restricted diffusion and blood-brain barrier disruption and suggested correlation with acute SBP reduction [39, 40]. Utilization of more advanced imaging modalities in patients with acute ICH can potentially assist the clinicians to identify a subset of ICH patients who may benefit from intensive SBP reduction and therefore provide more individualized SBP goal for those patients. Until future clinical trials provide further evidence on different aspects of acute SBP reduction in patients with ICH, standard SBP reduction to 140–160 mmHg seems safe and reasonable.

References

1. Ariesen MJ, Claus SP, Rinkel GJ, Algra A. Risk factors for intracerebral hemorrhage in the general population: a systematic review. Stroke. 2003;34(8):2060–5.
2. Britton M, Carlsson A, de Faire U. Blood pressure course in patients with acute stroke and matched controls. Stroke. Sep-Oct 1986;17(5):861–4.
3. Morfis L, Schwartz RS, Poulos R, Howes LG. Blood pressure changes in acute cerebral infarction and hemorrhage. Stroke. 1997;28(7):1401–5.
4. Qureshi AI, Ezzeddine MA, Nasar A, et al. Prevalence of elevated blood pressure in 563,704 adult patients with stroke presenting to the ED in the United States. Am J Emerg Med. 2007;25(1):32–8.

5. Ahmed N, Nasman P, Wahlgren NG. Effect of intravenous nimodipine on blood pressure and outcome after acute stroke. Stroke. Jun 2000;31(6):1250–5.
6. Lacy CR, Suh DC, Bueno M, Kostis JB. Delay in presentation and evaluation for acute stroke: stroke time registry for outcomes knowledge and epidemiology (S.T.R.O.K.E.). Stroke. 2001;32(1):63–9.
7. Qureshi AI, Geocadin RG, Suarez JI, Ulatowski JA. Long-term outcome after medical reversal of transtentorial herniation in patients with supratentorial mass lesions. Crit Care Med. 2000;28(5):1556–64.
8. Hilz MJ, Devinsky O, Szczepanska H, Borod JC, Marthol H, Tutaj M. Right ventromedial prefrontal lesions result in paradoxical cardiovascular activation with emotional stimuli. Brain. 2006;129(Pt 12):3343–55.
9. Nason MW Jr, Mason P. Modulation of sympathetic and somatomotor function by the ventromedial medulla. J Neurophysiol. 2004;92(1):510–22.
10. Kazui S, Minematsu K, Yamamoto H, Sawada T, Yamaguchi T. Predisposing factors to enlargement of spontaneous intracerebral hematoma. Stroke. 1997;28(12):2370–5.
11. Broderick JP, Brott TG, Tomsick T, Barsan W, Spilker J. Ultra-early evaluation of intracerebral hemorrhage. J Neurosurg. 1990;72(2):195–9.
12. Dandapani BK, Suzuki S, Kelley RE, Reyes-Iglesias Y, Duncan RC. Relation between blood pressure and outcome in intracerebral hemorrhage. Stroke. 1995;26(1):21–4.
13. Sakamoto Y, Koga M, Yamagami H, et al. Systolic blood pressure after intravenous antihypertensive treatment and clinical outcomes in hyperacute intracerebral hemorrhage: the stroke acute management with urgent risk-factor assessment and improvement-intracerebral hemorrhage study. Stroke. 2013;44(7):1846–51.
14. Sakamoto Y, Koga M, Todo K, et al. Relative systolic blood pressure reduction and clinical outcomes in hyperacute intracerebral hemorrhage: the SAMURAI-ICH observational study. J Hypertens. 2015;33(5):1069–73.
15. Ohwaki K, Yano E, Nagashima H, Hirata M, Nakagomi T, Tamura A. Blood pressure management in acute intracerebral hemorrhage: relationship between elevated blood pressure and hematoma enlargement. Stroke. 2004;35(6):1364–7.
16. Steiner T, Diringer MN, Schneider D, et al. Dynamics of intraventricular hemorrhage in patients with spontaneous intracerebral hemorrhage: risk factors, clinical impact, and effect of hemostatic therapy with recombinant activated factor VII. Neurosurgery. 2006;59(4):767–73. discussion 773–764
17. Mayer SA, Brun NC, Begtrup K, et al. Recombinant activated factor VII for acute intracerebral hemorrhage. N Engl J Med. 2005;352(8):777–85.
18. Mayer SA, Brun NC, Broderick J, et al. Safety and feasibility of recombinant factor VIIa for acute intracerebral hemorrhage. Stroke. 2005;36(1):74–9.
19. Mayer SA, Brun NC, Broderick J, et al. Recombinant activated factor VII for acute intracerebral hemorrhage: US phase IIA trial. Neurocrit Care. 2006;4(3):206–14.
20. Brott T, Broderick J, Kothari R, et al. Early hemorrhage growth in patients with intracerebral hemorrhage. Stroke. 1997;28(1):1–5.
21. Davis SM, Broderick J, Hennerici M, et al. Hematoma growth is a determinant of mortality and poor outcome after intracerebral hemorrhage. Neurology. 2006;66(8):1175–81.
22. Kazui S, Naritomi H, Yamamoto H, Sawada T, Yamaguchi T. Enlargement of spontaneous intracerebral hemorrhage. Incidence and time course. Stroke. 1996;27(10):1783–7.
23. Mayer SA, Brun NC, Begtrup K, et al. Efficacy and safety of recombinant activated factor VII for acute intracerebral hemorrhage. N Engl J Med. 2008;358(20):2127–37.
24. Mayer SA, Davis SM, Skolnick BE, et al. Can a subset of intracerebral hemorrhage patients benefit from hemostatic therapy with recombinant activated factor VII? Stroke. 2009;40(3):833–40.
25. Qureshi AI, Palesch YY. Antihypertensive treatment of acute cerebral hemorrhage (ATACH) II: design, methods, and rationale. Neurocrit Care. 2011;15(3):559–76.
26. Mayer SA, Sacco RL, Shi T, Mohr JP. Neurologic deterioration in noncomatose patients with supratentorial intracerebral hemorrhage. Neurology. 1994;44(8):1379–84.

27. Zazulia AR, Diringer MN, Videen TO, et al. Hypoperfusion without ischemia surrounding acute intracerebral hemorrhage. J Cereb Blood Flow Metab. 2001;21(7):804–10.
28. Butcher KS, Baird T, MacGregor L, Desmond P, Tress B, Davis S. Perihematomal edema in primary intracerebral hemorrhage is plasma derived. Stroke. 2004;35(8):1879–85.
29. Butcher KS, Jeerakathil T, Hill M, et al. The Intracerebral hemorrhage acutely decreasing arterial pressure trial. Stroke. 2013;44(3):620–6.
30. Qureshi AI, Mohammad YM, Yahia AM, et al. A prospective multicenter study to evaluate the feasibility and safety of aggressive antihypertensive treatment in patients with acute intracerebral hemorrhage. J Intensive Care Med. 2005;20(1):34–42.
31. Antihypertensive Treatment of Acute Cerebral Hemorrhage i. Antihypertensive treatment of acute cerebral hemorrhage. Crit Care Med. 2010;38(2):637–48.
32. Qureshi AI, Palesch YY, Martin R, et al. Effect of systolic blood pressure reduction on hematoma expansion, perihematomal edema, and 3-month outcome among patients with intracerebral hemorrhage: results from the antihypertensive treatment of acute cerebral hemorrhage study. Arch Neurol. May 2010;67(5):570–6.
33. Anderson CS, Huang Y, Wang JG, et al. Intensive blood pressure reduction in acute cerebral haemorrhage trial (INTERACT): a randomised pilot trial. Lancet Neurol. 2008;7(5):391–9.
34. Anderson CS, Heeley E, Huang Y, et al. Rapid blood-pressure lowering in patients with acute intracerebral hemorrhage. N Engl J Med. 2013;368(25):2355–65.
35. Wang X, Arima H, Heeley E, et al. Magnitude of blood pressure reduction and clinical outcomes in acute intracerebral hemorrhage: intensive blood pressure reduction in acute cerebral hemorrhage trial study. Hypertension. 2015;65(5):1026–32.
36. Sato S, Carcel C, Anderson CS. Blood pressure management after Intracerebral hemorrhage. Curr Treat Options Neurol. 2015;17(12):49.
37. Hemphill JC 3rd, Greenberg SM, Anderson CS, et al. Guidelines for the management of spontaneous intracerebral hemorrhage: a guideline for healthcare professionals from the American Heart Association/American Stroke Association. Stroke. 2015;46(7):2032–60.
38. Qureshi AI, Palesch YY, Barsan WG, et al. Intensive blood-pressure lowering in patients with acute cerebral hemorrhage. N Engl J Med. 2016;375(11):1033–43.
39. Prabhakaran S, Naidech AM. Ischemic brain injury after intracerebral hemorrhage: a critical review. Stroke. Aug 2012;43(8):2258–63.
40. Garg RK, Liebling SM, Maas MB, Nemeth AJ, Russell EJ, Naidech AM. Blood pressure reduction, decreased diffusion on MRI, and outcomes after intracerebral hemorrhage. Stroke. 2012;43(1):67–71.
41. Majidi S, Suarez JI, Qureshi AI. Management of acute hypertensive response in intracerebral hemorrhage patients after ATACH-2 trial. Neurocrit Care. 2016; https://doi.org/10.1007/s12028-016-0341-z. PMID: 28004328.

Chapter 5
Thromboprophylaxis and Seizure Management in Intracerebral Hemorrhage

Odysseas Kargiotis, Georgios Tsivgoulis, and Jose I. Suarez

Introduction

Intracerebral hemorrhage (ICH) is a common cause of death and disability in adults with an overall annual incidence of 24.6 cases per 100,000 people. The incidence is considerably higher in Asian populations (51.8 per 100,000 persons-years) and the elderly [1]. Mortality after ICH is high, exceeding 40% the first month and reaches 60% 1 year after insult. Interestingly, more than 50% of deaths occur within the first 48 h [2]. At least 75% of the survivors remain dependent at 6 months, with half of them having a modified Rankin score of 4 or 5 [3]. Surprisingly, mortality rates have remained unchanged over the last three decades [1]. Up to 50% of patients have advanced age and arterial hypertension as the most common risk factors for ICH [4]. In the present section, we review the available data regarding the prevention and treatment of common complications, namely, deep vein thrombosis (DVT), pulmonary embolism (PE), and seizures.

O. Kargiotis
Stroke Unit, Metropolitan Hospital, Piraeus, Greece

G. Tsivgoulis (✉)
Second Department of Neurology, "Attikon" Hospital, School of Medicine, University of Athens, Athens, Greece

Department of Neurology, The University of Tennessee Health Science Center, Memphis, TN, USA

J. I. Suarez
Division of Neurosciences Critical Care, Departments of Anesthesiology and Critical Care Medicine, Neurology, and Neurosurgery, The Johns Hopkins University School of Medicine, Baltimore, MD, USA

B. Ovbiagele, A. I. Qureshi (eds.), *Intracerebral Hemorrhage Therapeutics*,
https://doi.org/10.1007/978-3-319-77063-5_5

Thromboprophylaxis

Incidence of Venous Thromboembolism and Risk Factors

Patients with acute neurological insults and those undergoing major neurosurgical procedures are at increased risk for DVT and subsequent PE. The reported rates of these complications in different studies show substantial variation. The incidence of DVT and PE in stroke patients ranges from 1% to 10% (including asymptomatic patients) and from 0.5% to 1.6%, respectively [5–9]. It is estimated that, without preventive measures, 53% and 16% of stroke patients suffering from severe motor deficits will present with DVT or PE, respectively [10]. Neurosurgical patients might develop venous thromboembolism (VTE) even more often. Indeed, 16% to 25% of them suffer from such complications, whereas PE is associated with a 60% mortality [11, 12]. Prolonged immobility is a major risk factor that is determined mainly by the severity of the neurological deficit [5]. In cases with residual lower limp paralysis and without thromboprophylaxis, standard diagnostic tests may detect asymptomatic DVT in up to 75% of patients [13].

Among stroke patients, those with ICH have a fourfold increased risk of VTE compared with those with ischemic stroke [14]. Less aggressive thromboprophylaxis and more severe motor deficits in ICH might account for the higher rates of VTE compared with ischemic stroke [15]. The analysis of a large US-based national hospital discharge database comprising 1,606,000 cases with ICH revealed VTE rates of 1.93%, DVT of 1.37%, and PE of 0.68% [9]. In the FAST (Factor Seven for Acute Hemorrhagic Stroke) trial, the incidence of DVT and PE was 3% and 1%, respectively [16]. Smaller patient cohorts involving Asian patients have shown higher rates of DVT. Fourteen days after admission, DVT was diagnosed in the 21% of 81 Japanese patients, while 1 patient suffered PE. However it should be noted that no specific antithrombotic preventive measure was administered in this Japanese cohort of ICH patients [17]. Similarly, another study from Japan documented a 40.4% incidence of DVT among 52 ICH patients [18].

Eighty percent of DVTs develop between the second and the tenth day after ICH [7]. In addition, PE is responsible for 5% of deaths after ICH [19]. The emboli causing PE originate in the lower limbs in more than 90% of cases [20]. Factors associated with increased risk for DVT include older age, female sex, complete lower limb paralysis, severe neurological deficit with National Institute of Health Stroke Scale (NIHSS) score of more than 12, large hematoma volume and lobar location, obesity, cancer, prothrombotic state, hormonal therapy, and prolonged immobilization [14, 17, 18, 21, 22].

Practitioners may use one of several clinical predictive scores to assess the risk of developing DVT in hospitalized patients. The Padua Predictive Score (Table 5.1) was evaluated in a cohort of 1180 consecutive patients admitted to a department of internal medicine, with the most common diagnosis being active cancer, whereas stroke patients composed less than 5% of the study group. The patients were cat-

Table 5.1 The Padua risk assessment model for the identification of hospitalized medical patients at risk for venous thromboembolism [23]

Risk assessment model (high risk of VTE: ≥ 4)	
Baseline features	Score
Active cancer[a]	3
Previous VTE (with the exclusion of superficial vein thrombosis)	3
Reduced mobility[b]	3
Already known thrombophilic condition[c]	3
Recent (< 1 month) trauma and/or surgery	2
Elderly age (≥ 70 years)	1
Heart and/or respiratory failure	1
Acute myocardial infarction or ischemic stroke	1
Acute infection and/or rheumatologic disorder	1
Obesity (BMI ≥30)	1
Ongoing hormonal treatment	1

[a]Patients with local or distant metastases and/or in whom chemotherapy or radiotherapy had been performed in the previous 6 month

[b]Bed rest with bathroom privileges (either due to patient's limitations or physicians order) for at least 3 days

[c]Carriage of defects of antithrombin, protein C or S, factor V Leiden, G20210A prothrombin mutation, and antiphospholipid syndrome. From Barbar et al. [23], Table 1, with permission of John Wiley and Sons

egorized as either low or high risk for VTE according to a cutoff value of 4. The authors showed that only the 0.3% of low-risk patients developed VTE in comparison with the 11% of those at high risk but without thromboprophylaxis. Prophylactic treatment reduced VTE to 2.2% in high-risk patients [23]. According to this score, all patients with ICH and reduced mobility are at high thromboembolic risk. Among the other two predictive scores, Rogers score is applicable only to surgical patients, whereas Caprini's assessment model (Table 5.2), although validated also in surgical patients, appears practical and easy to use in nonsurgical patients, too, with all stroke patients being again categorized as at high thromboembolic risk [24–26].

Oral anticoagulant-related ICH is typically managed with the administration of prothrombin complex concentrates (PCCs), fresh frozen plasma (FFP), and vitamin K in order to reverse the anticoagulant effect [27]. Interestingly, these interventions might further increase the risk for VTE and DVT. A meta-analysis of 27 studies with 1032 ICH patients receiving acutely PCC found an 1.8% (95% CI 1.0–3.0) incidence of thromboembolic events in patients treated with 4-factor PCCs and 0.7% (95% CI 0.0–2.4) in patients treated with 3-factor PCCs [28]. The retrospective analysis of 54 ICH patients treated with rFVIIa (recombinant activated Factor VII) reported VTE rates of 5% [29]. However, these patients were not routinely screened for DVT, and the diagnosis was based on clinical suspicion. Of interest, the FAST clinical trial investigating the effect of rFVIIa administration in spontaneous, non-anticoagulation-related ICH found similar DVT and PE rates (3% and 1%, respec-

Table 5.2 The Caprini risk assessment model for the identification of hospitalized (surgical or medical) patients at risk for venous thromboembolism [25]

Clinical characteristics	Points[a]
Age	
Age 41–60	1
Age 61–74	2
Age ≥ 75	3
Surgery	
Minor surgery	1
Arthroscopic surgery	2
Major open surgery (> 45 min)	2
Laparoscopic surgery (> 45 min)	2
Elective arthroplasty	5
BMI > 25 kg/m^2	1
Lower limb edema	1
Lower limb varicose	1
Pregnancy or postpartum	1
History of spontaneous abortion	1
Oral contraceptives use	1
Recent sepsis (< 1 month)	1
Obstructive pulmonary disease	1
Recent pneumonia (< 1 month)	1
Abnormal pulmonary function tests	1
Acute myocardial infarction	1
Congestive heart failure	1
Inflammatory bowel disease	1
Bed rest	1
Bedridden (> 72 h)	2
Cancer	2
Immobilizing cast	2
Central venous catheter	2
Previous venous thromboembolism	3
Factor V (Leiden) mutation	3
Presence of lupus anticoagulant	3
Anticardiolipin antibodies	3
Homocysteinemia	3
Heparin-induced thrombocytopenia	3
Other congenital or acquired thrombophilia	3
Recent stroke (< 1 month)	5
Lower limb fracture	5
Recent spinal cord injury (< 1 month)	5
Maximum score	60 (medical patients), 65 (surgery patients)

Adapted from Caprini [25]

[a]The individual scores of each risk factor are summed to generate a cumulative risk score that defined the patient's venous thromboembolism risk level: very low risk 0–1, low risk 2, moderate risk 3–4, and high risk ≥5

tively) in the placebo and treated patients [16]. It is important to stress that after weighing all this evidence, patients presenting with anticoagulation-related ICH should undergo anticoagulation reversal upon admission [29].

Physicians who manage patients with ICH usually undertake a less aggressive approach concerning thromboprophylaxis, due to the possible enlargement of parenchymal hematoma secondary to ongoing bleeding. Indeed, a meta-analysis of 218 ICH cases demonstrated some degree of hematoma growth in 72.9% of them, which was associated with mortality and overall outcome [30]. Another prospective observational study of 103 patients found a significant association between early hematoma growth and clinical deterioration [31]. Thus, confirmation of bleeding cessation and hematoma volume stabilization is necessary before initiation of pharmacological thromboprophylaxis.

International Recommendations on Thromboprophylaxis Management in ICH

Since 2007, the American Heart Association/American Stroke Association (AHA/ASA) guidelines recommend low-dose unfractionated heparin (UH) or low-molecular-weight heparin (LMWH) after ICH for the prevention of VTE [32]. This initial weak recommendation suggested the use of anticoagulants after documentation of bleeding cessation in patients with hemiplegia but no earlier than 3–4 days after insult (Class IIb, Level of Evidence B). For the rest of the patients suffering from hemiparesis or hemiplegia, lower limb intermittent pneumatic compression (IPC) use was strongly recommended (Class I, Level of Evidence B). In 2015, the revised guidelines preserved the strong recommendation for IPC (Class I, Level of Evidence A) and recommended against the use of graduated compression stockings (Class III, Level of Evidence A). Moreover, the recommendation about low-dose anticoagulants allows for an earlier institution of prophylactic medication, even after 1 day from symptom onset, provided that bleeding cessation has been documented (Class IIb, Level of Evidence B) [27]. Despite these recommendations, a recent study depicted a less than 20% use of prophylactic anticoagulation in ICH patients (5395 out of 32,690), with almost half of them receiving treatment within 48 h [33].

Similarly, the most recent European Stroke Organization (ESO) guidelines for the management of spontaneous ICH include a strong recommendation for the use of IPC in immobile patients and overrule the application of short or long graduated compression stockings. Regarding UH or LMWH, they state that there is insufficient evidence to guide decisions about the details of its indication, so the recommendation for the prophylactic use of heparin is weak [34]. In line with AHA/ASA and ESO, the Japanese guidelines support the consideration of prophylactic low-dose anticoagulation [35]. The American College of Physicians and the American College of Chest Physicians recommend also the use of DVT pharmacoprophylaxis and discourage the application of graduated compression stockings [36, 37]. On the contrary, the United Kingdom and Australian authorities recommend against the prophylactic initiation of low-dose UH or LMWH in patients with ICH [38, 39].

Finally, the most recent guidelines from the Neurocritical Care Society regarding thromboprophylaxis for ICH patients requiring intensive care were based in the grade system [40]. The goal of this guideline was to provide clinicians with an evidence-based framework for the appropriate administration of thromboprophylaxis in patients with neurologic illness, with a focus on those requiring neurocritical care. The authors recommended the use of IPC and/or graduated compression stockings for VTE prophylaxis over no prophylaxis beginning at the time of hospital admission (strong recommendation and high-quality evidence). They also suggested using prophylactic doses of subcutaneous UFH or LMWH to prevent VTE in patients with stable hematomas and no ongoing coagulopathy beginning within 48 h of hospital admission (weak recommendation and low-quality evidence). Moreover, the authors recommended continuing mechanical VTE prophylaxis with IPCs in patients started on pharmacologic prophylaxis (weak recommendation low-quality evidence). As can be gathered from the evidence reviewed thus far, the inconsistency between the different expert's consensuses derives greatly from the lack of convincing, large-scale randomized trials on ICH pharmacologic thromboprophylaxis.

Studies on Non-pharmacologic Antithrombotic Measures

Calf IPC was originally investigated as a potential non-pharmacologic antithrombotic measure in surgical patients and in hospitalized patients with or without cancer in the early 1970s [41–43]. A few years later, the approach was studied on neurosurgical patients, including non-operated ones, with impressive results concerning VTE risk reduction [44, 45]. Subsequently, sequential compression devices were added to heparin plus elastic stockings (ES) in patients with ischemic stroke resulting in a significant 40-fold risk reduction of DVT [46]. The first strong evidence about the efficacy of IPC in the prevention of DVT in ICH patients came from a randomized trial by Lacut et al. The authors assigned 151 ICH patients to receive ES alone or combined with IPC, and after 10 days, they documented a substantial relative risk reduction of 71% in favor of the ES plus IPC treatment group [47]. Interestingly, asymptomatic DVT had a high incidence of 15.9% at 10 days in the group receiving only ES. Similar prophylactic effect of IPC in patients with ICH was also found in the CLOTS (Clots in Legs Or sTockings after Stroke) 3 trial, where a subgroup analysis verified a 10% absolute risk reduction of DVT in the group of patients randomized to IPC (6.7% versus 17.0%). CLOTS 3 trial was the largest to date randomized controlled clinical trial (RCT) that evaluated the safety and efficacy of IPC for DVT prophylaxis in a large sample of 2876 acute stroke patients including 376 cases with ICH [48].

The current evidence for the application of graduated compression stockings suggests that they do not afford substantial protection against DVT in stroke patients. In a small cohort of 99 randomized individuals suffering from stroke, elastic stockings did not reduce significantly the diagnosis of asymptomatic DVT (OR = 0.43, 95%

CI 0.14–1.36) [49]. Similarly, the large CLOTS 1 trial that was an outcome-blinded randomized controlled study, after having randomized 2518 stroke patients, including 232 cases with ICH, confirmed the lack of efficacy of graduated compression stockings for DVT prophylaxis in acute stroke. The nonsignificant absolute risk reduction of 0.5% for DVT was accompanied by significant local complications, such as skin breaks, ulcers, blisters, and skin necrosis, in the 5% of patients wearing stockings [7]. However, in the similarly designed CLOTS 2 trial, which allocated 3114 stroke patients, thigh-length graduated compression stockings were more efficient in reducing DVT risk than below-knee stockings, with an absolute risk reduction of 2.5% (95% CI, 0.7–4.4; $p = 0.008$) [50]. Thus, IPC is strongly recommended immediately after ICH, whereas graduated compression stockings should be avoided. In case of IPC unavailability, thigh-length, graduated compression stockings could be an alternative option, at least until the safe initiation of pharmacologic thromboprophylaxis treatment.

Studies on Pharmacologic Thromboprophylaxis

The prophylactic antithrombotic properties of low-dose UH or LMWH in hospitalized/immobilized patients have been investigated during the past 50 years. Initial studies showed that low-dose anticoagulation was very effective in reducing DVT occurrence in patients hospitalized for different etiologies, including myocardial infarction, orthopedic operations and hip replacement, urological surgery, and general surgery [51–56]. All studies used a control group and documented absolute percentage reductions of DVT rates ranging from 12% to more than 40%.

In stroke medicine, low-dose UH at first and LMWH at a later stage were studied as means of lower limb thromboprophylaxis [57]. In the initial studies, discrimination between ischemic and hemorrhagic stroke could only be made post-mortem. One such study with 305 patients achieved absolute DVT reduction rates of 50%, along with a significantly reduced mortality in the heparin group. Furthermore, PE detection was less frequent in patients that died during the follow-up and had been treated with heparin. Hemorrhagic stroke was subsequently found in 9.9% of the 84 deceased patients, with similar distribution between treatment groups [58]. Later, an absolute reduction in DVT incidence of 26–30% was demonstrated by different LMWH molecules compared to placebo in ischemic stroke patients [59, 60]. Again in patients with ischemic stroke, LMWH were compared in randomized trials with UH and were proven to be superior or non-inferior to UH in preventing DVT [61, 62]. The largest of these studies (PREVAIL Study) assigned 1762 patients with ischemic stroke to either enoxaparin 40 mg or UH 5000iu twice per day and found a risk reduction of DVT of 43% with enoxaparin (relative risk 0.57, 95% CI 0.44–0.76, $p = 0.0001$), without increase in intracranial hemorrhage incidence [63]. Finally, in a mixed population with both ischemic and hemorrhagic stroke patients in rehabilitation, the multivariate analysis showed that only therapeutic anticoagulation (OR = 0.37; 95% CI, 0.15–0.88) and then low-dose heparin (OR = 0.48; 95% CI, 0.23–0.98) protected against VTE, whereas antiplatelet agents had no effect (OR = 0.79; 95% CI, 0.40–1.57) [64].

It is well-documented and supported that pharmacologic thromboprophylaxis is warranted after ischemic stroke unless contraindications exist, whereas in cases with ICH there is still some controversy due to the limited available evidence from RCTs evaluating solely patients with acute ICH. The first prospective randomized study was conducted by Dickmann et al. and found that heparin did not offer substantial protection against VTE but neither increased the risk of bleeding [65]. The results of this study were incorporated to those of a subsequent randomized study, in which, an additional group of 22 ICH patients received very early heparin prophylaxis. Thus, the study compared the three groups of very early, early, and late pharmacoprophylaxis with UF (3 × 5000 IU/day subcutaneous on day 2, 4, and 10, respectively, after bleeding). There was a significant lowering of PE incidence in the group of very early treatment (odds ratio 9.2), without bleeding complications. DVTs were also reduced with very early heparin introduction, without the numbers reaching statistical significance [66]. Conversely, the use of heparinoids in 219 out of 988 ICH patients did not alter the risk of VTE [67].

The first report on the use of LMWH in ICH came from Kleindienst et al. that treated 238 patients with intracranial hemorrhage using prophylactic certoparin 3000 IU and observed no intracranial bleeding and very low rate of DVT and/or PE (0.8%) [68]. Subsequently, a retrospective analysis of 232 ICH patients treated with 20 mg of subcutaneous enoxaparin and 175 controls disclosed no difference in mortality or hematoma enlargement but also low VTE complication rates in both groups (3% and 2%, respectively) [69]. Heparin was also safe in another nonrandomized study of 200 ICH patients that received pharmacoprophylaxis in addition to elastic stockings and was compared with 258 patients that wore only elastic stockings [70]. Similar results were obtained from the randomization of 75 ICH patients to enoxaparin sodium 40 mg/day or compression stockings, 48 h after admission [71]. No hematoma growth and no fatal PE were reported in another cohort of 97 ICH patients receiving LMWH within 36 h after diagnosis [72]. Finally, two more studies verified the safety of early pharmacologic VTE prophylaxis after ICH [22, 73].

The only currently available meta-analysis of pharmacologic VTE prophylaxis in acute ICH included data from only four available studies (two randomized and two nonrandomized, total number of patients 1000) [66, 69–71]. The analysis found a significant reduction of PE events with low-dose anticoagulation (1.7% versus 2.9%; RR, 0.37; 95% CI, 0.17–0.80; $p = 0.01$). There was no difference in DVT rates (4.2% vs. 3.3%) or hematoma enlargement (8.0% vs. 4.0%) rates. A marginally nonsignificant reduction in mortality (16.1% vs. 20.9%; RR = 0.76; 95% CI, 0.57–1.03; $p = 0.07$) was observed in patients treated with low-dose anticoagulation [74].

Early Mobilization and Hydration for VTE Prophylaxis

Adequate hydration and early mobilization also have been studied for the prevention of VTE. Dehydration increases the risk for VTE in stroke patients, with odds ratios of 4.7, 2.8, and 3.4 for serum osmolality of >297 mOsm/kg, urea >7.5 mmol/l, and urea/creatinine ratio (mmol:mmol) >80, respectively [75]. The AHA/ASA guidelines for the management of spontaneous ICH adopt the same recommendations for the prehospital management with the AHA/ASA guidelines for the early management of ischemic stroke and state that euvolemia is desirable and hypovolemia should be corrected with intravenous normal saline (Class I; Level of Evidence C) [27, 76].

Early mobilization is considered an important element for the management of stroke patients hospitalized in specialized stroke units, as it can potentially limit the risk of complications, such as infections and thrombosis, and also accelerate clinical recovery through early augmentation of brain plasticity [77–79]. However, there is still uncertainty on the exact time of active physiotherapy initiation. A recent meta-analysis of 3 RCTs with 159 patients showed that initiation of mobilization within 24 h versus 48 h was associated with a nonsignificant increase in mortality (OR = 2.58; 95% CI, 0.98–6.79, $p = 0.06$), with no difference in other complications or outcomes. On the other hand, earlier transfer to rehabilitation centers improved outcomes in terms of physical independence [80]. Moreover, a small prospective RCT enrolling 52 patients that were subjected to mobilization within 24 or 48 h found no significant differences between groups with regard to month outcomes [81]. The largest RCT to date (AVERT) assigned 2104 patients (258 with ICH) to very early mobilization within 24 h or to standard care and reported worse functional outcomes in the group assigned to very early mobilization (adjusted OR = 0.73, 95% CI, 0.59–0.90; $p = 0.004$), but no significant differences in mortality or serious complications. Moreover, a subgroup analysis revealed that ICH patients might even be more vulnerable to very early mobilization when considering the 3-month outcome and death results [82]. Based mainly on the findings from AVERT, the mobilization of ICH patients should be avoided for the first 24 h, and physical rehabilitation should be applied with a progressively increased intensity taking into account the patient's clinical fragility. A simple algorithm referring our own clinical experience (after taking into account international recommendations) for ICH thromboprophylaxis is presented in Fig. 5.1.

Diagnosis of DVT and PE

Before the introduction of ultrasound, the diagnosis of DVT was based on venography, which could even visualize the distal veins with adequate detail. The diagnostic sensitivity of ultrasound for distal vein thrombosis is lower than that for proximal vein thrombosis and depends on the examination protocol [83]. However, in the hands of an experienced examiner, ultrasounds will miss only 0.5% of DVTs [84].

The diagnosis of PE frequently requires a high index of suspicion. Computed tomography pulmonary angiography (CTPA) is the gold standard to diagnose PE. Echocardiography, which can confirm right ventricular overload, as well as lower limb Doppler ultrasounds might be used as alternatives when CTPA is contraindicated, since up to 70% of patients with symptomatic PE have DVT [85]. In

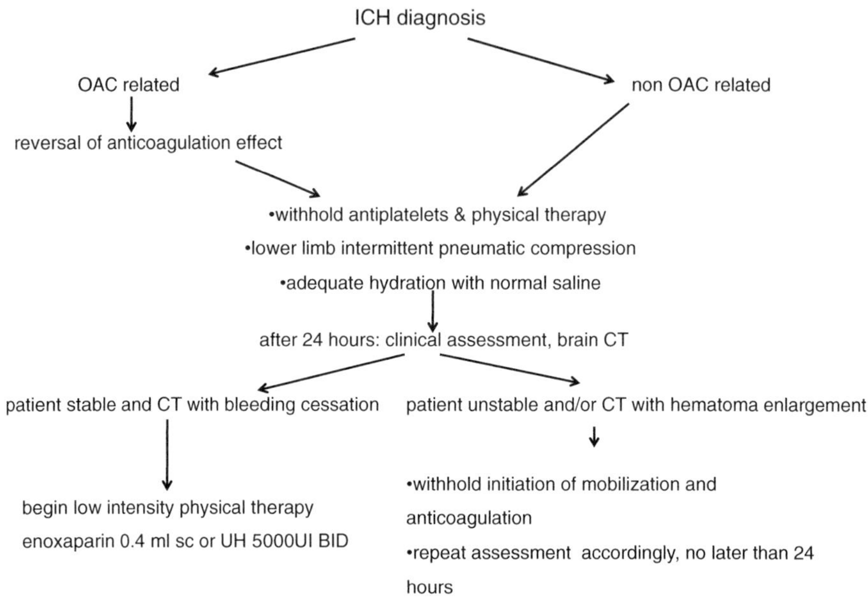

Fig. 5.1 A schematic algorithm of thromboprophylaxis in acute intracerebral hemorrhage (ICH). This algorithm reflects our clinical experience after taking into account current international recommendations. *CT, computed tomography; ICH, intracerebral hemorrhage; LMWH, low-molecular-weight heparin; OAC, oral anticoagulation; UH, unfractionated heparin*

addition, there are several clinical prediction scales for the diagnosis of PE, with sensitivity ranging from 88 to 96% [86]. The modified Wells score may distinguish between "likely PE" and "unlikely PE" and when combined with a D-dimer level < 0.50 μg/mL has a negative predictive value of 99.5% [87]. The score takes into account variables such as the clinical symptoms/signs suggestive of DVT, heart rate, duration of immobilization, and previous VTE [88].

D-dimers are very useful to exclude DVT, especially when applying a lower cutoff threshold of 0.5 mg/L which results in a sensitivity of 100% but with a specificity of only 46.2% in stroke patients with symptoms suggestive of DVT [89]. In low probability suspected PE, normal D-dimer values safely exclude PE, whereas increased values necessitate further investigation with CTPA [85].

Treatment of VTE in ICH Patients

Despite all prophylactic measures, physicians might be confronted with difficult treatment dilemmas when ICH is complicated by DVT or PE, especially early in the course of hospitalization. Current AHA/ASA guidelines recommend full dose anticoagulation or inferior vena cava (IVC) filter placement when ICH patients present with symptomatic DVT or PE (Class IIa; Level of Evidence C). It is also suggested that the decision to anticoagulated or place an IVC filter hinges on several clinical factors, such as the time from initiation of intracranial bleeding, hemorrhage cessation, cause and location of bleeding, and patient comorbidities (Class IIa; Level of Evidence C) [27]. For example, lobar hemorrhage has a twofold risk of rebleeding with the administration of therapeutic anticoagulation. Data from historical, non-treated case series with PE and proximal DVT, comprising of patients with various medical and surgical conditions, have shown mortality rates of 26.6% and 16.2%, respectively, whereas anticoagulation reduced the risk to 2.6% and 0.7%, respectively [90]. In stroke patients, untreated proximal DVT may be complicated by fatal PE in 10–20% of patients, and nonfatal PE may recur in 12–15% of untreated cases [27, 90]. Thus, symptomatic VTE in ICH patients should not be left untreated. However, there are no studies addressing important aspects of VTE treatment, such as timing after hemorrhage for the safe introduction of therapeutic anticoagulation, the indications of IVC filter placement as an alternative to anticoagulation, as well as when to remove the IVC filter.

Nieto et al. aimed to assess the effect of the location of a major hemorrhage to the subsequent risk for rebleeding, after the introduction of anticoagulation for symptomatic VTE. Their cohort included 94 ICH patients that had suffered VTE after hemorrhagic stroke. The mean time elapsed since bleeding was 20 days (SD 20 +/−9), and the majority of patients received LMWH (88%), a few patients UH (6.4%), and some IVC filter (30%). Surprisingly, there were no reports of rebleeding, whereas recurrence of VTE was documented in 5.3% of cases [91]. Although in this study VTE was a late complication after ICH, the results support the immediate use of therapeutic anticoagulation, which received the majority of the patients (94.4%) and underscores its safety and efficacy.

The main indications for IVC filter placement include a contraindication for anticoagulation and the recurrence of PE under therapeutic anticoagulation [92]. Although placement of IVC filters is a common practice, especially in high thromboembolic risk patients, a recent randomized open-label blinded end point trial (PREPIC2) of patients with DVT-related severe PE failed to show an additive prophylactic effect of IVC filter to anticoagulation during a 6-month follow-up period [93]. An earlier randomized trial of 400 patients with DVT, with or without PE, found a reduction of early PE occurrence in the group treated with both IVC filter and anticoagulation versus only anticoagulation. However, when taking into account only the symptomatic Pes, the difference was not significant [94]. More importantly, there is a lack of evidence from RCTs demonstrating the efficacy of IVC filter placement in the absence of concomitant anticoagulation.

In the event of VTE complicating ICH, we recommend full dose LMWH as long as the volume of hematoma has been stabilized on repeat brain imaging. IVC placement without anticoagulation can be reserved for cases with no evidence of bleeding cessation, VTEs occurring during the first 48 h following the index event and perhaps recent (<7 days) lobar hemorrhages. In case of PE recurrence despite full dose anticoagulation with documentation of adequate anticoagulant effect (anti-Xa assay), the addition of IVC filter may be considered.

Management of Seizures

Incidence and Predisposing Factors

Seizures are an important complication of spontaneous ICH. The incidence of early post-ICH seizures ranges from 2.7% to 7.3% and has been reported up to 12%–17%. Early seizures are generally more frequent than late ones [95–98]. The largest single center observational study of 1920 consecutive patients showed a 6.6% incidence of seizures after ICH, with early seizures (4.3%) being more common than late ones (2.3%). However, only the volume of hematoma increased the odds for recurrent seizures [99]. In a study using the US Nationwide Inpatient Sample database, there were 13,033 cases identified as ICH, of which 1430 (11%) received also a diagnosis of seizures [100]. In another study, among 761 patients with ICH, early seizures (at presentation or within 24 h) occurred in 32 cases (4.2%), whereas additional 25 (3.8%) patients had seizures after the first 24 h and within the first month. The 30-day post-ICH risk for seizures was 8.1%. In addition, among survivors with seizures, the risk of recurrence was 5.3% (95% CI, 1.6–8.9) in the first year and 27% (95% CI, 15.6–38.4) at 5 years [101]. Another prospective study of 562 consecutive ICH patients documented early seizures (within 1 week) in 71 patients (14%) [102]. In a smaller cohort consisting of 112 patients with nontraumatic, supratentorial ICH, early clinical seizures were reported in 19 cases (17%) [98]. Srinivasan et al. analyzed two different chronological cohorts comprising of 30 and 108 ICH patients and observed seizures in 6.6% and 13.0%, respectively [103]. Arntz et al. found a 31% cumulative risk of epilepsy and a 23% cumulative risk of epilepsy with recurrent seizures in ICH patients, with their mixed cohort consisting of 697 consecutive patients with ischemic stroke, transient ischemic attack, or ICH [104]. Similarly, it has been shown that the cumulative annual risk of experiencing a seizure after ICH was increased from 19.9% 1 year after insult to 26.1% after 5 years [105]. However, a minority of long-term ICH survivors suffer from chronic epilepsy at 5 years (6.5%) [106]. In studies with continuous electroencephalographic monitoring, seizures were recorded in 18–28% of patients with ICH within the first 48 and 72 h, respectively [107, 108]. The majority of seizures are simple partial or focal with secondary generalization [95].

Clinical and radiological characteristics may predict the risk of seizure occurrence. Early seizures correlate with lobar location, rebleeding, brain ischemia, hydrocephalus, and brain edema. In the study by Sung and Chu, 32% of patients with lobar ICH had seizures, and 62% of the 42 patients with lobar hematomas developed epilepsy [95]. Antiepileptic drugs (AEDs) reduce the risk of early seizures, and alcohol abuse predisposes to status epilepticus [101]. Frontal lobar hematomas are more epileptogenic, whereas individuals with seizures are younger and more frequently undergo craniectomy (2.1% vs. 1.2%, $p = 0.006$), ventriculostomy (8.5% vs. 6.0%, $p < 0.001$), intubation (32.2% vs. 25.9%, $p < 0.001$), and tracheostomy (6.4% vs. 4.2%, $p < 0.001$), probably in the context of a more severe ICH [100, 109]. Indeed, seizures are more frequent after neurological deterioration and midline shift in brain imaging [108]. Factors predisposing to the presentation of ICH with seizures include previous ICH (OR = 4.76; 95% CI, 1.53–14.84), cortical involvement (OR = 2.21; 95% CI, 1.11–4.43), younger age (OR = 0.97 per 1-year increase; 95% CI, 0.95–0.99), and increased NIHSS score at admission (OR:1.03 per 1 point increase; 95% CI, 1.01–1.06) [102]. Late onset seizures (2 weeks after hemorrhage) might predispose to recurrent seizures [95, 104], whereas others found only the volume of hematoma to be associated with recurrent seizures [99]. Higher NIHSS scores are also reported to predict epilepsy and epilepsy with recurrent seizures [104]. On the other hand, electrographic seizures are associated with more than 30% hematoma enlargement between the admission and the 24-h follow-up CT scan, whereas periodic epileptiform discharges (PEDs) are associated with hematomas located at least 1 mm from the cortex [107]. Collectively, large hematomas involving the cerebral cortex and those resulting in higher grades of neurological deficits exhibit an increased epileptogenic potential.

Seizures and Outcome

There are conflicting data regarding the influence of early or late seizures on the outcome of patients with ICH. Epilepsy might aggravate recovery of stroke survivors and reduce quality of life [104]. Theoretically, early seizures might predispose to hematoma enlargement due to transient increases of blood pressure and also accelerate the loss of stressed peri-hematomal neurons from increased metabolic demand or even cause aspiration-related infections. In addition, seizures after ICH might lead to epilepsy due to the promotion of aberrant neuronal networks [110].

In the study by Vespa et al., seizures were associated with higher neurological deficits and midline shift on CT scan but also with a nonstatistically significant trend toward poor outcome ($p < 0.06$) [108]. Furthermore, among 6044 patients with stroke, including 715 with ICH, those with early seizures had a twofold increase in the risk of 30-day mortality (32.1% vs. 13.3%; $p < 0.0001$). However, patients with early seizures had also higher NIHSS scores and lower Glasgow Coma Scale scores, a correlation that was even more powerful for the 60 (8.4%) patients with ICH and seizures. Further analysis did not confirm that seizures promote clinical deterioration nor that they are an independent factor of poor outcome, but it is rather argued that they reflect and are a consequence of severe brain damage [111]. In a Canadian multicenter cohort study of 5027 stroke patients, again seizures were associated with longer hospitalization, higher disability at discharge ($p < 0.001$), and increased mortality at 30 days (36.2% vs. 16.8%, $p < 0.0001$) and at 1-year poststroke (48.6% vs. 27.7%, $p < 0.001$) [112]. Also, among 1402 ICH patients, those with status epilepticus (11 patients) had slightly higher mortality rates (36%) than those without it (24%) [95]. Moreover, PEDs are shown to predict poor outcome after ICH [107].

Of interest, not all studies have shown an unfavorable outcome of ICH patients with seizures. Mortality of hospitalized patients was not affected by immediate or early seizures in the studies by Passero et al. and Labivitz et al., whereas Mullen et al. found that seizures were even associated with reduced odds of inhospital death (OR, 0.62, 95% CI, 0.52–0.75) [96, 100, 101]. In another study, early seizures did not affect outcome at 6 months after insult [102].

Based on the currently available data, it is not possible to draw safe conclusions regarding the impact of seizures on ICH outcome. Given the fact that seizures are more common in severely affected patients with less favorable prognosis due to the characteristics of the hematoma itself, one would expect an association of seizures with higher mortality and morbidity rates. This observation, however, is not sufficient to support a possible role of seizures in the expansion of brain injury.

International Recommendations on Prophylactic Antiepileptic Treatment in ICH

Current clinical practice is not consistent among different stroke units regarding the use of prophylactic AEDs in ICH patients. The most recent AHA/ASA guidelines recommend against prophylactic AED administration (Class III; Level of Evidence B) [27]. In contrast, the ESO guidelines do not make any recommendations on the same issue based on the lack of currently available trials [34]. Many physicians routinely prescribe preventive AEDs [27, 34].

Everyday Clinical Practice on Prophylactic Antiepileptic Treatment in ICH

Despite AHA recommendations advocating deferral of prophylactic AED, a large number of stroke physicians is using antiepileptic treatment for primary seizure prevention in patients with acute ICH. A prospective study of 744 ICH patients disclosed rates of 39% in the use of prophylactic AEDs, with levetiracetam being the most common treatment (89% of cases). Increased hematoma volume, lobar localization, as well as craniotomy were associated with more frequent use of preventive AEDs. These patients were obviously more severely affected and exhibited worse outcomes (OR, 1.40; 95% CI, 1.04–1.88; $p = 0.03$).. However, after adjusting for clinical and demographic characteristics, AED treatment was no longer significantly associated with outcome (odds ratio, 1.11; 95% confidence interval, 0.74–1.65; $p = 0.62$) [113]. A retrospective analysis of two chronological cohorts of patients with ICH, the first between 1/1/99 and 12/31/00 (30 patients) and the second between 1/1/09 and 12/31/10 (108 patients), revealed AED use in the 53.3% and 50%, respectively, although the 86.6% and 59.1% of patients discharged on AEDs did not exhibit clinical or electrographic seizures neither had epileptiform abnormalities in EEG [103]. A recent survey addressed to physicians managing ICH patients found that prophylactic AEDs were never used by only one third of the responders, whereas the rest of the physicians initiated treatment selectively, with the minority (9%) using AEDs in nearly all ICH cases. The duration of the prophylactic treatment was typically for less than 1 month, and levetiracetam was the most common medication prescribed (60%) [110]. The study highlights the significant heterogeneity that exists in the way different physicians approach and manage issues concerning the prevention of seizures in ICH patients.

Studies on Prophylactic Antiepileptic Treatment in ICH

An updated Cochrane review on primary and secondary prevention of seizures after stroke failed to provide sufficient evidence supporting the routine use of AEDs [114]. The review was based on the results of one available randomized placebo-controlled trial of valproic acid in 72 ICH patients. Treatment was maintained for 1 month, and follow-up was completed after 1 year. Valproic acid treatment failed to reduce long-term seizures. However, it decreased early seizures and improved the final neurological deficit, an effect that was not attributed to the antiepileptic action [115]. Short-term preventive AED treatment in lobar hematomas is also supported by another study of 761 ICH patients, 432 of whom received phenobarbital. The risk of early seizures was significantly reduced only in patients with lobar hematomas (OR, 0.62; 95% CI, 0.40–0.96; $p = 0.033$) [101].

However, the majority of the available studies conclude that prophylactic AEDs are not warranted in ICH patients. A retrospective cohort of 157 patients (29% on prophylactic AEDs) failed to demonstrate an association of treatment with the risk of early seizures, long-term epilepsy, disability, and death [116]. Similarly, the administration of prophylactic AED treatment in 216 ICH cases did not reduce the risk of early or late seizures [117].

Regarding the association between prophylactic anticonvulsants and outcome, the results of the available studies, the majority of which being nonrandomized, are inconsistent.. In a cohort of 295 patients, preventive AED use (and in particular phenytoin use) was associated with poor outcome, even after adjustment for other known risk factors after ICH (age, initial hematoma volume, presence of intraventricular blood, initial Glasgow Coma Scale score, and prior warfarin use) [118]. Moreover, prescription of phenytoin after ICH was associated with fever, worse NIHSS at 14 days, and worse modified Rankin Scale at 14 days, 28 days, and 3 months, whereas the exclusion of patients with seizures did not alter the results making seizures an unlike risk factor for poor outcome [119]. In the study by Woo et al., prophylactic AEDs were also linked to a worse modified Rankin score [117]. One randomized trial of 880 stroke patients treated with diazepam or placebo that included 95 ICH cases concluded that the incidences of pneumonia and death were increased in the diazepam group (35% versus 10% for pneumonia and 22% versus 12% for mortality, respectively) [120]. On the contrary, the randomized trial of valproic acid by Gilad et al. found a protective effect of the drug, as mentioned earlier [115]. Recently, the protocol of a randomized double-blind, placebo-controlled trial (SPICH) of short-duration valproate in ICH patients has been published. The trial will randomize 258 individuals and will assess seizure occurrence and outcome [121].

In clinical practice, prophylactic AED treatment is more likely to be introduced in patients with higher hematoma volumes and greater ICH scores, lobar hematomas, and craniotomy [113, 122, 123]. Thus, the adjustment for clinical and demographic characteristics is necessary in order to estimate the influence of AEDs on outcome. In this way, three recent studies that used mainly phenytoin and levetiracetam found an association of AEDs with poor outcome, but after multivariate adjustment, the relation was no longer statistically significant [113, 123, 124]. Thus, we cannot draw safe conclusions regarding the possible influence of anticonvulsants and especially as prophylactic treatment, on the outcome of ICH patients. The routine prophylactic use of AEDs is not justified, especially in patients with absence of cortical involvement [98]. In addition, and since nonconvulsive seizures may occur in about 20% of cases, continuous EEG recordings are recommended for patients with otherwise unexplained reduced level of consciousness [125].

Seizure Management in ICH

Current AHA recommendations advocate that patients with clinical seizures should be treated with AEDs (Class I, Level of Evidence A). Antiepileptic therapy should be also administered to patients with a change in mental status who are found to have electrographic seizures on electroencephalogram (Class I, Level of Evidence C) [27]. Since late seizures are related to increased risk of epilepsy, duration of treatment should be longer after late seizures, and the decision on treatment discontinuation should involve both clinical and electrophysiological data [27].

Regarding the choice of the AED, there are data supporting that levetiracetam appears to have a safer profile in critically ill patients, including ICH [113, 123, 126]. In stroke patients with late seizures, levetiracetam is well tolerated and effective, achieving seizure-freedom in the 77.1% to 82.4% of cases [127, 128]. Finally, a study comparing phenytoin and levetiracetam as prophylactic AEDs in ICH patients found greater efficacy and better cognitive performance of patients treated with levetiracetam [129]. A simple algorithm referring our own clinical experience (after taking into account international recommendations) for seizure management in ICH is shown in Fig. 5.2.

For those ICH patients experiencing status epilepticus (SE), prompt and emergent treatment is recommended to reduce morbidity and mortality [130]. The Neurocritical Care Society published guidelines for management of SE for all clinical conditions including ICH [130]. These guidelines recommend that the treatment of convulsive SE should occur rapidly and continue sequentially until clinical seizures are halted (strong recommendation, high quality). Critical care treatment and monitoring should be started simultaneously with emergent initial therapy and con-

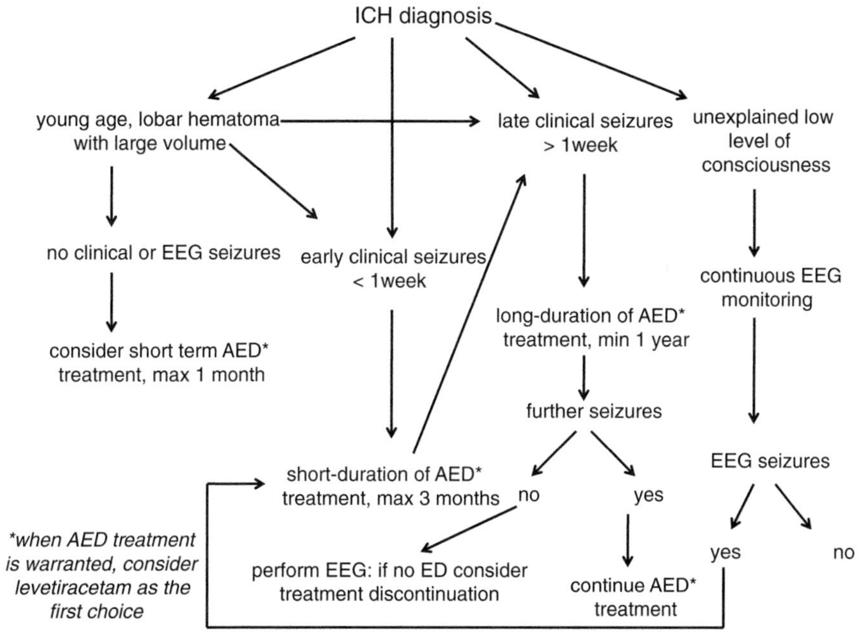

Fig. 5.2 A schematic algorithm of seizure prophylaxis and treatment in acute intracerebral hemorrhage (ICH). This algorithm reflects our clinical experience after taking into account current international recommendations. *AED, antiepileptic drug; ED, epileptiform discharges; EEG, electroencephalogram; ICH, intracerebral hemorrhage*

tinued until further therapy is consider successful or futile (strong recommendation, moderate quality). Benzodiazepines should be given as emergent initial therapy (strong recommendation, high quality). Urgent control AED therapy recommendations include the use of IV fosphenytoin/phenytoin, valproate sodium, or levetiracetam (strong recommendation, moderate quality). Finally, refractory SE therapy recommendations should consist of continuous infusion AEDs but vary by the patient's underlying condition (strong recommendation, low quality).

References

1. Van Asch C, Luitse MA, Rinkel GE, van der Tweel I, Klijn CM. Incidence, case fatality, and functional outcome of intracerebral haemorrhage over time, according to age, sex, and ethnic origin: a systematic review and meta-analysis. Lancet Neurol. 2010;9:167–76.
2. Morgenstern LB, Hemphill JC, Anderson C, et al. Guidelines for the management of spontaneous intracerebral hemorrhage: a guideline for healthcare professionals from the American Heart Association/American Stroke Association. Stroke. 2010;41:2108–29.
3. Dennis MS. Outcome after brain haemorrhage. Cerebrovasc Dis. 2003;16(Suppl 1):9–13.
4. Qureshi AI, Tuhrim S, Broderick JP, Batjer HH, Hondo H, Hanley DF. Spontaneous intracerebral hemorrhage. N Engl J Med. 2001;344:1450–60.

5. Gregory PC, Kuhlemeier KV. Prevalence of venous thromboembolism in acute hemorrhagic and thromboembolic stroke. Am J Phys Med Rehabil. 2003;82:364–9.
6. Amin AN, Lin J, Thompson S, Wiederkehr D. Rate of deep-vein thrombosis and pulmonary embolism during the care continuum in patients with acute ischemic stroke in the United States. BMC Neurol. 2013;13:17.
7. CLOTS Trials Collaboration, Dennis M, Sandercock PA, Reid J, et al. Effectiveness of thigh-length graduated compression stockings to reduce the risk of deep vein thrombosis after stroke (CLOTS trial 1): a multicentre, randomised controlled trial. Lancet. 2009;373:1958–65.
8. Pongmoragot J, Rabinstein AA, Nilanont Y, Swartz RH, Zhou L, Saposnik G. Pulmonary embolism in ischemic stroke: clinical presentation, risk factors, and outcome. J Am Heart Assoc. 2013;2:e000372.
9. Skaf E, Stein PD, Beemath A, Sanchez J, Bustamante MA, Olson RE. Venous thromboembolism in patients with ischemic and hemorrhagic stroke. Am J Cardiol. 2005;96:1731–3.
10. Warlow C, Ogston D, Douglas AS. Deep venous thrombosis of legs after strokes: part I – incidence and predisposing factors. Part II – natural history. Br Med J. 1976:1178–83.
11. Browd SR, Ragel BT, Davis GE, Scott AM, Skalabrin EJ, Couldwell WT. Prophylaxis for deep venous thrombosis in neurosurgery: a review of the literature. Neurosurg Focus. 2004;17:E1.
12. Khaldi A, Helo N, Schneck MJ, Origitano TC. Venous thromboembolism: deep venous thrombosis and pulmonary embolism in a neurosurgical population. J Neurosurg. 2011;114:40–6.
13. Andre` C, De Freitas GR, Fukujima MM. Prevention of deep venous thrombosis and pulmonary embolism following stroke: a systematic review of published articles. Eur J Neurol. 2007;14:21–32.
14. Albers GW, Amarenco P, Easton JD, Sacco RL, Teal P. Antithrombotic and thrombolytic therapy for ischemic stroke: American College of Chest Physicians Evidence-Based Clinical Practice Guidelines (8th edition). Chest. 2008;133:630S–69S.
15. Kappelle LJ. Preventing deep vein thrombosis after stroke: strategies and recommendations. Curr Treat Options Neurol. 2011;13:629–35.
16. Mayer SA, Brun NC, Begtrup K, et al. Efficacy and safety of recombinant activated factor VII for acute intracerebral hemorrhage. N Engl J Med. 2008;358:2127–37.
17. Kawase K, Okazaki S, Toyoda K, et al. Sex difference in the prevalence of deep-vein thrombosis in Japanese patients with acute intracerebral hemorrhage. Cerebrovasc Dis. 2009;27:313–9.
18. Ogata T, Yasaka M, Wakugawa Y, Inoue T, Ibayashi S, Okada Y. Deep venous thrombosis after acute intracerebral hemorrhage. J Neurol Sci. 2008;272:83–8.
19. Wijdicks EF, Scott JP. Pulmonary embolism associated with acute stroke. Mayo Clin Proc. 1997;72:297–300.
20. Agnelli G, Becattini C. Acute pulmonary embolism. N Engl J Med. 2010;363:266–74.
21. Goldstein JN, Fazen LE, Wendell L, et al. Risk of thromboembolism following intracerebral hemorrhage. Neurocrit Care. 2009;10:28–34.
22. Kim KS, Brophy GM. Symptomatc venous thromboembolism: incidence and risk factors in patients with spontaneous or traumatic intracranial hemorrhage. Neurocrit Care. 2009;11:28–33.
23. Barbar S, Noventa F, Rossetto V, et al. A risk assessment model for the identification of hospitalized medical patients at risk for venous thromboembolism: the Padua prediction score. J Thromb Haemost. 2010;8:2450–7.
24. Rogers SO Jr, Kilaru RK, Hosokawa P, Henderson WG, Zinner MJ, Khuri SF. Multivariable predictors of postoperative venous thromboembolic events after general and vascular surgery: results from the patient safety in surgery study. J Am Coll Surg. 2007;204:1211–21.
25. Caprini JA. Thrombosis risk assessment as a guide to quality patient care. Dis Mon. 2005;51:70–8.
26. Laryea J, Champagne B. Venous thromboembolism prophylaxis. Clin Colon Rectal Surg. 2013;26:153–9.

27. Hemphill JC 3rd, Greenberg SM, Anderson CS, et al. Guidelines for the management of spontaneous intracerebral hemorrhage: a guideline for healthcare professionals from the American Heart Association/American Stroke Association. Stroke. 2015;46:2032–60.
28. Dentali F, Marchesi C, Pierfranceschi MG, et al. Safety of prothrombin complex concentrates for rapid anticoagulation reversal of vitamin K antagonists. A meta-analysis. Thromb Haemost. 2011;106:429–38.
29. Robinson MT, Rabinstein AA, Meschia JF, Freeman WD. Safety of recombinant activated factor VII in patients with warfarin associated hemorrhages of the central nervous system. Stroke. 2010;41:1459–63.
30. Davis SM, Broderick J, Hennerici M, et al. Hematoma growth is a determinant of mortality and poor outcome after intracerebral hemorrhage. Neurology. 2006;66:1175–81.
31. Brott T, Broderick J, Kothari R, et al. Early hemorrhage growth in patients with intracerebral hemorrhage. Stroke. 1997;28:1–5.
32. Broderick J, Connolly S, Feldmann E, et al. Guidelines for the management of spontaneous intracerebral hemorrhage in adults 2007 update: a guideline from the American Heart Association/ American Stroke Association Stroke Council, High Blood Pressure Research Council, and the Quality of Care and Outcomes in Research Interdisciplinary Working Group. Stroke. 2007;38:2001–23.
33. Prabhakaran S, Herbers P, Khoury J, et al. Is prophylactic anticoagulation for deep venous thrombosis common practice after intracerebral hemorrhage? Stroke. 2015;46:369–75.
34. Steiner T, Al-Shahi Salman R, Beer R, et al. European Stroke Organisation (ESO) guidelines for the management of spontaneous intracerebral hemorrhage. Int J Stroke. 2014;9: 840–55.
35. Shinohara Y, Yanagihara T, Abe K, et al. III. Intracerebral hemorrhage. J Stroke Cerebrovasc Dis. 2011;20:S74–99.
36. Qaseem A, Chou R, Humphrey LL, Starkey M, Shekelle P. Venous thromboembolism prophylaxis in hospitalized patients: a clinical practice guideline from the American College of Physicians. Ann Intern Med. 2011;155:625–32.
37. Lansberg MG, O'Donnell MJ, Khatri P, et al. Antithrombotic and thrombolytic therapy for ischemic stroke: antithrombotic therapy and prevention of thrombosis, 9th ed: American College of Chest Physicians Evidence-Based Clinical Practice Guidelines. Chest. 2012;141(2 Suppl):e601S–36S.
38. National Stroke Foundation. Clinical guidelines for stroke management 2010. http://strokefoundation.com.au/health-professionals/tools-andresources/ clinical-guidelines-for-stroke-prevention-and-management/
39. National Institute for Health and Care Excellence (NICE). Reducing the risk of VTE (deep vein thrombosis and pulmonary embolism) in patients admitted to hospital. http://guidance.nice.org.uk/CG92
40. Nyquist P, Bautista C, Jichici D, et al. Prophylaxis of venous thrombosis in neurocritical care patients: an evidence-based guideline: a statement for healthcare professionals from the Neurocritical Care Society. Neurocrit Care. 2016;24:47–60.
41. Sabri S, Roberts VC, Cotton LT. Prevention of early postoperative deep vein thrombosis by intermittent compression of the leg during surgery. Br Med J. 1971;4:394–6.
42. Hills NH, Pflug JJ, Jeyasingh K, Boardman L, Calnan JS. Prevention of deep vein thrombosis by intermittent pneumatic compression of calf. Br Med J. 1972;1:131–5.
43. Roberts VC, Cotton LT. Prevention of postoperative deep vein thrombosis in patients with malignant disease. Br Med J. 1974;1:358–60.
44. Turpie AG, Gallus A, Beattie WS, Hirsh J. Prevention of venous thrombosis in patients with intracranial disease by intermittent pneumatic compression of the calf. Neurology. 1977;27:435–8.
45. Skillman JJ, Collins RE, Coe NP, et al. Prevention of deep vein thrombosis in neurosurgical patients: a controlled, randomized trial of external pneumatic compression boots. Surgery. 1978;83:354–8.

46. Kamran SI, Downey D, Ruff RL. Pneumatic sequential compression reduces the risk of deep vein thrombosis in stroke patients. Neurology. 1998;50:1683–8.
47. Lacut K, Bressollette L, Le Gal G, et al. Prevention of venous thrombosis in patients with acute intracerebral hemorrhage. Neurology. 2005;65:865–9.
48. Dennis M, Sandercock P, Reid J, Graham C, Forbes J, Murray G, et al. Effectiveness of intermittent pneumatic compression in reduction of risk of deep vein thrombosis in patients who have had a stroke (CLOTS 3): a multicentre randomised controlled trial. Lancet. 2013;382:516–24.
49. Muir KW, Watt A, Baxter G, Grosset DG, Lees KR. Randomized trial of graded compression stockings for prevention of deep-vein thrombosis after acute stroke. QJM. 2000;93:359–64.
50. CLOTS (Clots in Legs Or sTockings after Stroke) Trial Collaboration. Thigh-length versus below-knee stockings for deep venous thrombosis prophylaxis after stroke: a randomized trial. Ann Intern Med. 2010;153:553–62.
51. Handley AJ, Emerson PA, Fleming PR. Heparin in the prevention of deep vein thrombosis after myocardial infarction. Br Med J. 1972;2:436–8.
52. Abraham-Inpijn L, Vreeken J. Effect of low-dose heparin on incidence of postoperative thrombosis in orthopaedic patients. Arch Chir Neerl. 1975;27:63–8.
53. Sagar S, Nairn D, Stamatakis JD, et al. Efficacy of low-dose heparin in prevention of extensive deep-vein thrombosis in patients undergoing total-hip replacement. Lancet. 1976;1:1151–4.
54. Kutnowski M, Vandendris M, Steinberger R, Kraytman M. Prevention of postoperative deep-vein thrombosis by low-dose heparin in urological surgery. A double-blind, randomised study. Urol Res. 1977;5:123–5.
55. Dechavanne M, Ville D, Viala JJ, et al. Controlled trial of platelet anti-aggregating agents and subcutaneous heparin in prevention of postoperative deep vein thrombosis in high risk patients. Haemostasis. 1975;4:94–100.
56. Gallus AS, Hirsh J, O'Brien SE, McBride JA, Tuttle RJ, Gent M. Prevention of venous thrombosis with small, subcutaneous doses of heparin. JAMA. 1976;235:1980–2.
57. McCarthy ST, Turner JJ, Robertson D, Hawkey CJ, Macey DJ. Low-dose heparin as a prophylaxis against deep-vein thrombosis after acute stroke. Lancet. 1977;2:800–1.
58. McCarthy ST, Turner J. Low-dose subcutaneous heparin in the prevention of deep-vein thrombosis and pulmonary emboli following acute stroke. Age Ageing. 1986;15:84–8.
59. Turpie AG, Levine MN, Hirsh J, et al. Double-blind randomised trial of Org 10172 low-molecular-weight heparinoid in prevention of deep-vein thrombosis in thrombotic stroke. Lancet. 1987;1:523–6.
60. Prins MH, Gelsema R, Sing AK, van Heerde LR, den Ottolander GJ. Prophylaxis of deep venous thrombosis with a low-molecular-weight heparin (Kabi 2165/Fragmin) in stroke patients. Haemostasis. 1989;19:245–50.
61. Turpie AG, Gent M, Côte R, et al. A low-molecular-weight heparinoid compared with unfractionated heparin in the prevention of deep vein thrombosis in patients with acute ischemic stroke. A randomized, double-blind study. Ann Intern Med. 1992;117:353–7.
62. Diener HC, Ringelstein EB, von Kummer R, et al. Prophylaxis of thrombotic and embolic events in acute ischemic stroke with the low-molecular-weight heparin certoparin: results of the PROTECT trial. Stroke. 2006;37:139–44.
63. Sherman DG, Albers GW, Bladin C, et al. The efficacy and safety of enoxaparin versus unfractionated heparin for the prevention of venous thromboembolism after acute ischaemic stroke (PREVAIL study): an open-label randomised comparison. Lancet. 2007;369:1347–55.
64. Harvey RL, Lovell LL, Belanger N, Roth EJ. The effectiveness of anticoagulant and antiplatelet agents in preventing venous thromboembolism during stroke rehabilitation: a historical cohort study. Arch Phys Med Rehabil. 2004;85:1070–5.
65. Dickmann U, Voth E, Schicha H, Henze T, Prange H, Emrich D. Heparin therapy, deep-vein thrombosis and pulmonary embolism after intracerebral hemorrhage. Klin Wochenschr. 1988;66:1182–3.

66. Boeer A, Voth E, Henze T, Prange HW. Early heparin therapy in patients with spontaneous intracerebral haemorrhage. J Neurol Neurosurg Psychiatry. 1991;54:466–7.
67. Goldstein JN, Fazen LE, Wendell L, et al. Risk of thromboembolism following acute intracerebral hemorrhage. Neurocrit Care. 2009;10:28–34.
68. Kleindienst A, Harvey HB, Mater E, et al. Early antithrombotic prophylaxis with low molecular weight heparin in neurosurgery. Acta Neurochir. 2003;145:1085–90.
69. Tetri S, Hakala J, Juvela S, et al. Safety of low-dose subcutaneous enoxaparin for the prevention of venous thromboembolism after primary intracerebral haemorrhage. Thromb Res. 2008;123:206–12.
70. Wasay M, Khan S, Zaki KS, Khealani BA, Kamal A, Azam I, et al. A non-randomized study of safety and efficacy of heparin for DVT prophylaxis in intracerebral haemorrhage. J Pak Med Assoc. 2008;58:362–4.
71. Orken DN, Kenangil G, Ozkurt H, et al. Prevention of deep venous thrombosis and pulmonary embolism in patients with acute intracerebral hemorrhage. Neurologist. 2009;15:329–31.
72. Kiphuth IC, Staykov D, Köhrmann M, et al. Early administration of low molecular weight heparin after spontaneous intracerebral hemorrhage. A safety analysis. Cerebrovasc Dis. 2009;27:146–50.
73. Wu TC, Kasam M, Harun N, et al. Pharmacological deep vein thrombosis prophylaxis does not lead to hematoma expansion in intracerebral hemorrhage with intraventricular extension. Stroke. 2011;42:705–59.
74. Paciaroni M, Agnelli G, Venti M, Alberti A, Acciarresi M, Caso V. Efficacy and safety of anticoagulants in the prevention of venous thromboembolism in patients with acutecerebral hemorrhage: a meta-analysis of controlled studies. J Thromb Haemost. 2011;9:893–8.
75. Kelly J, Hunt BJ, Lewis RR, et al. Dehydration and venous thromboembolism after acute stroke. QJM. 2004;97:293–6.
76. Jauch EC, Saver JL, Adams HP Jr, American Heart Association Stroke Council, Council on Cardiovascular Nursing, Council on Peripheral Vascular Disease, et al. Guidelines for the early management of patients with acute ischemic stroke: a guideline for healthcare professionals from the American Heart Association/American Stroke Association. Stroke. 2013;44:870–947.
77. Govan L, Langhorne P, Weir CJ. Does the prevention of complications explain the survival benefi t of organized inpatient (stroke unit) care?: further analysis of a systematic review. Stroke. 2007;38:2536–40.
78. Allen C, Glasziou P, del Mar C. Bed rest: a potentially harmful treatment needing more careful evaluation. Lancet. 1999;354:1229–33.
79. Murphy TH, Corbett D. Plasticity during stroke recovery: from synapse to behaviour. Nat Rev Neurosci. 2009;10:861–72.
80. Lynch E, Hillier S, Cadilhac D. When should physical rehabilitation commence after stroke: a systematic review. Int J Stroke. 2014;9:468–78.
81. Sundseth A, Thommessen B, Rønning OM. Early mobilization after acute stroke. J Stroke Cerebrovasc Dis. 2014;23:496–9.
82. Bernhardt J, Langhorne P, Lindley RI, et al. Efficacy and safety of very early mobilisation within 24 h of stroke onset (AVERT): a randomised controlled trial. Lancet. 2015;386:46–55.
83. Palareti G, Schellong S. Isolated distal deep vein thrombosis: what we know and what we are doing. J Thromb Haemost. 2012;10:11–9.
84. Johnson SA, Stevens SM, Woller SC, et al. Risk of deep vein thrombosis following a single negative whole-leg compression ultrasound: a systematic review and meta-analysis. JAMA. 2010;303:438–45.
85. Limbrey R, Howard L. Developments in the management and treatment of pulmonary embolism. Eur Respir Rev. 2015;24:484–97.
86. Hendriksen JM, Geersing GJ, Lucassen WA, et al. Diagnostic prediction models for suspected pulmonary embolism: systematic review and independent external validation in primary care. BMJ. 2015;351:h4438.

87. Wells PS, Hirsh J, Anderson DR, et al. Accuracy of clinical assessment of deep-vein thrombosis. Lancet. 1995;345:1326–30.
88. Wells PS, Anderson DR, Rodger M, et al. Excluding pulmonary embolism at the bedside without diagnostic imaging: management of patients with suspected pulmonary embolism presenting to the emergency department by using a simple clinical model and d-dimer. Ann Intern Med. 2001;135:98–107.
89. Kong XL, Zhang X, Zhang SJ, Zhang L. Plasma level of D-dimer is an independent diagnostic biomarker for deep venous thrombosis in patients with ischemic stroke. Curr Neurovasc Res. 2016;13:100–6.
90. Kelly J, Hunt BJ, Lewis RR, Rudd A. Anticoagulation or inferior vena cava filter placement for patients with primary intracerebral hemorrhage developing venous thromboembolism? Stroke. 2003;34:2999–3005.
91. Nieto JA, Bruscas MJ, Ruiz-Ribo D, RIETE Investigators, et al. Acute venous thromboembolism in patients with recent major bleeding. The influence of the site of bleeding and the time elapsed on outcome. J Thromb Haemost. 2006;4:2367–72.
92. Hyers TM, Agnelli G, Hull RD. Antithrombotic therapy for venous thromboembolic disease. Chest. 1998;114(suppl):561S–78S.
93. Mismetti P, Laporte S, Pellerin O, PREPIC2 Study Group, et al. Effect of a retrievable inferior vena cava filter plus anticoagulation vs anticoagulation alone on risk of recurrent pulmonary embolism: a randomized clinical trial. JAMA. 2015;313:1627–35.
94. Decousus H, Leizorovicz A, Parent F, et al. A clinical trial of vena caval filters in the prevention of pulmonary embolism in patients with proximal deep-vein thrombosis. N Engl J Med. 1998;338:409–15.
95. Sung CY, Chu NS. Epileptic seizures in intracerebral haemorrhage. J Neurol Neurosurg Psychiatry. 1989;52:1273–6.
96. Labovitz DL, Hauser WA, Sacco RL. Prevalence and predictors of early seizure and status epilepticus after first stroke. Neurology. 2001;57:200–6.
97. Weisberg LA, Shamsnia M, Elliott D. Seizures caused by nontraumatic parenchymal brain hemorrhages. Neurology. 1991;41:1197–9.
98. Berger AR, Lipton RB, Lesser ML, Lantos G, Portenoy RK. Early seizures following intracerebral hemorrhage: implications for therapy. Neurology. 1988;38:1363–5.
99. Neshige S, Kuriyama M, Yoshimoto T, et al. Seizures after intracerebral hemorrhage; risk factor, recurrence, efficacy of antiepileptic drug. J Neurol Sci. 2015;359:318–22.
100. Mullen MT, Kasner SE, Messé SR. Seizures do not increase in-hospital mortality after intracerebral hemorrhage in the nationwide inpatient sample. Neurocrit Care. 2013;19:19–24.
101. Passero S, Rocchi R, Rossi S, Ulivelli M, Vatti G. Seizures after spontaneous supratentorial intracerebral hemorrhage. Epilepsia. 2002;43:1175–80.
102. De Herdt V, Dumont F, Hénon H, et al. Early seizures in intracerebral hemorrhage: incidence, associated factors, and outcome. Neurology. 2011;77:1794–800.
103. Srinivasan S, Shin H, Chou SH, Pennell PB, Dworetzky BA, Lee JW. Seizures and antiepileptic drugs in patients with spontaneous intracerebral hemorrhages. Seizure. 2013;22:512–6.
104. Arntz R, Rutten-Jacobs L, Maaijwee N, et al. Post-stroke epilepsy in young adults: a long-term follow-up study. PLoS One. 2013;8:e55498.
105. Burn J, Dennis M, Bamford J, Sandercock P, Wade D, Warlow C. Epileptic seizures after a first stroke: the Oxfordshire community stroke project. BMJ. 1997;315:1582–7.
106. Faught E, Peters D, Bartolucci A, Moore L, Miller PC. Seizures after primary intracerebral hemorrhage. Neurology. 1989;39:1089–93.
107. Claassen J, Jetté N, Chum F, Green R, et al. Electrographic seizures and periodic discharges after intracerebral hemorrhage. Neurology. 2007;69:1356–65.
108. Vespa PM, O'Phelan K, Shah M, et al. Acute seizures after intracerebral hemorrhage: a factor in progressive midline shift and outcome. Neurology. 2003;60:1441–6.
109. De Reuck J, Hemelsoet D, Van Maele G. Seizures and epilepsy in patients with a spontaneous intracerebral haematoma. Clin Neurol Neurosurg. 2007;109:501–14.

110. Jensen MB, Sattar A, Al Sherbini K. Survey of prophylactic antiseizure drug use for non-traumatic intracerebral hemorrhage. Neurol Res. 2013;35:984–7.
111. Szaflarski JP, Rackley AY, Kleindorfer DO, et al. Incidence of seizures in the acute phase of stroke: a population-based study. Epilepsia. 2008;49:974–81.
112. Burneo JG, Fang J, Saposnik G, Investigators of the Registry of the Canadian Stroke Network. Impact of seizures on morbidity and mortality after stroke: a Canadian multi-centre cohort study. Eur J Neurol. 2010;17:52–8.
113. Sheth KN, Martini SR, Moomaw CJ, et al. Prophylactic antiepileptic drug use and outcome in the ethnic/racial variations of intracerebral hemorrhage study. Stroke. 2015;46:3532–5.
114. Sykes L, Wood E, Kwan J. Antiepileptic drugs for the primary and secondary prevention of seizures after stroke. Cochrane Database Syst Rev. 2014:CD005398.
115. Gilad R, Boaz M, Dabby R, Sadeh M, Lampl Y. Are post intracerebral hemorrhage seizures prevented by anti-epileptic treatment? Epilepsy Res. 2011;95:227–31.
116. Reddig RT, Nixdorf KE, Jensen MB. The prophylactic use of an antiepileptic drug in intracerebral hemorrhage. Clin Neurol Neurosurg. 2011;113:895–7.
117. Woo KM, Yang SY, Cho KT. Seizures after spontaneous intracerebral hemorrhage. J Korean Neurosurg Soc. 2012;52:312–9.
118. Messé SR, Sansing LH, Cucchiara BL, Herman ST, Lyden PD, Kasner SE, et al. Prophylactic antiepileptic drug use is associated with poor outcome following ICH. Neurocrit Care. 2009;11:38–44.
119. Naidech AM, Garg RK, Liebling S, et al. Anticonvulsant use and outcomes after intracerebral hemorrhage. Stroke. 2009;40:3810–5.
120. Lodder J, van Raak L, Hilton A, Hardy E, Kessels A, EGASIS Study Group. Diazepam to improve acute stroke outcome: results of the early GABA-Ergic activation study in stroke trial. A randomized double-blind placebo-controlled trial. Cerebrovasc Dis. 2006;21:120–7.
121. Hu X, Fang Y, Li H. Protocol for seizure prophylaxis following intracerebral hemorrhage study (SPICH): a randomized, double-blind, placebo-controlled trial of short-term sodium valproate prophylaxis in patients with acute spontaneous supratentorial intracerebral hemorrhage. Int J Stroke. 2014;9:814–7.
122. Hemphill JC 3rd, Bonovich DC, Besmertis L, Manley GT, Johnston SC. The ICH score: a simple, reliable grading scale for intracerebral hemorrhage. Stroke. 2001;32:891–7.
123. Zandieh A, Messé SR, Cucchiara B, Mullen MT, Kasner SE, VISTA-ICH Collaborators. Prophylactic use of antiepileptic drugs in patients with spontaneous intracerebral hemorrhage. J Stroke Cerebrovasc Dis. 2016. pii: S1052-3057(16)30099-4.
124. Battey TW, Falcone GJ, Ayres AM, et al. Confounding by indication in retrospective studies of intracerebral hemorrhage: antiepileptic treatment and mortality. Neurocrit Care. 2012;17:361–6.
125. Gilmore E, Choi HA, Hirsch LJ, Claassen J. Seizures and CNS hemorrhage: spontaneous intracerebral and aneurysmal subarachnoid hemorrhage. Neurologist. 2010;16:165–75.
126. Dewolfe JL, Szaflarski JP. Levetiracetam use in the critical care setting. Front Neurol. 2013;4:121.
127. Belcastro V, Costa C, Galletti F, et al. Levetiracetam in newly diagnosed late-onset post-stroke seizures: a prospective observational study. Epilepsy Res. 2008;82:223–6.
128. Kutlu G, Gomceli YB, Unal Y, Inan LE. Levetiracetam monotherapy for late poststroke seizures in the elderly. Epilepsy Behav. 2008;13:542–4.
129. Taylor S, Heinrichs RJ, Janzen JM, Ehtisham A. Levetiracetam is associated with improved cognitive outcome for patients with intracranial hemorrhage. Neurocrit Care. 2011;15:80–4.
130. Brophy GM, Bell R, Claassen J, et al. Neurocritical Care Society Status Epilepticus Guideline Writing Committee. Guidelines for the evaluation and management of status epilepticus. Neurocrit Care. 2012;17:3–23.

Chapter 6
Surgical Treatment of Intracerebral Hemorrhage

Jan Vargas, Alejandro M. Spiotta, and Raymond D. Turner

Spontaneous Intracerebral Hemorrhage

Background and Demographics

Spontaneous intracerebral hemorrhage (ICH) is responsible for 10–15% of strokes, with an annual incidence of 10–30 per 100,000 and a 1-year mortality rate of more than 40% and a 5-year mortality rate of approximately 29.2% [1, 2]. When associated with intraventricular hemorrhage (IVH), the mortality rate increases to 50–80% [3–5]. Functional independent outcome (defined as an mRS of 0–2) is estimated at 16.7–24.6% at 1 year following ICH [1]. The long-term rate of recurrence is estimated to be 1.3–7.4% per year over an average follow-up of 1–7 years.

ICHs can be divided into supratentorial and infratentorial based on location, with considerable controversy concerning outcomes in patients with primary supratentorial ICH compared to infratentorial ICH.

Craniotomy for Supratentorial Intracranial Hemorrhages

Most ICHs are supratentorial, and spontaneous supratentorial ICH can be further subdivided into deep and superficial. Risk factors for mortality in the setting of ICH are increasing age, decreasing Glasgow Coma Scale score, increasing ICH volume, and presence of intraventricular hemorrhage [1]. The most recent guidelines for the management of spontaneous ICH suggest considering a standard craniotomy for

J. Vargas · A. M. Spiotta (✉) · R. D. Turner
Department of Neurosurgery, Medical University of South Carolina, Charleston, SC, USA
e-mail: spiotta@musc.edu

B. Ovbiagele, A. I. Qureshi (eds.), *Intracerebral Hemorrhage Therapeutics*,
https://doi.org/10.1007/978-3-319-77063-5_6

patients with supratentorial lobar hemorrhages within 1 cm of the cortical surface, with the goal being to prevent impending mortality [2].

For patients that do not meet these criteria, there is a lack of consensus on appropriate treatment despite the theoretical benefits of early hematoma evacuation and prevention of secondary insults following spontaneous ICH. The Surgical Trial in Traumatic Intracerebral Hemorrhage (STITCH) trial was a multicenter, randomized investigation that ultimately failed to show any overall benefit to early surgery versus medical management for patients with spontaneous, supratentorial ICH, with favorable outcomes observed in 26% of the surgical group compared to 24% in the medical group [6]. However, a subgroup analysis of the STITCH I data suggested that favorable outcomes were more likely with surgery performed on hematomas less than 1 cm from the cortical surface [7]. These findings lead to the STITCH II trial, which demonstrated similar results and did not show a benefit for the surgical evacuation of superficial lobar hemorrhages [8]. A subsequent meta-analysis of 14 trials of surgery for intracerebral hemorrhage demonstrated improved outcomes with surgery if randomization was performed within 8 h of hemorrhage, if the volume of hematoma was between 20 and 50 mL with a Glasgow Coma Scale of 9–12, or if patient age was between 50 and 69 years [9]. When the results of STITCH II were pooled with this data, the subgroup of patients with lobar intracranial hemorrhage and no IVH demonstrated a trend toward benefit with surgery, but this trend was not significant [8].

The STITCH trials suggested that while surgery may improve outcomes in some patients with superficial lobar hemorrhages, attempts at targeting deeper lesions may disrupt viable tissue and overcome any benefits yielded by hematoma removal. This has led to an interest in developing minimally invasive approaches for accessing and evacuating deep-seated hematomas.

Surgery for Infratentorial Intracranial Hemorrhages

The most recent guidelines for the management of spontaneous ICH published by the American Stroke Association in 2015 recommend immediate surgery for cerebellar hemorrhages with evidence of brainstem compression or hydrocephalus [2]. Despite lack of high-quality evidence, there is data to suggest that suboccipital decompressive craniectomy can reduce mortality when compared to medical therapy alone [10, 11]. These studies advocate for early decompression despite a low GCS in the setting of IVH and fourth ventricular obstruction, on the basis that non-surgical intervention carries with it a high mortality.

Craniectomy for Spontaneous Intracranial Hemorrhage

The neurological injury caused by spontaneous intracranial hemorrhage is felt to be not only due to the immediate mechanical disruption caused by the original hemorrhage but also from the accumulation of perihematoma edema (PHE) secondary to an inflammatory reaction incited by hemoglobin breakdown products such as iron, and the presence of thrombin. Additionally, there is some evidence that local mass effect limits regional perfusion, causing further secondary ischemic injury. This delayed, second phase of injury results in the extension of damage to potentially viable tissue [5, 12–18]. As a result, several studies have postulated that the addition of a decompressive craniectomy to hematoma evacuation can decrease ICP and increase cerebral blood perfusion, thus mitigating some of the delayed secondary injury and decreasing the morbidity and mortality [19–21]. There is limited evidence that hemicraniectomy can improve survival and recovery in patients with aneurysmal and spontaneous intracerebral hemorrhages [22–24].

A recent prospective controlled trial involving 40 patients with hypertensive ICHs randomized to hematoma evacuation with decompressive craniectomy with expansile duroplasty versus hematoma evacuation only found that adding decompressive craniectomy and duroplasty improved outcomes at 6 months (Fig. 6.1) [25]. In this study, patients with a hematoma volume of at least 60 ml and a GCS of 8 or less were included or if neurological deterioration resulted in surgical evacuation. The authors report that at 6 months, 70% of patients who underwent decompressive craniectomy and expansile duroplasty had a favorable outcome (mRS of 3 or less), compared to 20% in the hematoma-only group, a statistically significant difference. As a result of these data, the most recent American Stroke Association guidelines from 2015 state that craniectomy with or without hematoma evacuation might reduce mortality for patients with supratentorial ICH who are in a coma, have large hematomas with significant midline shift, or have elevated ICP refractory to medical management [2].

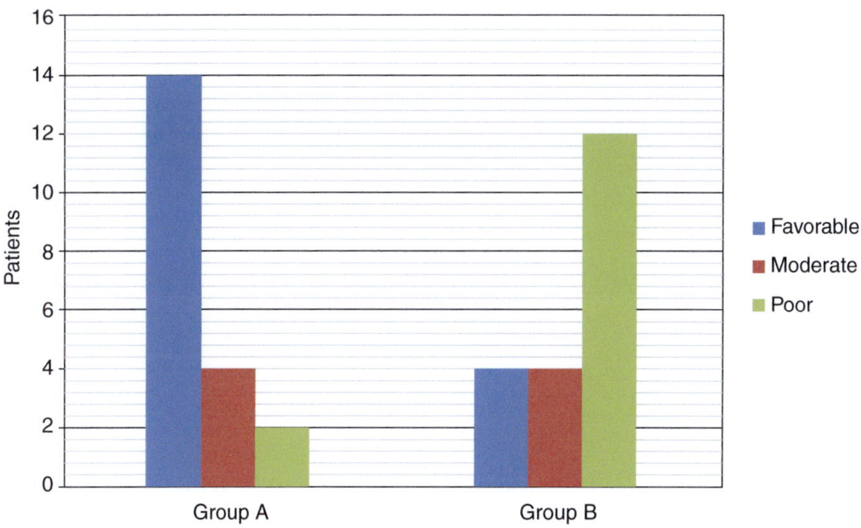

Fig. 6.1 Adapted from Moussa and Kheder, 2017. Group A received decompressive craniectomy and expansile duroplasty in addition to hematoma evacuation, whereas Group B only underwent hematoma evacuation. (From Moussa and Khedr [25], with permission of Springer)

Minimally Invasive Surgery for Spontaneous Intracranial Hemorrhage

History

A minimally invasive approach to the evacuation of intracranial hematomas has been a topic of interest for some time. In 1989, Auer et al. published their experiences in with early endoscopic irrigation and aspiration-based evacuation of ICH. This trial demonstrated a significant improvement in a 6-month mortality rate when compared to medical management [26].

There are several reports of the use of stereotactic minimally invasive techniques such as direct aspiration or mechanical clot disruption to safely remove deeper hemorrhages [26–30]. More recently, newer methods for hematoma disruption have been introduced, such as ultrasound or injection of recombinant tissue plasminogen activator directly into the hematoma [31, 32].

CLEAR Trials

The Clot Lysis Evaluating Accelerated Resolution of IVH Phase II (CLEAR II) trial aimed to investigate the benefit of clearing intraventricular blood in the setting of spontaneous ICH or subarachnoid hemorrhage [33]. IVH has been shown to be an independent risk factor for poor outcome and occurs in about 40–45% of ICH [7, 34, 35]. The patients who received intraventricular rtPA via an external ventricular drain showed a trend toward lower mortality at 30 days (18% vs. 23% in placebo groups); however this was not statistically significant. There was a significant relationship observed with respect to the rate of clot resolution and clinical improvement at 96 h. In addition, a greater percentage of patients treated with intraventricular tPA demonstrated mRS ≤ 4 (52% vs. 27%) and NIHSS <10 (54% vs. 29%) at 30 days. While the trial was not powered to assess functional outcomes, it demonstrated the safety of a minimally invasive approach to the treatment of IVH and paved the way for the launch of the CLEAR III trial.

MISTIE

The Minimally Invasive Surgery Plus Tissue-Type Plasminogen Activator for ICH Evacuation (MISTIE II) investigation was a controlled, phase II trial which included 123 patients randomized between medical management and minimally invasive

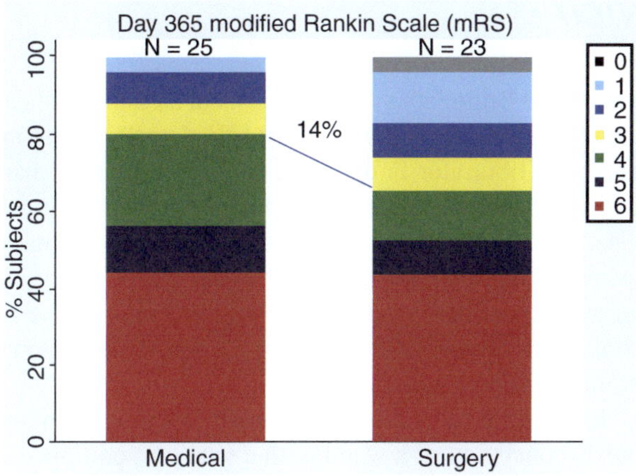

Fig. 6.2 The results of the MISTIE trial suggested improved outcomes and shorted hospital stay following minimally invasive catheter placement. Modified ranking shift at 1 year

surgery followed by catheter drainage with daily rtPA (recombinant tissue plasminogen activator) irrigation. The MISTIE II trial showed a strong trend toward clinical benefit in patients with ICH treated with minimally invasive surgery versus those which received medical management (Fig. 6.2). Surgical patients had a significant reduction in perihematoma edema volume, shorter hospital length of stay and reduced hospital costs, and greater gain activities of daily living scores on the Stroke Impact Scale [31].

New Techniques for MIS Evacuations

Apollo

The Penumbra Apollo (Penumbra Inc., Alameda CA) is an aspiration-irrigation system which allows the removal of hemorrhage via a wand with controlled aspiration. A vibrational element housed within the wand vibrates at high frequency to break down the hemorrhagic products inside of the wand and prevent clogging. The wand can be used in conjunction with commercially available endoscopes and is positioned in the hematoma under stereotactic guidance via a cranial burr hole with a small dural incision (Figs. 6.3, 6.4, 6.5, 6.6, and 6.7). Since its approval, the Apollo system has been used for the evacuation of both intraventricular and intracerebral hemorrhages, including those associated with ruptured aneurysms [36–39].

NICO

The NICO BrainPath system consists of a 13.5 mm sheath with an internal obturator that is placed stereotactically through a small craniotomy into intracranial hematomas. The obturator is designed to displace rather than disrupt brain parenchyma during placement, minimizing damage to underlying functional tissue. Once placed, the obturator is removed, allowing access to the hematoma which can be evacuated using conventional suction and bipolar cautery under the operating microscope or an exoscope which is aligned down the length of the BrainPath sheath. The NICO BrainPath sheath has been approved for visualization of the surgical field during brain and spinal surgery.

In addition to its BrainPath sheath, NICO also manufactures the Myriad handpiece, consisting of a wand with a side port equipped with a reciprocating cutting blade. The handpiece has an aspiration mechanism that pulls tissue into the side port. Using a foot pedal, the surgeon can both control the strength of aspiration

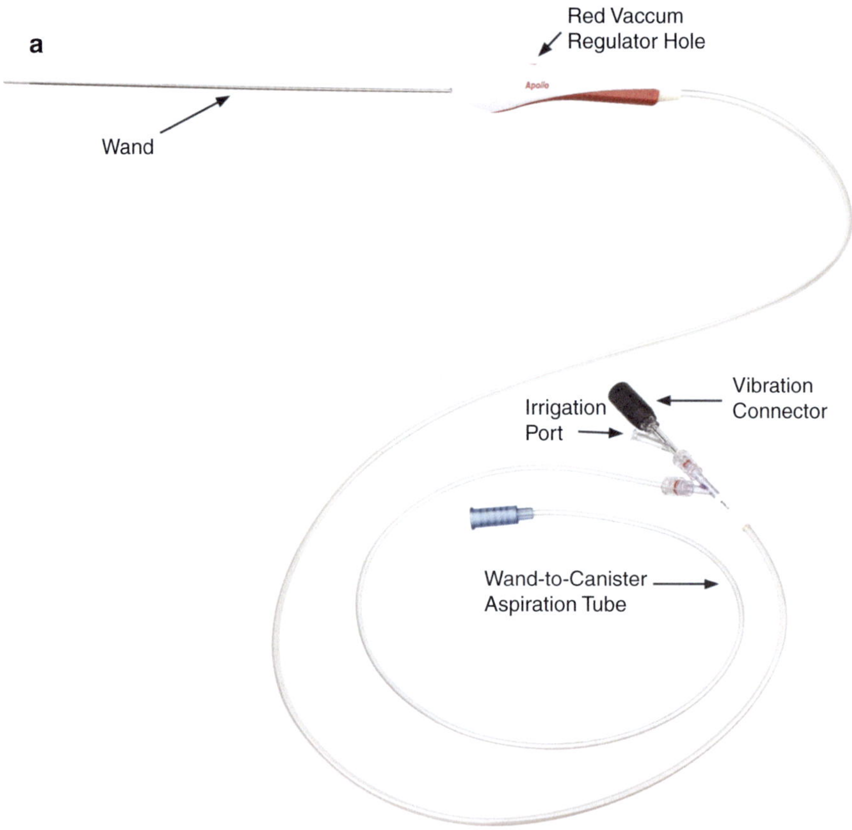

Fig. 6.3 (**a**) Apollo wand. (With permission of Penumbra, Inc.), (**b**) Apollo system. (With permission of Penumbra, Inc.)

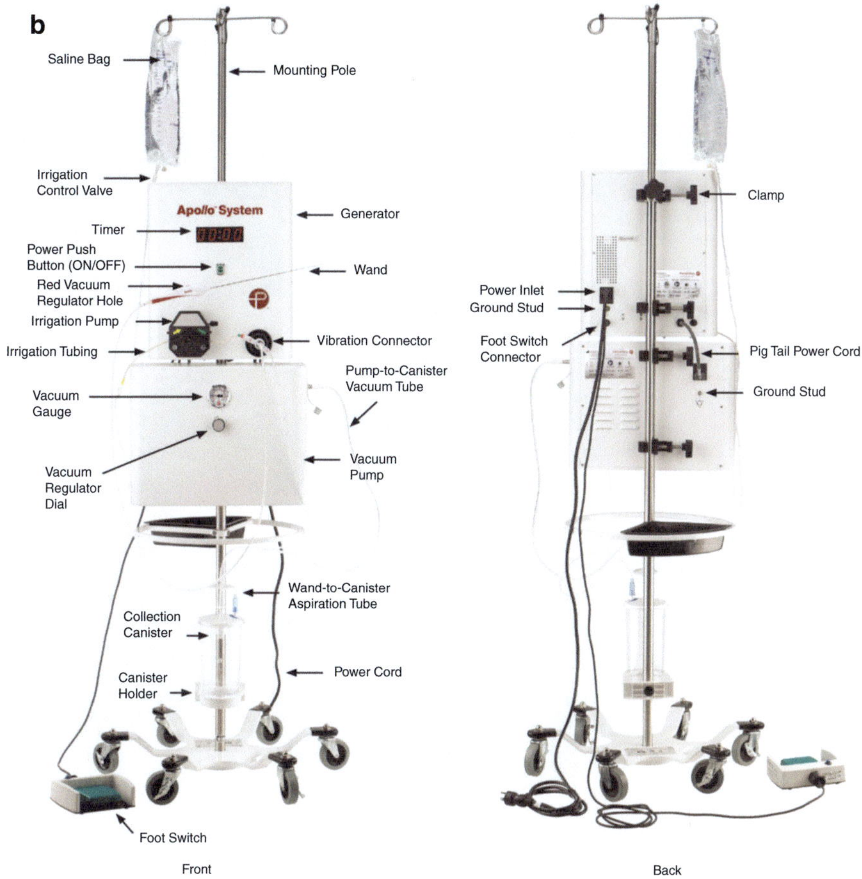

Fig. 6.3 (continued)

and turn the cutting blade on or off. The Myriad handpiece has been approved for the morcellation and removal of tissue during pelviscopic, laparoscopic, percutaneous, and open surgical procedures whenever access to the surgical site is limited.

The NICO BrainPath has been successfully used for the evacuation of intracerebral hematomas, with reported at least 87% reduction in hematoma volume, although 3 of the 11 patients (27%) suffered postoperative complications including a fatal hemorrhage [40, 41] (Fig. 6.8).

Upcoming Trials

The encouraging findings of recent case series have led to the development of several randomized controlled trials to investigate MIS techniques.

Fig. 6.4 Setup with endoscope

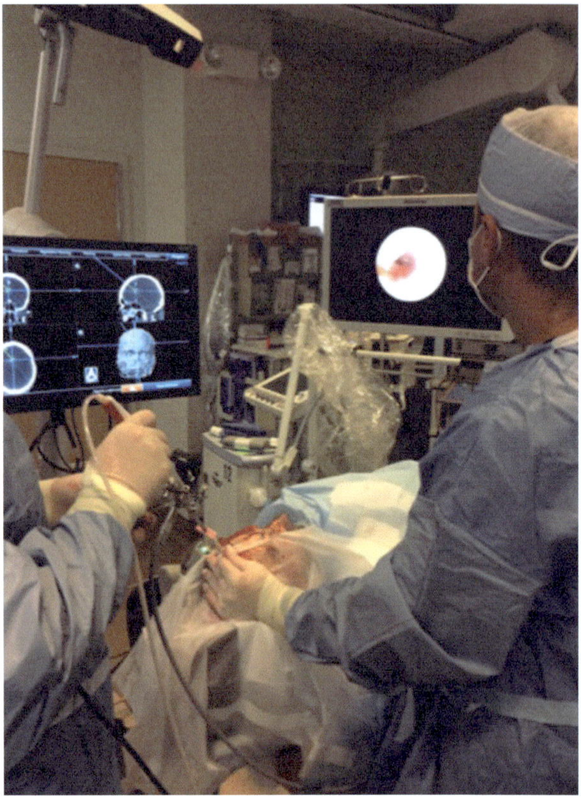

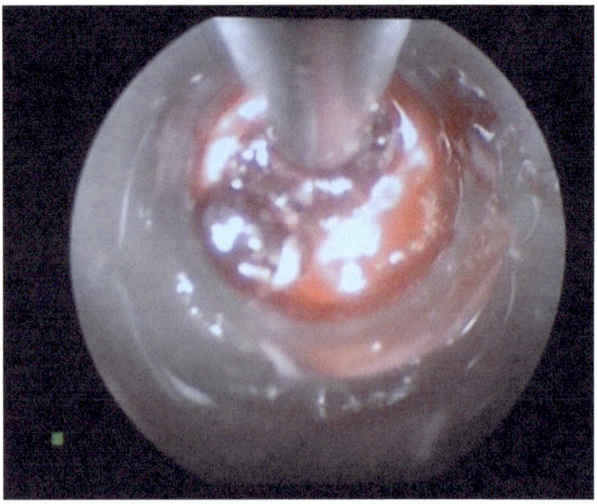

Fig. 6.5 Endoscopic view of hematoma and/or ICH evac cavity

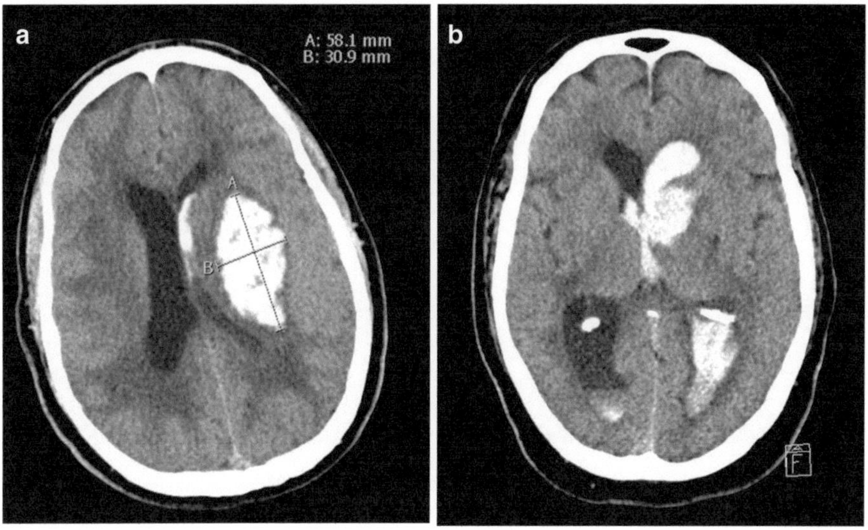

Fig. 6.6 (**a**, **b**) Pre-Apollo evac examples

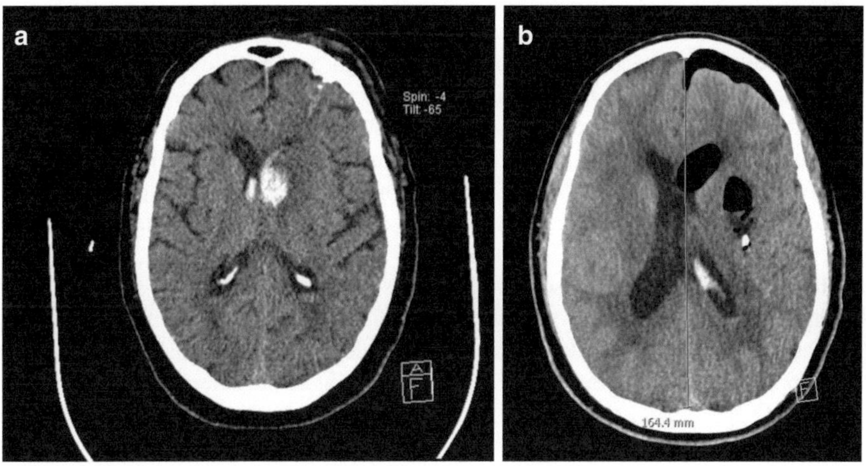

Fig. 6.7 (**a**, **b**) Post-Apollo evac samples

Minimally Invasive Endoscopic Surgical Treatment with Apollo Versus Medical Management for Supratentorial ICH (INVEST) trial is a phase II trial which will compare ICH evacuation using the Apollo system to medical management in 222 patients with moderate to large (30–80 cm^3) spontaneous supratentorial hemorrhages [42]. The NICO BrainPath system will also be part of a randomized controlled trial, which will include up to 10 centers.

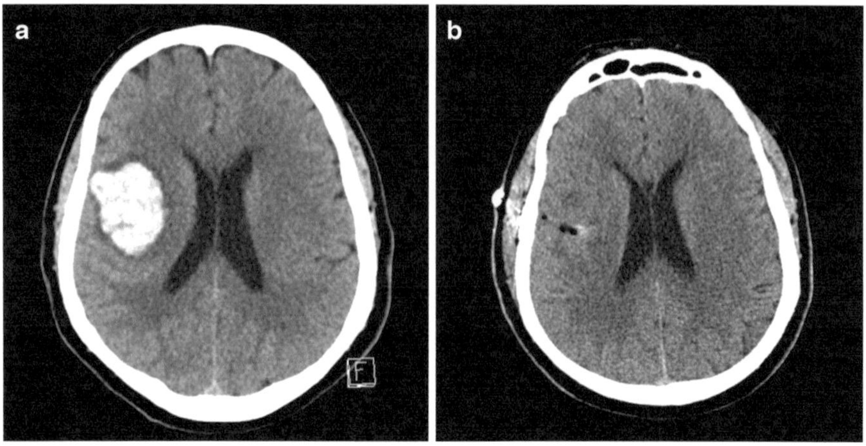

Fig. 6.8 (ICH pre and post MIS evacuation). (**a**) Large right ICH hemorrhage approaching the cortical surface. (**b**) Post-NICO evacuation of the hemorrhage

Timing of Surgery

The current American Stroke Association guidelines from 2015 do not have any recommendations regarding early evacuation versus waiting for a neurological decline, reflecting the significant controversy regarding the timing of surgery for spontaneous intracranial hemorrhage [2]. However, there is data suggesting that approximately 50% of deaths from spontaneous ICH occur within the first 48 h [43]. Although the STITCH I trial failed to demonstrate added benefit for early surgery, a subgroup analysis of STITCH II demonstrated that there may be a benefit of surgery if performed before 21 h of ictus [8]. Additionally, there is data suggesting that surgery within the first 12–24 h improves neurologic function [44, 45]. A meta-analysis performed by Gregson et al. suggested that operation on supratentorial spontaneous ICH within 8 h of ictus was beneficial with an OR of 0.59 [9].

Despite the lack of evidence, currently guidelines suggest that supratentorial hematoma evacuation in deteriorating patients might be considered as a life-saving measure [37].

References

1. Poon MT, Fonville AF, Al-Shahi Salman R. Long-term prognosis after intracerebral haemorrhage: systematic review and meta-analysis. J Neurol Neurosurg Psychiatry. 2014;85(6):660–7.
2. Hemphill JC 3rd, Greenberg SM, Anderson CS, Becker K, Bendok BR, Cushman M, et al. Guidelines for the management of spontaneous intracerebral hemorrhage: a guideline for healthcare professionals from the American Heart Association/American Stroke Association. Stroke. 2015;46(7):2032–60.
3. Dennis MS. Outcome after brain haemorrhage. Cerebrovasc Dis. 2003;16(Suppl 1):9–13.

4. Labovitz DL, Halim A, Boden-Albala B, Hauser WA, Sacco RL. The incidence of deep and lobar intracerebral hemorrhage in whites, blacks, and Hispanics. Neurology. 2005;65(4):518–22.
5. Qureshi AI, Mendelow AD, Hanley DF. Intracerebral haemorrhage. Lancet. 2009;373(9675):1632–44.
6. Mendelow AD, Gregson BA, Fernandes HM, Murray GD, Teasdale GM, Hope DT, et al. Early surgery versus initial conservative treatment in patients with spontaneous supratentorial intracerebral haematomas in the International Surgical Trial in Intracerebral Haemorrhage (STICH): a randomised trial. Lancet. 2005;365(9457):387–97.
7. Bhattathiri PS, Gregson B, Prasad KS, Mendelow AD, Investigators S. Intraventricular hemorrhage and hydrocephalus after spontaneous intracerebral hemorrhage: results from the STICH trial. Acta Neurochir Suppl. 2006;96:65–8.
8. Mendelow AD, Gregson BA, Rowan EN, Murray GD, Gholkar A, Mitchell PM, et al. Early surgery versus initial conservative treatment in patients with spontaneous supratentorial lobar intracerebral haematomas (STICH II): a randomised trial. Lancet. 2013;382(9890):397–408.
9. Gregson BA, Broderick JP, Auer LM, Batjer H, Chen XC, Juvela S, et al. Individual patient data subgroup meta-analysis of surgery for spontaneous supratentorial intracerebral hemorrhage. Stroke. 2012;43(6):1496–504.
10. Luney MS, English SW, Longworth A, Simpson J, Gudibande S, Matta B, et al. Acute posterior cranial fossa hemorrhage-is surgical decompression better than expectant medical management? Neurocrit Care. 2016;25(3):365–70.
11. Kirollos RW, Tyagi AK, Ross SA, van Hille PT, Marks PV. Management of spontaneous cerebellar hematomas: a prospective treatment protocol. Neurosurgery. 2001;49(6):1378–86; discussion 86-7
12. Xi G, Wagner KR, Keep RF, Hua Y, de Courten-Myers GM, Broderick JP, et al. Role of blood clot formation on early edema development after experimental intracerebral hemorrhage. Stroke. 1998;29(12):2580–6.
13. Lee KR, Kawai N, Kim S, Sagher O, Hoff JT. Mechanisms of edema formation after intracerebral hemorrhage: effects of thrombin on cerebral blood flow, blood-brain barrier permeability, and cell survival in a rat model. J Neurosurg. 1997;86(2):272–8.
14. Lee KR, Colon GP, Betz AL, Keep RF, Kim S, Hoff JT. Edema from intracerebral hemorrhage: the role of thrombin. J Neurosurg. 1996;84(1):91–6.
15. Wang G, Shao A, Hu W, Xue F, Zhao H, Jin X, et al. Changes of ferrous iron and its transporters after intracerebral hemorrhage in rats. Int J Clin Exp Pathol. 2015;8(9):10671–9.
16. Wang G, Hu W, Tang Q, Wang L, Sun XG, Chen Y, et al. Effect comparison of both iron chelators on outcomes, iron deposit, and iron transporters after intracerebral hemorrhage in rats. Mol Neurobiol. 2016;53(6):3576–85.
17. Qing WG, Dong YQ, Ping TQ, Lai LG, Fang LD, Min HW, et al. Brain edema after intracerebral hemorrhage in rats: the role of iron overload and aquaporin 4. J Neurosurg. 2009;110(3):462–8.
18. Xi G, Keep RF, Hoff JT. Erythrocytes and delayed brain edema formation following intracerebral hemorrhage in rats. J Neurosurg. 1998;89(6):991–6.
19. Diringer MN, Edwards DF, Zazulia AR. Hydrocephalus: a previously unrecognized predictor of poor outcome from supratentorial intracerebral hemorrhage. Stroke. 1998;29(7):1352–7.
20. Gebel JM Jr, Jauch EC, Brott TG, Khoury J, Sauerbeck L, Salisbury S, et al. Natural history of perihematomal edema in patients with hyperacute spontaneous intracerebral hemorrhage. Stroke. 2002;33(11):2631–5.
21. Xi G, Fewel ME, Hua Y, Thompson BG Jr, Hoff JT, Keep RF. Intracerebral hemorrhage: pathophysiology and therapy. Neurocrit Care. 2004;1(1):5–18.
22. Schirmer CM, Hoit DA, Malek AM. Decompressive hemicraniectomy for the treatment of intractable intracranial hypertension after aneurysmal subarachnoid hemorrhage. Stroke. 2007;38(3):987–92.
23. Dierssen G, Carda R, Coca JM. The influence of large decompressive craniectomy on the outcome of surgical treatment in spontaneous intracerebral haematomas. Acta Neurochir. 1983;69(1–2):53–60.

24. Ziai WC, Port JD, Cowan JA, Garonzik IM, Bhardwaj A, Rigamonti D. Decompressive craniectomy for intractable cerebral edema: experience of a single center. J Neurosurg Anesthesiol. 2003;15(1):25–32.
25. Moussa WM, Khedr W. Decompressive craniectomy and expansive duraplasty with evacuation of hypertensive intracerebral hematoma, a randomized controlled trial. Neurosurg Rev. 2017;40(1):115–27.
26. Auer LM, Deinsberger W, Niederkorn K, Gell G, Kleinert R, Schneider G, et al. Endoscopic surgery versus medical treatment for spontaneous intracerebral hematoma: a randomized study. J Neurosurg. 1989;70(4):530–5.
27. Backlund EO, von Holst H. Controlled subtotal evacuation of intracerebral haematomas by stereotactic technique. Surg Neurol. 1978;9(2):99–101.
28. Barrett RJ, Hussain R, Coplin WM, Berry S, Keyl PM, Hanley DF, et al. Frameless stereotactic aspiration and thrombolysis of spontaneous intracerebral hemorrhage. Neurocrit Care. 2005;3(3):237–45.
29. Higgins AC, Nashold BS, Cosman E. Stereotactic evacuation of primary intracerebral hematomas: new instrumentation. Appl Neurophysiol. 1982;45(4–5):438–42.
30. Marquardt G, Wolff R, Janzen RW, Seifert V. Basal ganglia haematomas in non-comatose patients: subacute stereotactic aspiration improves long-term outcome in comparison to purely medical treatment. Neurosurg Rev. 2005;28(1):64–9.
31. Mould WA, Carhuapoma JR, Muschelli J, Lane K, Morgan TC, McBee NA, et al. Minimally invasive surgery plus recombinant tissue-type plasminogen activator for intracerebral hemorrhage evacuation decreases perihematomal edema. Stroke. 2013;44(3):627–34.
32. Newell DW, Shah MM, Wilcox R, Hansmann DR, Melnychuk E, Muschelli J, et al. Minimally invasive evacuation of spontaneous intracerebral hemorrhage using sonothrombolysis. J Neurosurg. 2011;115(3):592–601.
33. Naff N, Williams MA, Keyl PM, Tuhrim S, Bullock MR, Mayer SA, et al. Low-dose recombinant tissue-type plasminogen activator enhances clot resolution in brain hemorrhage: the intraventricular hemorrhage thrombolysis trial. Stroke. 2011;42(11):3009–16.
34. Daverat P, Castel JP, Dartigues JF, Orgogozo JM. Death and functional outcome after spontaneous intracerebral hemorrhage. A prospective study of 166 cases using multivariate analysis. Stroke. 1991;22(1):1–6.
35. Hallevi H, Albright KC, Aronowski J, Barreto AD, Martin-Schild S, Khaja AM, et al. Intraventricular hemorrhage: anatomic relationships and clinical implications. Neurology. 2008;70(11):848–52.
36. Fiorella D, Gutman F, Woo H, Arthur A, Aranguren R, Davis R. Minimally invasive evacuation of parenchymal and ventricular hemorrhage using the Apollo system with simultaneous neuronavigation, neuroendoscopy and active monitoring with cone beam CT. J Neurointerv Surg. 2015;7(10):752–7.
37. Spiotta AM, Fiorella D, Vargas J, Khalessi A, Hoit D, Arthur A, et al. Initial multicenter technical experience with the Apollo device for minimally invasive intracerebral hematoma evacuation. Neurosurgery. 2015;11(Suppl 2):243–51; discussion 51.
38. Tan LA, Lopes DK, Munoz LF, Shah Y, Bhabad S, Jhaveri M, et al. Minimally invasive evacuation of intraventricular hemorrhage with the Apollo vibration/suction device. J Clin Neurosci Off J Neurosurg Soc Australas. 2016;27:53–8.
39. Turner RD, Vargas J, Turk AS, Chaudry MI, Spiotta AM. Novel device and technique for minimally invasive intracerebral hematoma evacuation in the same setting of a ruptured intracranial aneurysm: combined treatment in the neurointerventional angiography suite. Neurosurgery. 2015;11(Suppl 2):43–50; discussion -1.
40. Ding D, Przybylowski CJ, Starke RM, Sterling Street R, Tyree AE, Webster Crowley R, et al. A minimally invasive anterior skull base approach for evacuation of a basal ganglia hemorrhage. J Clin Neurosci Off J Neurosurg Soc Australas. 2015;22(11):1816–9.

41. Przybylowski CJ, Ding D, Starke RM, Webster Crowley R, Liu KC. Endoport-assisted surgery for the management of spontaneous intracerebral hemorrhage. J Clin Neurosci Off J Neurosurg Soc Australas. 2015;22(11):1727–32.
42. Fiorella D, Arthur AS, Mocco JD. 305 The INVEST trial: a randomized, controlled trial to investigate the safety and efficacy of image-guided minimally invasive endoscopic surgery with Apollo vs best medical management for supratentorial intracerebral hemorrhage. Neurosurgery. 2016;63(Suppl 1):187.
43. Broderick JP, Brott TG, Duldner JE, Tomsick T, Huster G. Volume of intracerebral hemorrhage. A powerful and easy-to-use predictor of 30-day mortality. Stroke. 1993;24(7):987–93.
44. Wang YF, Wu JS, Mao Y, Chen XC, Zhou LF, Zhang Y. The optimal time-window for surgical treatment of spontaneous intracerebral hemorrhage: result of prospective randomized controlled trial of 500 cases. Acta Neurochir Suppl. 2008;105:141–5.
45. Maila SK. Factors affecting the outcome of surgical evacuation of spontaneous deep intra cerebral bleeds. Br J Neurosurg. 2015;29(5):668–71.

Chapter 7
Intracerebral Hemorrhage Prognosis

Craig A. Williamson and Venkatakrishna Rajajee

Clinical Case

A 78-year-old woman with a history of mild cognitive impairment, hypertension, and chronic kidney disease is found down by her husband with altered mental status and left-sided weakness. She is brought in by an ambulance to the emergency room where, on initial examination, her Glasgow Coma Scale (GCS) is 13 (E3M6V4) and National Institute of Health Stroke Scale (NIHSS) is 21, with a neurological exam notable for disorientation, right gaze preference, dysarthria, left-sided neglect, left facial droop, and hemiparesis. A head CT reveals an approximately 60 cc right parietal intraparenchymal hematoma without intraventricular extension. As the treating provider, you sit down for an initial meeting to review the physical exam and head CT findings with the patient's family. The patient's husband asks about prognosis and shows you an advance directive that states that "In the event of permanent coma or vegetative state, as determined by the treating physician," the patient would not wish to receive life-prolonging treatments, such as mechanical ventilation and artificial nutrition.

Introduction

Outcomes for spontaneous intracerebral hemorrhage (ICH) remain stubbornly poor in comparison with ischemic stroke, despite a possible reduction in 30-day mortality in the last three decades [1]. Addressing questions related to prognosis, within the limits of accurate prediction, is a core component of ICH care. It is also one of the most challenging tasks providers are called upon to do, with enormous potential

C. A. Williamson (✉) · V. Rajajee
Departments of Neurosurgery and Neurology, University of Michigan, Ann Arbor, MI, USA
e-mail: craigaw@med.umich.edu

B. Ovbiagele, A. I. Qureshi (eds.), *Intracerebral Hemorrhage Therapeutics*,
https://doi.org/10.1007/978-3-319-77063-5_7

impact on patient outcome. Families use prognostic information to inform decision-making about early treatment interventions, such as intubation, ventriculostomy placement, and surgery, taking into consideration the known or inferred wishes of patients who typically cannot speak for themselves. Advance directives sometimes exist, but these are often too vaguely worded to directly apply to the complex situations providers and families confront.

There are numerous population- and hospital-based publications on short- and long-term prognosis after ICH. Multiple predictive models have also been described, the most widely used of which remains the ICH score. However, completely accurate prognostic data remains elusive. The overwhelming majority of deaths in ICH result from early withdrawal of life-sustaining treatment, therefore creating potential for a "self-fulfilling prophecy," where perceived prognosis directly affects survival and thus confounds truly objective determination of prognosis [2, 3].

This chapter will first review epidemiological data in order to provide a general overview of prognosis after ICH. It will then discuss individual factors that are known to most strongly influence prognosis. Next, common prognostic models will be reviewed, while being mindful of the limits of applying population-based models to individual patients. Finally, current guidelines and recommendations for prognostication will be covered.

Overview of ICH Prognosis

Most assessments of outcome following ICH estimate a substantial short-term mortality rate, ranging from 28% to greater than 50%. One meta-analysis of 36 population-based studies from 1980 to 2008 identified a median 30-day mortality rate of 40.4% and did not find that mortality rates were decreasing with time [4]. In contrast, Ovbiagele et al., in a US study using the Nationwide Inpatient Sample, found that in-hospital mortality rates for ICH experienced a slight but statistically significant decline between 1997 and 2006, from 30.4% to 28.3% [5]. Using another US administrative database, Adeoye et al. identified a significant decrease in in-hospital mortality from 34.5% in 2000 to 28.5% in 2008 [6]. Recent population-based assessments have shown similarly varying results. In a study of stroke incidence and outcomes in Corpus Christi, TX, Zahuranec et al. found that while ICH incidence declined between 2000 and 2010, there was no decrease in 30-day case-adjusted mortality rate between 2000 and 2010 [7]. In contrast, in the Dijon Stroke Registry, 30-day mortality rates were noted to decrease significantly over time, from 48.9% during 1985–1993 to 29.6% during 2003–2011 [1]. In a national Dutch ICH registry, since 2003 ICH mortality was found to substantially decrease for individuals less than 75, but no change was noted in older patients [8].

Less data is available regarding long-term survival following ICH. However, multiple studies have documented an increase in mortality rates among ICH survivors. In a population-based study of all ICH patients in a region of Central Finland, from 1985 to 1991, the 28-day mortality rate was 50.6%. Among survivors, the annual mortality rate was 4.5 times higher than the general population during the first year and then 2.2 times higher between years 2 and 6 before declining to below the population rate [9]. In a later Finnish study, among 3-month ICH survivors, the 7-year mortality was 32.9% versus 19.4% in age- and sex-matched controls, though there was no difference among survivors with a good functional recovery at 3 months [10]. Flaherty et al. assessed long-term survival in ICH patients in 1988 and then in 2002–2003. They reported 12-month mortality rates of 59% and 53%, respectively. Ten-year survival in the 1988 cohort was 18%, and survival analysis did not find a significant difference in mortality rate between the two cohorts [11]. In another study of a predominantly rural Italian population, ICH mortality rate was 50.3% at 30 days and 59.0% at 1 year, with a 10-year survival rate of 24.1% [12]. A recent meta-analysis of published cohort studies found pooled survival estimate of 46% at 1 year and 29% at 5 years [13].

In general, outcomes after ICH are thought to be significantly worse in comparison to those for ischemic stroke. There clearly is a higher mortality rate among ICH patients, but studies differ regarding whether ICH independently leads to worse long-term functional outcome. In a large multicenter neuroprotection trial that enrolled both ischemic stroke and ICH patients, mortality rates were similar, but ICH patients had significantly worse functional outcomes at 3 months [14]. In a South London population-based stroke registry, ICH patients experienced worse functional outcomes at 3 months and 1 year, but functional status was equivalent at 5 years [15]. However, other studies have reported similar functional outcomes upon controlling for initial stroke severity [16, 17].

It is important to note that different pathophysiological mechanisms affect initial severity in ICH and ischemic stroke patients. Whereas ischemia immediately leads to bioenergetic failure causing cell dysfunction and rapid cell death, early neuronal dysfunction in ICH is largely mediated by tissue displacement and direct compression. These pathophysiological differences may result in potential for a greater and more rapid recovery among ICH survivors, as has been noted in several studies [18, 19]. For example, in a case-control study of 270 stroke patients admitted to a single rehabilitation center, ICH patients showed larger and more rapid improvements than ischemic stroke patients [20]. In another population-based stroke registry, ICH patients had a significantly greater rate of improvement between baseline and 3 months in comparison to ischemic stroke patients [15].

In summary, ICH is associated with high overall mortality, with 1-month mortality rates ranging from 28 to over 50% in multiple studies. While some studies suggest that the mortality rate may be declining over time, other studies have failed to identify any trend toward decreasing mortality. Withdrawal of medical care is the most common cause of death in ICH, and it is not possible to quantify the degree to which the self-fulfilling prophecy may contribute to early mortality rates. When disability is present in ICH survivors, the mortality rate remains well above that of the general population for many years. Overall functional outcomes appear to be worse for ICH patients in comparison to ischemic stroke, but studies of whether this effect is independent of baseline stroke severity differ. Among ICH survivors, there does appear to be a more rapid early recovery in comparison to ischemic stroke sufferers, along with potential for greater gains in rehabilitation.

Individual Factors Associated with Prognosis

Numerous factors have been reported to be associated with outcome after ICH, and it is not our intention to review all of them. However, several key features have been identified in multiple studies and are included as components of various predictive models. Other predictors have been more recently identified and may be incorporated into future predictive models. Overall, in the absence of any definitive evidenced-based treatment, outcome is primarily determined by patient and disease factors, with some emerging evidence that specialized care and the absence of care limitations may improve outcome.

Imaging and Clinical Features

Numerous clinical studies have found a worse outcome to be significantly associated with increasing age and decreasing Glasgow Coma Scale (GCS). Coagulopathy, iatrogenic and otherwise, is consistently associated with hematoma expansion and worse outcome, while platelet dysfunction has also been implicated. Studies after the widespread adoption of CT scans in routine practice showed a strong association with ICH volume and outcome [21], and multiple more recent studies have confirmed this finding. Additional radiographic features with strong evidence for an association with worse outcome include deep or infratentorial location, the presence of intraventricular hemorrhage, and hematoma expansion. Visualization of contrast extravasation on CT scans – the "spot sign" – has been shown to be associated with greater likelihood of hematoma expansion and worse outcome [22]. Some studies have also suggested that the presence of white matter lesions on CT scan is associated with greater initial severity and is an independent predictor of worse outcome [23, 24]. Electroencephalography (EEG) is not widely utilized as a prognostic tool in ICH, but an association between periodic discharges and worse outcomes has been reported [25]. Whether seizures independently predict worse outcome is unclear based on current studies.

Treatment Factors

Though there is no definitive treatment for ICH, the provision of high-quality supportive care clearly has the potential to improve outcomes. Increasingly, ICH patients are cared for in specialized neurocritical care and stroke units, which may be associated with better outcomes. Multiple clinical trials have found that outcomes improve when ischemic stroke patients receive care in specialized stroke units [26]. A systematic review and meta-analysis of trials that include hemorrhagic stroke patients suggest that hemorrhagic patients experience the same reduction in death and disability as ischemic stroke patients, with a nonsignificant trend toward a further mortality reduction [27].

Compared with ischemic stroke, hemorrhagic stroke patients are more likely to be admitted to an intensive care unit (ICU). Increasingly, this care is provided in specialized neurological ICUs. Several studies have evaluated whether outcomes are better for patients treated in specialized neurocritical care units, in comparison with general ICUs. Diringer and Edwards, in a 2001 study utilizing a prospectively collected ICU database from multiple institutions, found that admission to a specialized neurological ICU was associated with a significantly lower inpatient mortality rate [28]. Subsequent studies have had slightly differing results. Varelas et al. found that introduction of a neurointensivist into an existing neuro ICU resulted in significantly reduced LOS and overall significant increase in the percentage of stroke patients well enough to be discharged home, although there was no statistical difference in adjusted mortality for ICH patients [29]. In another recent study, specialized neurocritical care was associated with decreased ICU and hospital length of stay but did not affect mortality rate or 3- and 12-month functional outcomes [30]. In contrast, Damian et al., using a national ICU database sample in England and Wales, noted a temporal trend of increasing ICH admission to specialized neurocritical care units between 1996 and 2009. For ICH patients admitted to neurological ICUs during this period, mean LOS was longer, but mortality was decreased, and there was a significant decrease in the mortality rate over time in comparison to patients admitted to non-neurological ICUs [31].

Impact of Withdrawal of Care and DNR Orders

As mentioned previously, the overwhelming majority of patients with ICH die shortly after cessation of life-sustaining treatments, so decisions about withdrawal of care can dramatically affect prognosis. This also results in difficulty obtaining a truly objective understanding of clinical correlates of poor outcome that are truly independent of goals-of-care decisions. Becker et al., in a 2001 study, were the first to bring attention to the impact of a "self-fulfilling prophecy" on hospital mortality following ICH. In their single-center ICH cohort, the overall mortality was 34.5%. Twenty-three of 30 deaths occurred as a result of withdrawal of medical care. The strength of association between withdrawal of care and mortality was such that when introduced as a covariate in a logistic regression model, no other prognostic factor achieved statistical significance. Based on a survey, the authors also concluded that practitioners tended to be overly pessimistic about the prognosis for functional recovery after ICH [32].

Since only a small minority of ICH patients die following unexpected cardiac arrest, "do not resuscitate" (DNR) orders might reasonably be expected to have a correspondingly low impact on mortality rates. However, in actual practice DNR orders are often viewed as a waypoint on a continuum progressing toward withdrawal of life-sustaining treatments and therefore may serve as a surrogate marker for less aggressive care. Hemphill et al., in a statewide study of 234 California hospitals, found that there were significant differences in the rate at which hospitals implemented early (<24 h) DNR orders. Hospitals with a higher rate of early DNR orders had a significantly higher case-adjusted mortality rate, and this effect occurred independent of the DNR order itself, suggesting early DNR status may be a proxy for less aggressive early resuscitation that then increases mortality [33]. These findings were corroborated by results from a study of a population-based cohort of ICH patients, in which early limitations on treatment were associated with a more than doubling of the hazard for short- and long-term mortality, independent from other clinical predictors [34].

As described previously, survivors of ICH have increased overall mortality and often significantly impaired quality of life. Therefore, it is very appropriate for practitioners and families to be concerned about long-term prognosis and together arrive at treatment goals that are consistent with a patient's wishes, either spoken or unspoken. Unwarranted early pessimism may, however, inadvertently result in a poor outcome for a patient who might otherwise have potential for recovery [35–37]. Making prognostication more difficult is the fact that patients with the most severe injury may occasionally demonstrate delayed neurological recovery. In a single-center study by Rajajee et al. of long-term recovery in patients whose surrogates decided to pursue long-term supportive care following severe acute brain injury requiring the placement of tracheostomy and percutaneous gastrostomy, 29 patients with ICH were identified in a 5-year period [38]. Of these, 20 (71%) were unable to ambulate 1–3 months following injury. Of these 20, however, 5 (25%) were able to ambulate independently, and 3 (15%) were able to independently perform activities of daily living 6–12 months following injury. In select patients with a good premorbid functional status whose families are inclined to pursue long-term supportive care, a period of at least many months may be necessary before the full potential for recovery is realized.

Prognostic Models

Multiple predictive models, most utilizing logistic regression, have been developed to predict ICH prognosis. One early model in the post-CT era used GCS, hematoma size, and intraventricular extension to predict outcome at last follow-up in a cohort of 112 patient [39]. Another model used the combination of GCS, hematoma size, and widened pulse pressure to predict 30-day mortality in a single-center cohort with a high degree of accuracy [40]. In 2001, Hemphill et al. published the "ICH score" – the first simple, numeric, prognostic grading system. In its first derivation, the ICH score used GCS, hematoma volume, interventricular extension, posterior fossae location, and age to predict 30-day mortality in a cohort of 152 patients. Mortality was most strongly associated with GCS, so this factor was given the greatest weight: 2 points for GCS 3–4 and 1 point for a GCS 5–12. For all other factors, 1 point was assigned for a given binary outcome: hematoma volume ≥ 30 ml, intraventricular extension, posterior fossae location, and age ≥ 80, for a maximum score of 6 [41]. External validation was subsequently performed in multiple populations [42–45], and the ICH score remains the most widely used grading scale.

The ICH score was criticized because it was developed to predict early mortality, rather than functional outcome, which is arguably of greater interest to families and providers. In 2008, Rost et al. published the FUNC score, which was derived to predict functional independence, defined as Glasgow Outcome Scale (GOS) ≥ 4 3 months after disease onset, in a large single-center prospective cohort. This 11-point scale uses the following components to predict increasing probability of functional independence: hematoma volume, location (lobar, deep, infratentorial), age, GCS, and presence of premorbid cognitive dysfunction [46]. With inclusion of these variables, IVH was found to no longer be statistically significant and so was not included in the final model. In a subsequent validation study, the ICH score was tested and found to correlate with 12-month functional outcomes, in addition to early mortality [47].

Several modifications of the ICH score have also been described. The modified ICH score substitutes the NIHSS for GCS, with the primary intention of more accurately stratifying aphasic patients [42]. The ICH grading score (ICH-GS) includes the same components as the original ICH score but contains more numerous and different cut points for scoring, as well as rating IVH volume and including different volume cut points for infratentorial and supratentorial hemorrhages [48]. Chuang et al. proposed a simplified ICH score (sICH), which includes only patient factors such as age, GCS, serum glucose, as well a history of hypertension and dialysis dependency [49]. Other scores with varying combinations of patient and imaging factors have also been proposed [50, 51]. Bruce et al. confirmed that all of these grading scales demonstrated excellent discrimination in predicting mortality and that they generally performed well at predicting functional outcomes in a cohort of 97 patients with ICH [52]. In a larger comparison of >2500 patients from the multicenter INTERACT 2 trial, the ICH score, modified ICH score, and ICH-GS scores were compared. All scores showed good discrimination for 30-day mortality, with the modified ICH score performing slightly better than the ICH score or ICH grading scale (*c*-statistic 0.78, 0.75, 0.75, respectively). The modified ICH score also showed slightly better discrimination for predicting poor 3-month outcome (*c*-statistic 0.75) in comparison to the ICH score (0.68) and ICH-GS (0.69) [53].

Several investigators have further examined the impact of limitations of life-sustaining treatment on various prognostic models. Zahuranec et al. examined the performance of several commonly used predictive models after patients were stratified based on the presence of DNR orders within the first 24 h. In general, there were statistically significant deviations between observed and protected mortalities for all models assessed. However, after stratification, the models substantially underestimated mortality for patients with early DNR orders while overestimating mortality when an early DNR order was not placed [54]. Creutzfeld et al. found similar results in another cohort of ICH patients. They determined that their newly developed logistic regression model and the ICH score became poorly calibrated when stratifying by DNR status, again overestimating mortality when an early DNR was not present and underestimating mortality when early DNR was placed [55]. These studies underscore the difficulties of applying prognostic models to patients without considering the impact of decisions to limit treatment.

The Approach to Prognostication in ICH

Since current prognostic models cannot account for the influence of decisions to limit life support and the self-fulfilling prophecy, the 2015 Emergency Neurological Life Support (ENLS) module for management of ICH specifically recommends against the use of grading scales to guide early decisions to limit the use of supportive care or therapeutic intervention [56]. The 2015 ENLS guidelines suggest that the ICH score may be best utilized as a communication tool to convey severity of illness between providers, as well as during discussions with patients and families. Similarly, the American Heart Association's (AHA) 2015 ICH guidelines recommend that aggressive, guideline-concordant therapy be used in the early phase of care (about the first 24 h), for all ICH patients without an advance directive that specifically limits such treatment [57]. The optimal duration of observation while aggressive supportive care is provided is unclear. Factors such as premorbid functional status, surrogates' recall of statements by patients on what might constitute an acceptable quality of life, and the clinical course following admission often guide subsequent conversations between providers and families. Providing accurate information and supporting families struggling to make treatment decisions in the face of prognostic uncertainty remains one of the most challenging aspects of ICH care. A willingness to pursue early aggressive care, constant emotional support to families, and objective, evidence-based estimates of the potential for recovery are all cornerstones of the management of the patient with ICH.

References

1. Bejot Y, Grelat M, Delpont B, Durier J, Rouaud O, Osseby G-V, et al. Temporal trends in early case-fatality rates in patients with intracerebral hemorrhage. Neurology. 2017;88:985–90.
2. Naidech AM, Bernstein RA, Bassin SL, Garg RK, Liebling S, Bendok BR, et al. How patients die after intracerebral hemorrhage. Neurocrit Care. 2009;11(1):45–9.
3. Zuransky JA, Aiyagari V, Zazulia AR, Shackelford A, Diringer MN. Early mortality following spontaneous intracerebral hemorrhage. Neurology. 2005;64:725–7.
4. van Asch CJJ, Luitse MJA, Rinkel GJE, van der Tweel I, Algra A, Klijn CJM. Incidence, case fatality, and functional outcome of intracerebral haemorrhage over time, according to age, sex, and ethnic origin: a systematic review and meta-analysis. The Lancet Neurology. 2010;9(2):167–76.
5. Ovbiagele B. Nationwide trends in in-hospital mortality among patients with stroke. Stroke. 2010;41(8):1748–54.
6. Adeoye O, Ringer A, Hornung R, Khatri P, Zuccarello M, Kleindorfer D. Trends in surgical management and mortality of intracerebral hemorrhage in the United States before and after the STICH trial. Neurocrit Care. 2010;13(1):82–6.
7. Zahuranec DB, Lisabeth LD, Sanchez BN, Smith MA, Brown DL, Garcia NM, et al. Intracerebral mortality is not changing despite declining evidence. Neurology. 2014;82: 2180–6.
8. Jolink WMT, Klijn CJM, Brouwers PJAM, Kappelle LJ, Vaartjes I. Time trends in incidence, case fatality, and mortality of intracerebral hemorrhage. Neurology. 2015;85:1318–24.

9. Fogelholm R, Murros K, Rissanen A, Avikainen S. Long term survival after primary intracerebral haemorrhage: a retrospective population based study. J Neurol Neurosurg Psychiatry. 2005;76(11):1534–8.
10. Saloheimo P, Lapp TM, Juvela S, Hillbom M. The impact of functional status at three months on long-term survival after spontaneous intracerebral hemorrhage. Stroke. 2006;37(2):487–91.
11. Flaherty ML, Haverbusch M, Sekar P, Kissela B, Kleindorfer D, Moomaw CJ, et al. Long term mortality after intracerebral hemorrhage. Neurology. 2006;66:1182–6.
12. Sacco S, Marini C, Toni D, Olivieri L, Carolei A. Incidence and 10-year survival of intracerebral hemorrhage in a population-based registry. Stroke. 2009;40(2):394–9.
13. Poon MT, Fonville AF, Al-Shahi SR. Long-term prognosis after intracerebral haemorrhage: systematic review and meta-analysis. J Neurol Neurosurg Psychiatry. 2014;85(6):660–7.
14. Chiu D, Peterson L, Elkind MS, Rosand J, Gerber LM, Silverstein MD, et al. Comparison of outcomes after intracerebral hemorrhage and ischemic stroke. J Stroke Cerebrovasc Dis. 2010;19(3):225–9.
15. Bhalla A, Wang Y, Rudd A, Wolfe CD. Differences in outcome and predictors between ischemic and intracerebral hemorrhage: the South London Stroke Register. Stroke. 2013;44(8):2174–81.
16. Barber M. Poor outcome in primary intracerebral haemorrhage: results of a matched comparison. Postgrad Med J. 2004;80(940):89–92.
17. Nadeau JO, Phillips S, Shi HS, Kapral MK, Gladstone DJ, Silver FL, et al. Intracerebral hemorrhage: outcomes and eligibility for factor VIIa treatment in a National Stroke Registry. Cerebrovasc Dis. 2006;22(4):271–5.
18. Kelly PJ, Furie KL, Shafqat S, Rallis N, Chang Y, Stein J. Functional recovery following rehabilitation after hemorrhagic and ischemic stroke. Arch Phys Med Rehabil. 2003;85:968–72.
19. Wei JW, Heeley EL, Wang JG, Huang Y, Wong LK, Li Z, et al. Comparison of recovery patterns and prognostic indicators for ischemic and hemorrhagic stroke in China: the ChinaQUEST (QUality Evaluation of Stroke Care and Treatment) Registry study. Stroke. 2010;41(9):1877–83.
20. Paolucci S, Antonucci G, Grasso MG, Bragoni M, Coiro P, De Angelis D, et al. Functional outcome of ischemic and hemorrhagic stroke patients after inpatient rehabilitation: a matched comparison. Stroke. 2003;34(12):2861–5.
21. Broderick JP, Brott TG, Duldner JE, Toemsick T, Huster G. Volume of intracerebral hemorrhage. A powerful and easy-to-use predictor of 30-day mortality. Stroke. 1993;24:987–93.
22. Delgado Almandoz JE, Yoo AJ, Stone MJ, Schaefer PW, Oleinik A, Brouwers HB, et al. The spot sign score in primary intracerebral hemorrhage identifies patients at highest risk of in-hospital mortality and poor outcome among survivors. Stroke. 2010;41(1):54–60.
23. Lou M, Al-Hazzani A, Goddeau RP Jr, Novak V, Selim M. Relationship between white-matter hyperintensities and hematoma volume and growth in patients with intracerebral hemorrhage. Stroke. 2010;41(1):34–40.
24. Lee SH, Kim BJ, Ryu WS, Kim CK, Kim N, Park BJ, et al. White matter lesions and poor outcome after intracerebral hemorrhage. Neurology. 2010;74:1502–10.
25. Claassen J, Jette N, Chum F, Green R, Schmidt M, Choi H, et al. Electrographic seizures and periodic discharges after intracerebral hemorrhage. Neurology. 2007;69:1356–65.
26. Collaboration SUT. Organized inpatient (stroke unit) care for stroke. Cochrane Database Syst Rev. 2013;9
27. Langhorne P, Fearon P, Ronning OM, Kaste M, Palomaki H, Vemmos K, et al. Stroke unit care benefits patients with intracerebral hemorrhage: systematic review and meta-analysis. Stroke. 2013;44(11):3044–9.
28. Diringer MN, Edwards DF. Admission to a neurologic/neurosurgical intensive care unit is associated with reduced mortality rate after intracerebral hemorrhage. Crit Care Med. 2001;29:635–40.
29. Varelas PN, Schultz L, Conti M, Spanaki M, Genarrelli T, Hacein-Bey L. The impact of a neuro-intensivist on patients with stroke admitted to a neurosciences intensive care unit. Neurocrit Care. 2008;9(3):293–9.

30. Knopf L, Staff I, Gomes J, McCullough L. Impact of a neurointensivist on outcomes in critically ill stroke patients. Neurocrit Care. 2012;16(1):63–71.
31. Damian MS, Ben-Shlomo Y, Howard R, Bellotti T, Harrison D, Griggs K, et al. The effect of secular trends and specialist neurocritical care on mortality for patients with intracerebral haemorrhage, myasthenia gravis and Guillain-Barre syndrome admitted to critical care: an analysis of the Intensive Care National Audit and Research Centre (ICNARC) national United Kingdom database. Intensive Care Med. 2013;39:1405–12.
32. Becker KJ, Baxter AB, Cohen WA, Bybee HM, Tirschwll DI, Newell DW, et al. Withdrawal of support in intracerebral hemorrhage may lead to self-fulfilling prophecies. Neurology. 2001;56:766–72.
33. Hemphill JC 3rd, Newman J, Zhao S, Johnston SC. Hospital usage of early do-not-resuscitate orders and outcome after intracerebral hemorrhage. Stroke. 2004;35(5):1130–4.
34. Zahuranec DB, Brown DL, Lisabeth LD, Gonzales NR, Longwell PJ, Smith MA, et al. Early care limitations independently predict mortality after intracerebral hemorrhage. Neurology. 2007;68:1651–7.
35. Hemphill JC. Do-not-resuscitate orders, unintended consequences, and the ripple effect. Critical Care. 2007;11(2):121.
36. Hemphill JC 3rd, White DB. Clinical nihilism in neuroemergencies. Emerg Med Clin North Am. 2009;27(1):27–37. vii–viii
37. Rabinstein AA, Diringer MN. Withholding care in intracerebral hemorrhage: realistic compassion or self-fulfilling prophecy. Neurology. 2007;68:1647–8.
38. Abstracts of the Neurocritical Care Society 11th Annual Meeting. October 1–4, 2013. Philadelphia, Pennsylvania, USA. Neurocrit Care. 2013;19 Suppl 1:S5–331.
39. Portenoy RK, Lipton RB, Berger AR, Lesser ML, Lantos G. Intracerebral hemorrhage: a model for the prediction of outcome. J Neurol Neurosurg Psychiatry. 1987;50:976–9.
40. Tuhrim S, Dambrosia JM, Price TR, Mohr JP, Wolf PA, Heyman A, et al. Prediction of intracerebral hemorrhage survival. Ann Neurol. 1988;24:258–63.
41. Hemphill JC, Bonovich DC, Besmertis L, Manley GT, Johnston SC, Tuhrim S. The ICH score : a simple, reliable grading scale for intracerebral hemorrhage editorial comment: a simple, reliable grading scale for intracerebral hemorrhage. Stroke. 2001;32(4):891–7.
42. Cheung RT, Zou LY. Use of the original, modified, or new intracerebral hemorrhage score to predict mortality and morbidity after intracerebral hemorrhage. Stroke. 2003;34(7):1717–22.
43. Clarke JL, Johnson SC, Farrant M, Bernstein R, Tong D, Hemphill JC. External validation of the ICH score. Neurocrit Care. 2004;1:53–60.
44. Fernandes H, Gregson BA, Siddique MS, Mendelow AD. Testing the ICH score. Stroke. 2002;33:1455–6.
45. Jamora RD, Kishi-Generao EM, Bitanga FS, Gan RN, Apaga NE, San Jose MC. The ICH score: predicting mortality and functional outcome in an Asian population. Stroke. 2003;34:6–7.
46. Rost NS, Smith EE, Chang Y, Snider RW, Chanderraj R, Schwab K, et al. Prediction of functional outcome in patients with primary intracerebral hemorrhage: the FUNC score. Stroke. 2008;39(8):2304–9.
47. Hemphill JC III, Farrant M, Neill TA Jr. Prospective validation of the ICH score for 12-month functional outcome. Neurology. 2009;73:1088–94.
48. Ruiz-Sandoval JL, Chiquete E, Romero-Vargas S, Padilla-Martinez JJ, Gonzalez-Cornejo S. Grading scale for prediction of outcome in primary intracerebral hemorrhages. Stroke. 2007;38(5):1641–4.
49. Chuang Y-C, Chen Y-M, Peng S-K, Peng S-Y. Risk stratification for predicting 30-day mortality of intracerebral hemorrhage. Int J Qual Health Care. 2009;21:441–7.
50. Godoy DA, Pinero G, Di Napoli M. Predicting mortality in spontaneous intracerebral hemorrhage: can modification to original score improve the prediction? Stroke. 2006;37(4):1038–44.
51. Weimar C, Benemann J, Diener HC, German Stroke Study C. Development and validation of the Essen Intracerebral Haemorrhage Score. J Neurol Neurosurg Psychiatry. 2006;77(5):601–5.

52. Bruce SS, Appelboom G, Piazza M, Hwang BY, Kellner C, Carpenter AM, et al. A comparative evaluation of existing grading scales in intracerebral hemorrhage. Neurocrit Care. 2011;15(3):498–505.
53. Heeley E, Anderson CS, Woodward M, Arima H, Robinson T, Stapf C, et al. Poor utility of grading scales in acute intracerebral hemorrhage: results from the INTERACT2 trial. Int J Stroke. 2015;10(7):1101–7.
54. Zahuranec DB, Morgenstern LB, Sanchez BN, Resnicow K, White DB, Hemphill JC III. Do-not-resuscitate orders and predictive models after intracerebral hemorrhage. Neurology. 2010;75:626–33.
55. Creutzfeldt CJ, Becker KJ, Weinstein JR, Khot SP, McPharlin TO, Ton TG, et al. Do-not-attempt-resuscitation orders and prognostic models for intraparenchymal hemorrhage. Crit Care Med. 2011;39(1):158–62.
56. Jauch EC, Pineda JA, Hemphill JC. Emergency neurological life support: intracerebral hemorrhage. Neurocrit Care. 2015;23(Suppl 2):S83–93.
57. Hemphill JC 3rd, Greenberg SM, Anderson CS, Becker K, Bendok BR, Cushman M, et al. Guidelines for the management of spontaneous intracerebral hemorrhage: a guideline for healthcare professionals from the American Heart Association/American Stroke Association. Stroke. 2015;46(7):2032–60.

Chapter 8
Prevention of Recurrent Intracerebral Hemorrhage

Chirantan Banerjee and Bruce Ovbiagele

Introduction

Spontaneous non-traumatic intracerebral hemorrhage (ICH) accounts for 10–15% of strokes worldwide, with an annual incidence of 24.6 per 100,000 [1]. In low and middle-income countries, it accounts for ~20% of all strokes [2]. ICH is associated with a high 30-day mortality rate that has remained unchanged over the past couple of decades, hovering around ~40% [1]. A recent meta-analysis found no improvement in 1-year survival between years 1983 and 2004, as well as no change in 5-year survival rates between 1983 and 1997 either [3]. Similarly, the overall incidence of ICH has disappointingly remained roughly constant over the past three decades, as observed in data from community-based cohorts in the UK and France [4, 5]. However, a closer look at these data revealed that while on one hand there was a reduction in hypertension-related ICH due to improved blood pressure control, on the other hand, this was offset by an increase in cases of ICH among the elderly, which mainly comprised amyloid-related lobar hemorrhages associated with use of antithrombotic drugs [4, 5].

Beyond its association with a high mortality rate, survivors of an initial ICH are also at elevated risk of secondary strokes including recurrent ICH and ischemic stroke [6]. This chapter will focus on evidence-based strategies to prevent the occurrence of recurrent ICH, taking into consideration the challenge that several patients who survive a first-time ICH are also at risk of a future ischemic stroke, which raises an important question for providers taking care of ICH patients about the potential benefits and hazards of antithrombotic (antiplatelet and anticoagulant) drugs in these high-risk patients.

C. Banerjee (✉)
Department of Neurology, Medical University of South Carolina, Charleston, SC, USA
e-mail: banerjeec@musc.edu

B. Ovbiagele
University of California, San Francisco Medical Center, San Francisco, CA, USA
e-mail: Bruce.Ovbiagele@va.gov

B. Ovbiagele, A. I. Qureshi (eds.), *Intracerebral Hemorrhage Therapeutics*,
https://doi.org/10.1007/978-3-319-77063-5_8

Table 8.1 Risk of recurrent intracerebral hemorrhage (ICH) after index ICH

Study	Cohort size	Mean duration (years)	Recurrence risk/proportion
Passero et al. (1995) [11]	112	1	7.2
Arakawa et al. (1998) [12]	74	5.6	2.0
Bae et al. (1999) [13]	933	1	1.8
Hill et al. (2000) [14]	423	3.6	2.4
Vermeer et al. (2002) [15]	243	5.5	2.1
Inagawa et al. (2005) [10]	279	3	2.3
Cheung et al. (2007) [16]	108	1	7.4
Azarpazhooh et al. (2008) [17]	191	2	2.6
Zia et al. (2009) [18]	353	3	2.3
Schmidt et al. (2016) [8]	15,270	5	13.7

Risk of Stroke Recurrence After Intracerebral Hemorrhage

Risk of ICH recurrence has been assessed in both hospital-based and population-based cohorts over the years. The proportion of patients having a recurrent ICH by 1 year varies from 1.8% to 8.9% in various studies, as listed in Table 8.1. This variation is likely secondary to differences in study methodology, population characteristics, as well as different durations. A systematic review of the risks of recurrent ICH and ischemic stroke among ICH survivors was conducted in 2007, which pooled data from patients in heterogeneous studies and reported a higher annual risk of recurrent ICH (2.3%) than ischemic stroke (1.1%) [7]. A more recent meta-analysis conducted in 2014 identified 13 studies which reported the risk of recurrent ICH at 1 year. The annualized rate of ICH recurrence was 2.0–2.4%, and the proportion of patients having a recurrent ICH in the first year varied from 1.8% to 7.4% [3]. In this study, the authors analyzed data from four studies and found that ischemic stroke incidence was at least as common as recurrent ICH over 3 years [3]. A Danish cohort of 15,270 primary ICH patients between 1996 and 2011 had 2053 recurrences, with a cumulative recurrence risk of 8.9% at 1 year and 13.7% after 5 years [8]. The risk of ICH recurrence is highest in the first year after the index bleed but can extend several years out [7–9]. Table 8.1 summarizes the risk of recurrent ICH after index ICH in various studies. As far as location of ICH is concerned, most of the initial and recurrent hemorrhages tend to be lobar among Caucasians. On the other hand, deep hemorrhages (both initial and recurrent) are more common in Asians [7, 10].

Risk Factors for Recurrence of ICH

The most important risk factors of ICH recurrence are hypertension, older age, and location of the initial hemorrhage (lobar versus deep) [3, 7, 8]. Hypertension is associated with an increase in the recurrence of ICH, irrespective of whether the initial hemorrhage was deep or lobar [3, 7, 8, 19]. In a prospective study of Italian ICH survivors, during follow-up, poor control of hypertension was found in 47% of hypertensive patients with rebleeding, as opposed to 7% of hypertensive patients without rebleeding [11].

Increased age is also attributed to a higher risk of recurrence. This may be secondary to higher prevalence of lobar ICH and cerebral amyloid angiopathy (CAA) and increased use of antithrombotic medications with accumulating comorbidities among the elderly [19, 20].

Lobar location has been associated with a higher risk of ICH recurrence as compared to deep hemorrhages, with the recurrent ICH also more likely to occur in a lobar location [7, 11, 14]. As compared to nonlobar index hemorrhages, patients with lobar hemorrhage were 3.8–4.9 times more likely to have a recurrent bleed in the first year in two distinct cohorts [11, 21]. In a prospective, longitudinal study of consecutive elderly ICH survivors with lobar ICH, the 2-year cumulative rate of ICH recurrence was 21% [22]. In the same study, apolipoprotein E genotype was significantly associated with the risk of recurrence. Carriers of the ε2 or ε4 allele had a 3.8 times higher risk of recurrence as compared to patients with the common apolipoprotein E ε3/ε3 genotype (28% versus 10%) [22].

CAA is a recognized risk factor for recurrent ICH. Pooled data from ten studies including 1306 patients were meta-analyzed to assess the significance of CAA [presumed based on lobar distribution of cerebral microbleeds (CMBs)], as well as the number of CMBs [23]. The annual recurrent ICH risk was higher in CAA-related ICH vs CAA-unrelated ICH (7.4% vs 1.1%). Among patients with lobar CMBs, presence of ≥2 CMBs increased the risk of recurrent ICH. In CAA-unrelated ICH, however, only >10 CMBs (versus none) were associated with recurrent ICH (OR 5.6).

Lacunar ischemic stroke has a shared pathophysiology with ICH. A history of prior lacunar stroke has been found to be associated with ICH recurrence in a couple of Caucasian cohorts [17, 24].

A significantly increased recurrence risk has also been observed for patients who underwent surgical evacuation of the primary ICH compared to medically managed patients, with 1-year cumulative recurrence risk of 21.2% for surgically treated patients compared to 8.3% for conservatively managed patients [8]. In the same cohort, patients with renal insufficiency had a significantly increased recurrence risk with a 1-year cumulative recurrence risk of 16.1% versus 8.7% for other cohort members [8]. Among the preceding risk factors, hypertension and the use of antithrombotic agents are modifiable.

Management of Blood Pressure

As discussed briefly in the previous section, hypertension is a key risk factor for ICH and ICH recurrence, with hypertensive patients having a 5.7 times increased risk of ICH compared with those without hypertension [25]. Untreated hypertension further increases the risk of ICH, with these patients having a 2.5–3.5 times increased risk of ICH when compared to persons on hypertension treatment [26, 27]. This increased risk is also noted among patients who ceased taking their antihypertensive treatment [27]. With regard to recurrent ICH risk, antihypertensive treatment is associated with a significantly reduced risk (RR 0.82) with 1-year cumulative recurrence risk for patients treated for hypertension of 7.5% as compared to 9.7% for others [8].

In the Perindopril Protection Against Recurrent Stroke Study (PROGRESS) [28], patients with ischemic stroke or ICH and with or without hypertension were randomized to antihypertensive medications perindopril (an angiotensin-converting enzyme inhibitor) and indapamide (a thiazide diuretic) or placebo. Over 3.9 years of follow-up, patients with ICH treated with the antihypertensive agents had a 50% relative risk reduction in the absolute rates of recurrent ICH from 2% to 1%. This effect was more robust than in patients with ischemic stroke where a 24% relative risk reduction was achieved in the rate of recurrent stroke. This underscores the notion that patients with ICH are particularly likely to benefit from blood pressure reduction as a measure of secondary prevention, even more so than patients with ischemic stroke. Combination therapy with perindopril and indapamide reduced blood pressure by 12/5 mm Hg as compared to 5/3 mm Hg by single-drug therapy in the trial. Only combination therapy produced a discernable reduction in risk of stroke [29].

The SPS3 trial randomized patients with a recent lacunar infarct to a SBP target of 130–149 mm Hg or less than 130 mm Hg [30]. The primary end point was reduction in occurrence of any stroke (ischemic stroke and intracranial hemorrhage). After 1 year, the mean systolic blood pressure was 138 mm Hg in the higher-target group and 127 mm Hg in the lower-target group. Nonsignificant rate reductions were seen for all stroke and the composite outcome of myocardial infarction or vascular death in the lower target group. But there was a robust and significant reduction in the rate of ICH (HR 0.37, 95% CI 0.15–0.95) [30]. As lacunar strokes and most ICH share a pathogenesis, this would suggest that ICH patients should have their BP lowered to or beyond the targets currently recommended in other high-risk groups (<130 mm Hg SBP and 80 mm Hg DBP in the presence of diabetes mellitus, heart failure, or chronic kidney disease) [31].

In a retrospective analysis of prospectively collected data on a cohort consisting of 15,270 individuals diagnosed with a primary ICH in Denmark between 1996 and 2011, antihypertensive treatment was associated with a significantly reduced recurrence risk (RR 0.82, 95% CI 0.74–0.91). The 1-year cumulative recurrence risk for patients treated for hypertension was 7.5% compared to 9.7% for others [8].

In a single-site observational study of 2197 consecutive patients with ICH presenting between July 1994 and December 2013 [32], 1145 patients with ICH survived at least 90 days and were followed up for a mean duration of 36.8 months. The event rates for both lobar and nonlobar ICHs were significantly higher among patients with inadequate BP control as compared to patients with adequate BP control (84 versus 49 per 1000 person-years for lobar and 52 versus 27 per 1000 person-years for nonlobar ICH). Both systolic and diastolic BP during follow-up were associated with increased risk of lobar ICH recurrence, but only diastolic BP was associated with increased risk of nonlobar ICH recurrence. Inadequate BP control was associated with higher risk of recurrence of both lobar ICH (HR 3.53, 95% CI 1.65–7.54]) and nonlobar ICH (HR 4.23, 95% CI 1.02–17.52) [32].

An ongoing English pilot trial, Prevention of Hypertensive Injury to the Brain by Intensive Treatment after Intracerebral Hemorrhage (PROHIBIT-ICH), will assess whether home telemetry-guided treatment can improve ICH recurrence rates by randomly allocating ICH survivors to either home BP monitoring using telemetry (sending BP information to a study coordinating center) to allow treatment adjustments to improve BP control or to standard care [33].

Finally, the actual optimal timing for initiating BP lowering after ICH to prevent recurrence is unknown, but post hoc analyses of the CATIS [34] and COSSACS [35] trials suggested that early initiation of antihypertensives was associated with better BP control at 2 weeks.

Antithrombotic Medications

Oral anticoagulants (OAC) are increasingly used for long-term primary and secondary prevention of stroke and systemic embolism in patients with atrial fibrillation and mechanical heart valves due to proven efficacy [36]. ICH is probably the most feared complication of OAC and accounts for >50% of all deaths associated with hemorrhage in anticoagulated patients [37]. One fourth of all ICH were related to OAC in a German prospective cohort study [38]. Also, OAC-related ICHs have higher hematoma volume, worse functional outcome [39], and higher mortality [40] as compared to non-OAC ICH. Novel OACs (NOACs) such as dabigatran, rivaroxaban, apixaban, and edoxaban are safer than vitamin K antagonists (VKA) in terms of risk of major hemorrhage and have half the risk of intracranial hemorrhage compared to VKA [41]. Furthermore, NOAC-associated ICH has smaller hematoma volume and better functional outcome as compared to warfarin-associated ICH [42, 43].

There have been no randomized clinical trials or prospective cohort studies to assess the risk of ICH recurrence with anticoagulation post-ICH versus the benefit toward lowering risk of thromboembolism. A nationwide observational cohort study among patients with atrial fibrillation and warfarin-related ICH in Denmark between 1998 and 2016 found that resuming warfarin therapy was associated with a lower rate of ischemic stroke or systemic embolism (adjusted HR 0.49; 0.24–1.02) and an increased rate of recurrent ICH (adjusted HR, 1.31; 0.68–2.50) compared with not resuming warfarin therapy, but these differences did not reach statistical significance [44]. A systematic review and meta-analysis to summarize the associations of anticoagulation resumption with the subsequent risk of ICH recurrence and thromboembolism were published in 2017 [45]. It included 5306 ICH patients from 8 retrospective cohort studies. 1899 (35.8%) patients were restarted on anticoagulation therapy, with a total follow-up for 3494 person-years, and 3407 patients (64.2%) were not, who were followed for a total of 7030 person-years. Recurrence of ICH was observed in 166 (8.7%) patients on anticoagulation and in 267 (7.8%) not on antithrombotic agents (pooled RR, 1.01; 0.58–1.77). There was heterogeneity however between the included studies. Sensitivity analyses were carried out, and significant heterogeneity was found with the inclusion of studies that used NOACs. After the exclusion of these studies, the pooled RR was 1.18 (0.83–1.70). Thus, there was no significant difference in ICH recurrence between the two groups. To assess the risk of thromboembolic events, data from 6 of the 8 retrospective studies with 2044 patients were analyzed. The rate of thromboembolic events in patients on anticoagulation therapy was 6.7% compared with 17.6% for patients not restarted on anticoagulation therapy (pooled RR, 0.34; 0.25–0.45). There are several inherent limitations of this analysis, however, the main one being the lack of detailed data on hematoma location and volume, as it may have been a possibility that anticoagulation was more likely to be reinstated in patients with smaller hematomas. Also, ICHs were not classified as being index or recurrent, as recurrent hemorrhages are more likely to be lobar and secondary to amyloid angiopathy. The reason this is important is because a prior Markov decision analysis [46] stratified by ICH location estimated a 1-year risk of ICH recurrence of 15% after lobar ICH versus 2.1% for deep ICH and found that withholding anticoagulation improved quality-adjusted life year (QALY) expectancy by 1.9 QALYs after lobar ICH and 0.3 QALYs after deep ICH. The authors concluded that anticoagulation should be avoided after lobar ICH but can be considered in patients with deep hemorrhage if the risk of thromboembolism is particularly high [46]. Another systematic review and meta-analysis of studies reporting recurrent ICH and ischemic stroke in ICH survivors with atrial fibrillation compared recurrent ICH and ischemic stroke risk among patients restarted on VKA versus antiplatelet agents (APAs) and no antithrombotic agents. The pooled RR estimates for ischemic stroke were lower for VKA compared to APAs (RR 0.45; 0.27–0.74) and no antithrombotic (RR 0.47; 0.29–0.77). At the same time, pooled RR estimates for ICH recurrence were not significantly increased across treatment groups (VKA vs APA: RR 1.34; 0.79–2.30, VKA vs no antithrombotic: RR 0.93; 0.45–1.90) [47]. There is no data to evaluate the utility of use of NOACs among warfarin-related ICH survivors with atrial fibrillation.

Among patients where resumption of anticoagulation after ICH is necessary, the optimal timing is also uncertain. The above meta-analysis found a wide variation in the timing of anticoagulation resumption in the included studies, with a range from 10 days up to 6 months [45]. Two single-center retrospective studies with small sample sizes between 1998 and 2001 reported low rates of cardioembolic events among patients with prosthetic heart valves while not receiving anticoagulation therapy or recurrent ICH when anticoagulation was reinitiated at median 7 and 15 days, respectively, and the patients were followed for 23.5 months and 6 months [48, 49]. A study of patients with warfarin-related ICH were followed up for a median of 69 weeks found that the combined risk of recurrent intracranial hemorrhage or ischemic stroke reached a nadir if warfarin was resumed after approximately 10–30 weeks [50].

Resumption of antiplatelet agents (APAs) after ICH has never been evaluated in a randomized clinical trial. The ongoing randomized controlled REstart or STop Antithrombotic Randomized Trial (NCT02966119, http://www.RESTARTtrial.org/) is assessing whether a policy of starting APA after ICH results in a net reduction in serious vascular events compared with a policy of avoiding APA. Meta-analyses evaluating the efficacy of aspirin for primary and secondary prevention of ischemic stroke and myocardial infarction have noted a significant increase in the risk of ICH (12 events per 10,000 persons), but this is superseded by a larger 15–34% reduction in risk of stroke, myocardial infarction, and death [51, 52]. A Chinese study found a twofold reduction (52 per 1000 patient-aspirin years versus 113 per 1000 patient-years; $P = 0.04$) in all vascular events (combined ischemic and hemorrhagic) among patients who restarted aspirin after any ICH [53]. There was no difference in the risk of recurrent ICH alone (22.7/1000 patient-aspirin years vs 22.4/1000 patient-aspirin years, $P = 70$) as well.

About one third of non-anticoagulated ICH patients in the Get with the Guideline Database were already taking a single or dual antiplatelet agent [54], and those on combination antiplatelet therapy had higher in-hospital mortality (adjusted OR 1.50; 1.39–1.63), but not those on single APA. In a multivariable analysis of patients in the placebo arm of the randomized Cerebral Hemorrhage and NXY-059 Treatment (CHANT) trial, there was no association of use of APAs with ICH expansion or clinical outcome at 90 days [55].

In a prospective German study of 496 ICH patients followed for 2 years, APAs were used in 28.4% and were not associated with increased risk of ICH recurrence [9]. Another single-center prospective study found that antiplatelet use in 22% of ICH survivors was not associated with an increase in the risk of ICH recurrence among both lobar and deep hemorrhage patients [56]. In a subsequent study by the same group that focused solely on lobar ICH, aspirin was not associated with ICH recurrence in univariate analysis, but after adjusting for baseline clinical predictors, it independently increased the risk of recurrent ICH (adjusted HR 3.95; 1.6–8.3) [20]. This, however, may have been secondary to overfitting of the multivariable model [57].

In the same Markov decision analysis described above, aspirin was found to be the preferred treatment among patients with deep ICH who had moderate ischemic stroke risk and recurrent ICH relative risk less than ~1.3. Among patients with lobar ICH, aspirin was preferred when the risk of ischemic stroke was average (4.5% per year) and the relative risk of recurrent ICH was less than ~1.04 [46].

Statins

Conflicting data exists pertaining to use of statins post-ICH. A number of studies have found an inverse relationship between total and LDL cholesterol and the risk of ICH [58]. In the Stroke Prevention by Aggressive Reduction in Cholesterol Levels (SPARCL) trial, the benefit of high-dose atorvastatin in reducing ischemic stroke recurrence was accompanied by an increased risk of ICH, without differences in overall mortality [59]. In a subsequent sub-analysis of the trial, in addition to atorvastatin, ICH was more frequent in those with ICH as entry event, men, those with increased age, and those with stage 2 hypertension [60]. An increase in the rate of hemorrhagic stroke was not observed in the previously conducted Heart Protection Study, which included patients with prior stroke randomized to simvastatin or placebo [61]. A Markov decision analysis evaluated the risks and benefits of statin therapy in patients with prior ICH and found that in survivors of lobar ICH without prior cardiovascular events, avoiding statins yielded a life expectancy gain of 2.2 QALYs compared with statin use. In patients with lobar ICH who had prior cardiovascular events, the annual recurrence risk of myocardial infarction would have to exceed 90% to favor statin therapy [62]. Avoiding statin therapy was also favored, although by a smaller margin, in secondary prevention for survivors of deep ICH [62]. On the other hand, a meta-analysis of 31 randomized controlled trials which included 91,588 statin-treated patients found no significant association between statin use and ICH (OR 1.08; 0.88–1.32); all strokes and all-cause mortality were in fact significantly reduced with statin therapy [63]. Continued statin use after ICH was associated with early neurological improvement and reduced 6-month mortality in a small retrospective study [64]. Hydrophilic statin therapy was associated with a reduced risk of recurrent ICH in post-ICH patients in a Taiwanese cohort [65]. It therefore remains unclear whether statins should be continued or discontinued in ICH patients, and the decision should be individualized based on the patient's cardiovascular profile, ICH location, and presence of CMBs.

Other Risk Factors

Several other factors, such as the presence of obstructive sleep apnea (OSA), alcohol use, smoking, recreational drug abuse, and other lifestyle modifications, should also be considered in prevention of ICH recurrence despite the lack of systematic data regarding their effect on ICH secondary prevention.

As discussed above, untreated hypertension is a robust predictor of recurrent ICH. Hypertension is considered resistant when the blood pressure remains above goal despite lifestyle modification and administration of three antihypertensive agents of different classes including a diuretic. Large population-based studies have suggested that OSA is a risk factor for resistant hypertension [66]. In a small study among noncomatose hypertensive ICH patients, OSA occurred acutely in >50% of patients and was associated with perihematoma edema [67].

An Australian case-control study reported an increase in ICH risk (OR 3.4; 1.4–8.4) with heavy drinking (>60 g/day of alcohol for men and >40 g/day of alcohol for women) [68]. Similarly, a Japanese study documented an increased risk of ICH in those who drink heavily (defined as drinking 450 g of alcohol or more per week), a finding that was significant despite controlling for hypertension (RR 2.07; 1.12–3.83) [69]. In the standardized INTERSTROKE case-control study in 22 countries,

>30 drinks per month was associated with ICH (OR 1.51; 1.18–1.92), as was binge drinking [70].

Tobacco use is also associated with increased ICH risk in several epidemiologic studies [70, 71]. Data from the Women's Health Study showed that as compared to nonsmokers, women who smoked ≥15 cigarettes/day had 2.67 times higher risk of ICH [72]. Current male smokers of ≥20 cigarettes/day had a relative risk for ICH of 2.06 (1.08–3.96) as compared to never smokers in the Physician's Health Study over 17.8 years of follow-up [73].

Several recreational drugs, including cocaine, methamphetamine, and dimethylamylamine (DMAA), have been associated with ICH [74–76]. Drug cessation counseling and treatment is very important for secondary prevention of ICH in patients with identified drug abuse.

Nonmodifiable risk factors such as apolipoprotein E2 or E4 [77] as well as modifiable lifestyle risk factors such as body mass index, waist hip ratio, diet (vegetable consumption), and physical activity [70, 78] have been associated with ICH in epidemiological studies.

References

1. van Asch CJ, Luitse MJ, Rinkel GJ, van der Tweel I, Algra A, Klijn CJ. Incidence, case fatality, and functional outcome of intracerebral haemorrhage over time, according to age, sex, and ethnic origin: a systematic review and meta-analysis. Lancet Neurol. 2010;9(2):167–76.
2. Feigin VL, Lawes CM, Bennett DA, Barker-Collo SL, Parag V. Worldwide stroke incidence and early case fatality reported in 56 population-based studies: a systematic review. Lancet Neurol. 2009;8(4):355–69.
3. Poon MT, Fonville AF, Al-Shahi SR. Long-term prognosis after intracerebral haemorrhage: systematic review and meta-analysis. J Neurol Neurosurg Psychiatry. 2014;85(6):660–7.
4. Lovelock CE, Molyneux AJ, Rothwell PM. Change in incidence and aetiology of intracerebral haemorrhage in Oxfordshire, UK, between 1981 and 2006: a population-based study. Lancet Neurol. 2007;6(6):487–93.
5. Bejot Y, Cordonnier C, Durier J, Aboa-Eboule C, Rouaud O, Giroud M. Intracerebral haemorrhage profiles are changing: results from the Dijon population-based study. Brain. 2013;136(Pt 2):658–64.
6. Wani M, Nga E, Navaratnasingham R. Should a patient with primary intracerebral haemorrhage receive antiplatelet or anticoagulant therapy? BMJ. 2005;331(7514):439–42.
7. Hanger HC, Wilkinson TJ, Fayez-Iskander N, Sainsbury R. The risk of recurrent stroke after intracerebral haemorrhage. J Neurol Neurosurg Psychiatry. 2007;78(8):836–40.
8. Schmidt LB, Goertz S, Wohlfahrt J, Melbye M, Munch TN. Recurrent intracerebral hemorrhage: associations with comorbidities and medicine with antithrombotic effects. PLoS One. 2016;11(11):e0166223.
9. Weimar C, Benemann J, Terborg C, Walter U, Weber R, Diener HC. Recurrent stroke after lobar and deep intracerebral hemorrhage: a hospital-based cohort study. Cerebrovasc Dis. 2011;32(3):283–8.
10. Inagawa T. Recurrent primary intracerebral hemorrhage in Izumo City, Japan. Surg Neurol. 2005;64(1):28–35. discussion –6
11. Passero S, Burgalassi L, D'Andrea P, Battistini N. Recurrence of bleeding in patients with primary intracerebral hemorrhage. Stroke. 1995;26(7):1189–92.

12. Arakawa S, Saku Y, Ibayashi S, Nagao T, Fujishima M. Blood pressure control and recurrence of hypertensive brain hemorrhage. Stroke. 1998;29(9):1806–9.
13. Bae H, Jeong D, Doh J, Lee K, Yun I, Byun B. Recurrence of bleeding in patients with hypertensive intracerebral hemorrhage. Cerebrovasc Dis. 1999;9(2):102–8.
14. Hill MD, Silver FL, Austin PC, Tu JV. Rate of stroke recurrence in patients with primary intracerebral hemorrhage. Stroke. 2000;31(1):123–7.
15. Vermeer SE, Algra A, Franke CL, Koudstaal PJ, Rinkel GJ. Long-term prognosis after recovery from primary intracerebral hemorrhage. Neurology. 2002;59(2):205–9.
16. Cheung CM, Tsoi TH, Hon SF, Au-Yeung M, Shiu KL, Lee CN, et al. Outcomes after first-ever stroke. Hong Kong Med J. 2007;13(2):95–9.
17. Azarpazhooh MR, Nicol MB, Donnan GA, Dewey HM, Sturm JW, Macdonell RA, et al. Patterns of stroke recurrence according to subtype of first stroke event: the North East Melbourne Stroke Incidence Study (NEMESIS). Int J Stroke. 2008;3(3):158–64.
18. Zia E, Engstrom G, Svensson PJ, Norrving B, Pessah-Rasmussen H. Three-year survival and stroke recurrence rates in patients with primary intracerebral hemorrhage. Stroke. 2009;40(11):3567–73.
19. Izumihara A, Suzuki M, Ishihara T. Recurrence and extension of lobar hemorrhage related to cerebral amyloid angiopathy: multivariate analysis of clinical risk factors. Surg Neurol. 2005;64(2):160–4. discussion 4
20. Biffi A, Halpin A, Towfighi A, Gilson A, Busl K, Rost N, et al. Aspirin and recurrent intracerebral hemorrhage in cerebral amyloid angiopathy. Neurology. 2010;75(8):693–8.
21. Yen CC, et al. Recurrent primary intracerebral hemorrhage: a hospital based study. Acta Neurol Taiwan. 2007;16(2):74–80.
22. O'Donnell HC, Rosand J, Knudsen KA, Furie KL, Segal AZ, Chiu RI, et al. Apolipoprotein E genotype and the risk of recurrent lobar intracerebral hemorrhage. N Engl J Med. 2000;342(4):240–5.
23. Charidimou A, Imaizumi T, Moulin S, Biffi A, Samarasekera N, Yakushiji Y, et al. Brain hemorrhage recurrence, small vessel disease type, and cerebral microbleeds: a meta-analysis. Neurology. 2017;89(8):820–9.
24. Huhtakangas J, Lopponen P, Tetri S, Juvela S, Saloheimo P, Bode MK, et al. Predictors for recurrent primary intracerebral hemorrhage: a retrospective population-based study. Stroke. 2013;44(3):585–90.
25. Feldmann E, Broderick JP, Kernan WN, Viscoli CM, Brass LM, Brott T, et al. Major risk factors for intracerebral hemorrhage in the young are modifiable. Stroke. 2005;36(9):1881–5.
26. Woo D, Haverbusch M, Sekar P, Kissela B, Khoury J, Schneider A, et al. Effect of untreated hypertension on hemorrhagic stroke. Stroke. 2004;35(7):1703–8.
27. Thrift AG, McNeil JJ, Forbes A, Donnan GA. Three important subgroups of hypertensive persons at greater risk of intracerebral hemorrhage. Melbourne Risk Factor Study Group. Hypertension. 1998;31(6):1223–9.
28. Chapman N, Huxley R, Anderson C, Bousser MG, Chalmers J, Colman S, et al. Effects of a perindopril-based blood pressure-lowering regimen on the risk of recurrent stroke according to stroke subtype and medical history: the PROGRESS trial. Stroke. 2004;35(1):116–21.
29. Randomised trial of a perindopril-based blood-pressure-lowering regimen among 6,105 individuals with previous stroke or transient ischaemic attack. Lancet. 2001;358(9287):1033–41.
30. Benavente OR, Coffey CS, Conwit R, Hart RG, McClure LA, Pearce LA, et al. Blood-pressure targets in patients with recent lacunar stroke: the SPS3 randomised trial. Lancet. 2013;382(9891):507–15.
31. Broderick J, Connolly S, Feldmann E, Hanley D, Kase C, Krieger D, et al. Guidelines for the management of spontaneous intracerebral hemorrhage in adults: 2007 update: a guideline from the American Heart Association/American Stroke Association Stroke Council, High Blood Pressure Research Council, and the Quality of Care and Outcomes in Research Interdisciplinary Working Group. Stroke. 2007;38(6):2001–23.
32. Biffi A, Anderson CD, Battey TW, Ayres AM, Greenberg SM, Viswanathan A, et al. Association between blood pressure control and risk of recurrent intracerebral hemorrhage. JAMA. 2015;314(9):904–12.

33. Protecting the brain after a bleed with home monitored blood pressure control 2016 [updated 2016-04-28]. Available from: https://www.stroke.org.uk/research/protecting-brain-after-bleed-home-monitored-blood-pressure-control.
34. Xu T, Zhang Y, Bu X, Wang D, Sun Y, Chen CS, et al. Blood pressure reduction in acute ischemic stroke according to time to treatment: a subgroup analysis of the China Antihypertensive Trial in Acute Ischemic Stroke trial. J Hypertens. 2017;35(6):1244–51.
35. Robinson TG, Potter JF, Ford GA, Bulpitt CJ, Chernova J, Jagger C, et al. Effects of antihypertensive treatment after acute stroke in the Continue or Stop Post-Stroke Antihypertensives Collaborative Study (COSSACS): a prospective, randomised, open, blinded-endpoint trial. Lancet Neurol. 2010;9(8):767–75.
36. Hart RG, Pearce LA, Aguilar MI. Meta-analysis: antithrombotic therapy to prevent stroke in patients who have nonvalvular atrial fibrillation. Ann Intern Med. 2007;146(12):857–67.
37. Gomez-Outes A, Lagunar-Ruiz J, Terleira-Fernandez AI, Calvo-Rojas G, Suarez-Gea ML, Vargas-Castrillon E. Causes of death in anticoagulated patients with atrial fibrillation. J Am Coll Cardiol. 2016;68(23):2508–21.
38. Horstmann S, Rizos T, Lauseker M, Mohlenbruch M, Jenetzky E, Hacke W, et al. Intracerebral hemorrhage during anticoagulation with vitamin K antagonists: a consecutive observational study. J Neurol. 2013;260(8):2046–51.
39. Falcone GJ, Biffi A, Brouwers HB, Anderson CD, Battey TW, Ayres AM, et al. Predictors of hematoma volume in deep and lobar supratentorial intracerebral hemorrhage. JAMA Neurol. 2013;70(8):988–94.
40. Hanger HC, Fletcher VJ, Wilkinson TJ, Brown AJ, Frampton CM, Sainsbury R. Effect of aspirin and warfarin on early survival after intracerebral haemorrhage. J Neurol. 2008;255(3):347–52.
41. Ruff CT, Giugliano RP, Braunwald E, Hoffman EB, Deenadayalu N, Ezekowitz MD, et al. Comparison of the efficacy and safety of new oral anticoagulants with warfarin in patients with atrial fibrillation: a meta-analysis of randomised trials. Lancet. 2014;383(9921):955–62.
42. Wilson D, Charidimou A, Shakeshaft C, Ambler G, White M, Cohen H, et al. Volume and functional outcome of intracerebral hemorrhage according to oral anticoagulant type. Neurology. 2016;86(4):360–6.
43. Hagii J, Tomita H, Metoki N, Saito S, Shiroto H, Hitomi H, et al. Characteristics of intracerebral hemorrhage during rivaroxaban treatment: comparison with those during warfarin. Stroke. 2014;45(9):2805–7.
44. Nielsen PB, Larsen TB, Skjoth F, Lip GY. Outcomes associated with resuming warfarin treatment after hemorrhagic stroke or traumatic intracranial hemorrhage in patients with atrial fibrillation. JAMA Intern Med. 2017;177(4):563–70.
45. Murthy SB, Gupta A, Merkler AE, Navi BB, Mandava P, Iadecola C, et al. Restarting anticoagulant therapy after intracranial hemorrhage: a systematic review and meta-analysis. Stroke. 2017;48(6):1594–600.
46. Eckman MH, Rosand J, Knudsen KA, Singer DE, Greenberg SM. Can patients be anticoagulated after intracerebral hemorrhage? A decision analysis. Stroke. 2003;34(7):1710–6.
47. Korompoki E, Filippidis FT, Nielsen PB, Del Giudice A, GYH L, Kuramatsu JB, et al. Long-term antithrombotic treatment in intracranial hemorrhage survivors with atrial fibrillation. Neurology. 2017;89(7):687–96.
48. Butler AC, Tait RC. Restarting anticoagulation in prosthetic heart valve patients after intracranial haemorrhage: a 2-year follow-up. Br J Haematol. 1998;103(4):1064–6.
49. Ananthasubramaniam K, Beattie JN, Rosman HS, Jayam V, Borzak S. How safely and for how long can warfarin therapy be withheld in prosthetic heart valve patients hospitalized with a major hemorrhage? Chest. 2001;119(2):478–84.
50. Majeed A, Kim YK, Roberts RS, Holmstrom M, Schulman S. Optimal timing of resumption of warfarin after intracranial hemorrhage. Stroke. 2010;41(12):2860–6.
51. He J, Whelton PK, Vu B, Klag MJ. Aspirin and risk of hemorrhagic stroke: a meta-analysis of randomized controlled trials. JAMA. 1998;280(22):1930–5.
52. Collaborative overview of randomised trials of antiplatelet therapy – I: prevention of death, myocardial infarction, and stroke by prolonged antiplatelet therapy in various categories of patients. Antiplatelet Trialists' Collaboration. BMJ. 1994;308(6921):81–106.

53. Chong BH, Chan KH, Pong V, Lau KK, Chan YH, Zuo ML, et al. Use of aspirin in Chinese after recovery from primary intracranial haemorrhage. Thromb Haemost. 2012;107(2):241–7.
54. Khan NI, Siddiqui FM, Goldstein JN, Cox M, Xian Y, Matsouaka RA, et al. Association between previous use of antiplatelet therapy and intracerebral hemorrhage outcomes. Stroke. 2017;48(7):1810–7.
55. Sansing LH, Messe SR, Cucchiara BL, Cohen SN, Lyden PD, Kasner SE. Prior antiplatelet use does not affect hemorrhage growth or outcome after ICH. Neurology. 2009;72(16):1397–402.
56. Viswanathan A, Rakich SM, Engel C, Snider R, Rosand J, Greenberg SM, et al. Antiplatelet use after intracerebral hemorrhage. Neurology. 2006;66(2):206–9.
57. Al-Shahi Salman R, Dennis MS. Antiplatelet therapy may be continued after intracerebral hemorrhage. Stroke. 2014;45(10):3149–50.
58. Wang X, Dong Y, Qi X, Huang C, Hou L. Cholesterol levels and risk of hemorrhagic stroke: a systematic review and meta-analysis. Stroke. 2013;44(7):1833–9.
59. Amarenco P, Bogousslavsky J, Callahan A 3rd, Goldstein LB, Hennerici M, Rudolph AE, et al. High-dose atorvastatin after stroke or transient ischemic attack. N Engl J Med. 2006;355(6):549–59.
60. Goldstein LB, Amarenco P, Szarek M, Callahan A 3rd, Hennerici M, Sillesen H, et al. Hemorrhagic stroke in the Stroke Prevention by Aggressive Reduction in Cholesterol Levels study. Neurology. 2008;70(24 Pt 2):2364–70.
61. Collins R, Armitage J, Parish S, Sleight P, Peto R. Effects of cholesterol-lowering with simvastatin on stroke and other major vascular events in 20536 people with cerebrovascular disease or other high-risk conditions. Lancet. 2004;363(9411):757–67.
62. Westover MB, Bianchi MT, Eckman MH, Greenberg SM. Statin use following intracerebral hemorrhage: a decision analysis. Arch Neurol. 2011;68(5):573–9.
63. McKinney JS, Kostis WJ. Statin therapy and the risk of intracerebral hemorrhage: a meta-analysis of 31 randomized controlled trials. Stroke. 2012;43(8):2149–56.
64. Tapia-Perez JH, Rupa R, Zilke R, Gehring S, Voellger B, Schneider T. Continued statin therapy could improve the outcome after spontaneous intracerebral hemorrhage. Neurosurg Rev. 2013;36(2):279–87. discussion 87
65. Tai SY, Lin FC, Lee CY, Chang CJ, Wu MT, Chien CY. Statin use after intracerebral hemorrhage: a 10-year nationwide cohort study. Brain Behav. 2016;6(8):e00487.
66. Khan A, Patel NK, O'Hearn DJ, Khan S. Resistant hypertension and obstructive sleep apnea. Int J Hypertens. 2013;2013:193010.
67. Pontes-Neto OM, Fernandes RM, Sander HH, da Silva LA, Mariano DC, Nobre F, et al. Obstructive sleep apnea is frequent in patients with hypertensive intracerebral hemorrhage and is related to perihematoma edema. Cerebrovasc Dis. 2010;29(1):36–42.
68. Thrift AG, Donnan GA, McNeil JJ. Heavy drinking, but not moderate or intermediate drinking, increases the risk of intracerebral hemorrhage. Epidemiology. 1999;10(3):307–12.
69. Iso H, Baba S, Mannami T, Sasaki S, Okada K, Konishi M, et al. Alcohol consumption and risk of stroke among middle-aged men: the JPHC Study Cohort I. Stroke. 2004;35(5):1124–9.
70. O'Donnell MJ, Xavier D, Liu L, Zhang H, Chin SL, Rao-Melacini P, et al. Risk factors for ischaemic and intracerebral haemorrhagic stroke in 22 countries (the INTERSTROKE study): a case-control study. Lancet. 2010;376(9735):112–23.
71. Ariesen MJ, Claus SP, Rinkel GJ, Algra A. Risk factors for intracerebral hemorrhage in the general population: a systematic review. Stroke. 2003;34(8):2060–5.
72. Kurth T, Kase CS, Berger K, Gaziano JM, Cook NR, Buring JE. Smoking and risk of hemorrhagic stroke in women. Stroke. 2003;34(12):2792–5.
73. Kurth T, Kase CS, Berger K, Schaeffner ES, Buring JE, Gaziano JM. Smoking and the risk of hemorrhagic stroke in men. Stroke. 2003;34(5):1151–5.
74. Gee P, Tallon C, Long N, Moore G, Boet R, Jackson S. Use of recreational drug 1,3 Dimethylamylamine (DMAA) [corrected] associated with cerebral hemorrhage. Ann Emerg Med. 2012;60(4):431–4.

75. Aggarwal SK, Williams V, Levine SR, Cassin BJ, Garcia JH. Cocaine-associated intracranial hemorrhage: absence of vasculitis in 14 cases. Neurology. 1996;46(6):1741–3.
76. Pozzi M, Roccatagliata D, Sterzi R. Drug abuse and intracranial hemorrhage. Neurol Sci. 2008;29(Suppl 2):S269–70.
77. Woo D, Sauerbeck LR, Kissela BM, Khoury JC, Szaflarski JP, Gebel J, et al. Genetic and environmental risk factors for intracerebral hemorrhage: preliminary results of a population-based study. Stroke. 2002;33(5):1190–5.
78. Zhang Y, Tuomilehto J, Jousilahti P, Wang Y, Antikainen R, Hu G. Lifestyle factors on the risks of ischemic and hemorrhagic stroke. Arch Intern Med. 2011;171(20):1811–8.

Chapter 9
Special Disease Management Considerations

Nabeel A. Herial and Magdy Selim

Intraventricular Hemorrhage (IVH)

Case A 76-year-old woman with history of untreated hypertension developed sudden vomiting and loss of consciousness. She was intubated at the scene for airway protection. Blood pressure upon arrival to the hospital was 222/125 mm Hg. Plain head CT scan (Fig. 9.1a) showed a large left basal ganglionic hemorrhage extending into both lateral, third, fourth ventricles and obstructive hydrocephalus with enlargement of the occipital and temporal horns of the left lateral ventricle. She was started on nicardipine infusion. Routine laboratory studies were all within normal limits, and toxicology screen was negative. On examination, eyes were closed. There were no spontaneous movements or response to voice. Pupils were equal and minimally reactive to light. Eyes were down in the resting position. Corneal and gag reflexes were active. She withdrew the left side and has extensor posturing of the right arm to painful stimulation. Toes were upgoing bilaterally. Neurosurgery was consulted. A right frontal external ventricular drain (EVD) terminating near the right foramen of Monroe was placed (Fig. 9.1b), and 1 mg of intraventricular t-PA was administered. The patient's exam remained unchanged without evidence of radiological improvement of hydrocephalus after 4 doses of t-PA. A second left frontal EVD was

N. A. Herial (✉)
Departments of Neurology and Neurosurgery, Sidney Kimmel Medical College, Thomas Jefferson University, Philadelphia, PA, USA
e-mail: nabeel.herial@jefferson.edu

M. Selim
Department of Neurology, Stroke Division, Beth Israel Deaconess Medical Center, Boston, MA, USA
e-mail: mselim@bidmc.harvard.edu

B. Ovbiagele, A. I. Qureshi (eds.), *Intracerebral Hemorrhage Therapeutics*,
https://doi.org/10.1007/978-3-319-77063-5_9

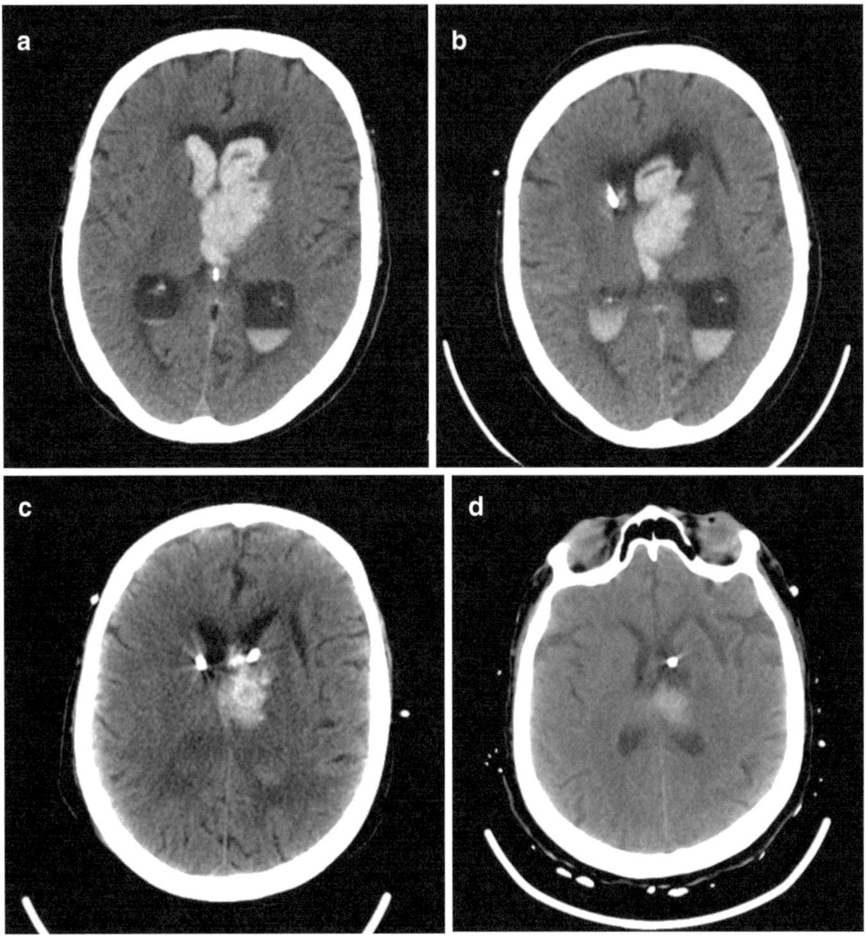

Fig. 9.1 (**a**) Non-contrast CT head showing large left basal ganglionic hemorrhage extending into both lateral and ventricles with enlarged occipital horns. (**b**) A right frontal external ventricular drain entering the right lateral ventricle. (**c**) CT head without contrast with evidence of bilateral external ventricular drains in the lateral ventricles. (**d**) A follow-up CT head showing improvement in ventricular hemorrhage

placed (Fig. 9.1c) with some radiological improvement (Fig. 9.1d). The patient's examination remained unchanged. Family ultimately decided to withdraw supportive care, and the patient died.

Discussion

The management of patients with IVH involves two important steps that should be carried out in parallel: (1) identifying the underlying etiology of IVH and (2) prevention and management of complications, in particular the development of obstructive hydrocephalus and associated risks of increased intracranial pressure and herniation, which could be potentially fatal. Intraventricular hemorrhage commonly occurs in the setting of deep intracerebral hemorrhage (ICH), which is often attributed to hypertension, or aneurysmal subarachnoid hemorrhage, and is referred to as secondary IVH, in contrast to primary IVH, where IVH is isolated, not associated with ICH or SAH, and confined to the ventricles. Primary IVH is relatively uncommon; it may complicate traumatic head injury or use of anticoagulant therapy, but the most common etiology is vascular malformations.

Secondary IVH is an independent risk factor for poor outcomes. It is associated with high morbidity and mortality [1, 2]. Mortality is reported to be greater than 50%, and more than 75% of survivors have poor functional outcomes [1, 2]. Patients with IVH are at risk of neurological deterioration as a result of hydrocephalus and its sequelae. The presence of blood in the 3rd or 4th ventricles is often associated with higher risk for the development of obstructive hydrocephalus, which can be potentially fatal [3]. Patients may also develop a delayed communicating hydrocephalus after IVH. IVH expansion/extension may also occur, particularly in patients with an underlying vascular lesion or in the setting of a coagulopathy.

Although plain head CT scan is often sufficient to determine the presence and extent of IVH, to monitor its progression, and to identify hydrocephalus, we recommend that patients with IVH undergo further imaging with MRI and MRA or CTA during the early days of hospitalization to rule out an underlying vascular malformation particularly when an obvious cause such as trauma, concomitant use of anticoagulation therapy, or a hypertensive deep ICH is absent. Repeat imaging including MRI with gadolinium and/or a conventional cerebral angiogram may be warranted in some cases [4], where the suspicion for an underlying lesion is high, after approximately 4–8 weeks to allow for reabsorption of the IVH.

The treatment of IVH should focus on prevention of IVH expansion, early detection and treatment of hydrocephalus and high intracranial pressure, and prevention and treatment of medical complications of ICH such as aspiration and deep vein thrombosis. The latter conforms to the general recommendations of the American Heart Association/American Stroke Association Guidelines for management of spontaneous ICH [5]. The insertion of an EVD to facilitate the drainage of blood and cerebrospinal fluid has been the standard initial treatment strategy for acute hydrocephalus resulting from IVH. However, difficulty in maintaining EVD patency led to a rising interest in the use of intraventricular thrombolysis, i.e., administration of thrombolytic agents such as tissue plasminogen activator (t-PA) through EVD, as an effective way to maintain EVD patency to remove IVH in order to relieve obstructive hydrocephalus and to reduce the toxic effects of blood product in the ventricles with the hope of improving survival and long-term functional outcomes. Indeed, animal studies and small clinical series, largely open-label or retrospective, have reported that intraventricular administration of fibrinolytic agents, including t-PA, is safe and may reduce morbidity and mortality after IVH by accelerating blood clearance and clot lysis [6–10].

The efficacy of intraventricular fibrinolysis in IVH, however, has been debatable. While a Cochrane review in 2002 found no sufficient good quality evidence from randomized trials to determine whether this approach does more good than harm [11], a subsequent meta-analysis in 2014 of 8 randomized and 16 observational studies found that intraventricular thrombolysis reduces mortality, decreases the need for ventriculoperitoneal (VP) shunt placement, and improves functional outcome after IVH [12]. However, the included trials were underpowered to support concrete recommendations about the use of intraventricular t-PA in IVH. Most recently, the largest, randomized, placebo-controlled trial of intraventricular t-PA in IVH (CLEAR III trial) was completed [13].

In this trial, 500 patients with stable, non-traumatic, spontaneous ICH less than 30 ml with secondary IVH obstructing the 3rd or 4th ventricles were randomized to receive up to 12 doses (8 h apart) of 1 mg of t-PA or normal saline via an EVD. It is important to point out that patients with coagulopathy-associated ICH/IVH and those with suspected underlying vascular malformation were not included in this trial. Expectedly, treatment with t-PA led to greater end-of-treatment IVH removal compared with saline; 33% of t-PA vs. 10% of the saline-treated patients had 80% of the IVH removed by the end of treatment. However, there was a wide variability in the number and location of EVDs and number of treatment doses within the trial, which may have impacted the removal of IVH. The primary efficacy outcome was good functional outcome, defined as modified Rankin Scale score (mRS) of ≤3 after 6 months. The primary efficacy outcome was similar in the t-PA- and saline-treated groups; 48% of t-PA-treated patients vs. 45% of saline-treated patients achieved good outcome at 6 months (risk ratio 1.06; 95% CI 0.88–1.28; $p = 0.55$), even after adjustment for IVH volume and thalamic location of ICH (risk ratio 1.98; 95% CI 0.90–1.29; $p = 0.42$). However, a reduction in the odds of death after 6 months by 50% was noted in the group treated with t-PA (adjusted odds ratio 0.50; 95% CI 0.31–0.80; $p = 0.55$). Mortality at 6 months was significantly lower (18% vs. 29%) in the t-PA treated group compared to the saline-treated group (hazard ratio 0.60; 95% CI 0.41–0.86; $p = 0.006$). In secondary post hoc analyses, faster and greater removal of IVH with t-PA was associated with mRS ≤3 (adjusted odds ratio 0.96; 95% CI 0.94–0.97; $p < 0.0001$) and lower case fatality (adjusted hazard ratio 1.03; 95% CI 1.02–1.04; $p < 0.0001$). Patients with initial IVH volume ≥ 20 ml also achieved better functional outcomes with t-PA, and the probability of good functional recovery increased when IVH clearance was >80%.

Most recently, we conducted a meta-analysis of six randomized-controlled trials, including CLEAR III, involving a total of 607 IVH patients, and found similar results; the use of intraventricular thrombolysis in IVH patients reduced all-cause mortality (risk ratio 0.63; 95% CI 0.47–0.83). However, the use of t-PA did not reduce the proportion of survivors with poor functional outcome (risk ratio 1.39; 95% CI 1.04–1.77), the composite end point of death and poor functional outcome (risk ratio 0.96; 95% CI 0.83–1.11), and the need for VP shunt placement (risk ratio 1.06; 95% CI 0.75–1.49) after secondary IVH [14].

Conclusion

The above data suggest that in most patients with IVH, local administration of t-PA (1 mg up to 12 doses 8 h apart) via an EVD is unlikely to benefit their functional recovery. While IVF appears to be safe, its benefit is limited to a reduction in mortality at the expense of increased number of survivors with moderately severe to severe disability. There is insufficient data to determine if this approach is more beneficial in a subset of IVH patients with thalamic ICH or IVH ≥20 ml. There is also no data to determine whether t-PA doses >1 ml or > 12 doses are safe. The decision to use intraventricular thrombolysis in IVH patients should take into account the patients'/family's attributes toward survival and dependency. Obviously, the use of t-PA should be restricted to patients who do not have an underlying vascular malformation and cautiously considered or if not avoided in patients with a large ICH or an associated coagulopathy. If the decision is made to use t-PA, experience from CLEAR III provides some helpful insights: (1) greater clot clearance is achieved with EVD placed ipsilateral to the dominant IVH; (2) in patients with IVH ≥20 ml, greater clot removal is achieved with multiple EVDs than with a single EVD; and (3) higher number of t-PA doses (up to 12) facilitates better IVH removal.

The Use of Recombinant Factor VII A (rFVIIa) in ICH

Case A 63-year-old man presented with sudden onset of aphasia and right-sided weakness within 3 h of symptom onset. Head CT scan revealed a 20 ml left fronto-temporal ICH and subdural hemorrhage. Head CTA was noted for the presence of a "spot sign" within the hematoma. His past medical history was noted for coronary artery disease. His medications included aspirin and atorvastatin. Routine laboratory studies, including coagulation studies, were within normal limits. He was treated with rFVIIa at a dose of 80 μg per kilogram.

Discussion

Early hematoma expansion is one of the most consistent predictors of poor outcome and mortality after ICH [15]. Hematoma growth after ICH is a common phenomenon; an increase in ICH volume > 33% is noted in approximately 38% of ICH patients initially scanned within 3 h of ICH onset [16]. This is attributed to continued bleeding or re-bleeding within the hematoma region or in its vicinity.

Recombinant activated factor VII (rFVIIa), which is used to treat hemophilia, has eluded us since the early 2000s as a potential hemostatic therapeutic strategy to stop bleeding in order to limit ICH growth. In 2005, a phase 2A trial of 399 patients with spontaneous ICH randomized patients to receive placebo or 40 μg of rFVIIa per kilogram of body weight, 80 μg per kilogram, or 160 μg per kilogram within 4 h after ICH onset [17]. The primary outcome measure was the percent change in the volume of ICH at 24 h. Clinical outcomes were assessed at 90 days. Treatment with rFVIIa limited the growth of the hematoma, reduced mortality, and improved functional outcomes at 90 days relative to placebo. The mean increase in ICH volume after 24 h was 29% in the placebo group, compared with 16%, 14%, and 11% in the rFVIIa groups ($p = 0.01$). At day 90, 61% of placebo-treated patients died or were severely disabled (as defined by mRS score of 4–6), compared with 55%, 49%, and 54% of the patients who were treated with rFVIIa ($p = 0.004$). In a subsequent phase 3 trial involving 841 patients with spontaneous ICH, treatment with rFVIIa did not improve survival or functional outcome despite reducing hematoma expansion [18]. The mean increase in ICH volume at 24 h was 26% in the placebo group, compared with 18% in the group receiving 20 μg of rFVIIa per kilogram ($p = 0.09$) and 11% in the group receiving 80 μg ($p < 0.001$). However, there was no significant difference among the three groups in the proportion of patients with mRS <4 between the three groups. Furthermore, arterial thromboembolic and myocardial adverse events were more frequent in the group receiving 80 μg/kg of rFVIIa than in the placebo group (9% vs. 4%; $p = 0.04$). A subsequent post hoc subgroup analysis of the trials' datasets investigated whether rFVIIa might be beneficial in a particular subset of ICH patients. This analysis indicated that patients ≤70 years of age with baseline ICH volume < 60 ml and IVH volume < 5 ml who were treated with 80 μg of rFVIIa within ≤2.5 h of ICH onset had an adjusted odds ratio of 0.28 (95% CI 0.08–1.06) for poor outcome and doubling in the reduction of ICH growth (7.3 ± 3.2 vs. 3.8 ± 1.5 ml; $p = 0.02$) [19].

Most recently, two collaborative trials, the SPOTLIGHT trial in Canada and STOP-IT in the United States, utilized contrast extravasation on CT angiogram, termed "the spot sign," to improve patient selection and to identify ICH patients at greater risk for hematoma expansion for treatment with rFVIIa [20]. A total of 69 spot sign-positive patients were randomly assigned within 6.5 h of ICH onset to receive 80 μg/kg of rFVIIa or placebo, while 73 spot sign-negative patients were enrolled into a prospective observational cohort with the same inclusion criteria. The primary outcome was the ICH volume on 24-h CT scan. In spot sign-positive patients, the median baseline ICH volume in rFVIIa-treated group was 16 ml and 22 ml on 24 h scan vs. 20 and 29 ml, respectively, in placebo-treated patients ($p = 0.9$). At 90 days, there was no difference in the proportion of patients with mRS 5–6 between rFVIIa and placebo groups (20% vs. 21%; $p = 0.6$). It has been argued, however, that poor enrollment which led to a small sample size and late ICH onset to treatment time might have contributed to these disappointing results.

Conclusion

In light of the above data, we do not recommend the use of rFVIIa as a treatment for spontaneous ICH at this time. Although its use can limit hematoma growth, it is also associated with an increase, albeit small, in thromboembolic and myocardial adverse events with no benefit on functional outcome. We also do not recommend routine use of rFVIIa as the sole hemostatic agent for reversal of coagulopathy in warfarin-associated ICH. Although rFVIIa can rapidly normalize international normalized ratio (INR), it does not replenish all vitamin K-dependent factors and may not restore thrombin generation and clotting despite lowering INR [21].

ICH Related to Brain Arteriovenous Malformation (BAVM) and Dural Arteriovenous Fistula (DAVF)

Case A 50-year-old woman presented with headache of sudden onset with associated nausea and vomiting. Headache was reported as left frontal in location and severity of pain rated as 10 (on a 10-point scale). She had no associated visual disturbance, weakness, tingling or numbness, or speech impairment at headache onset. Patient had a long-standing history of headaches diagnosed as migraines, occurring in the left frontal area, associated with nausea and blurred vision. Duration of headaches reported as several hours to a day. Headache frequency has decreased over the years to 1 headache day every 3–4 months. At current presentation, characteristics of headache reported as different include sudden onset of headache and severity worse than any of her prior episodes. She also had a history of an untreated brain arteriovenous malformation (bAVM), first diagnosed approximately 24 years ago.

Initial CT head without contrast revealed acute left parieto-occipital intraparenchymal hemorrhage measuring about 2.7 cm in diameter, subdural hematoma in the left frontal convexity measuring 9 mm, and a midline shift to the right measuring 8.3 mm (Fig. 9.2a). Extra-axial extension of hemorrhage was noted along the interhemispheric fissure and left tentorial leaflet to overly the frontal and temporal lobes. CT angiogram of the head indicated a large arteriovenous malformation in the left parietal-occipital region with arterial feeders from the left posterior cerebral artery (PCA), left anterior cerebral artery (ACA), and left middle cerebral artery (MCA). Venous drainage involved both the superficial and the deep cortical veins. A repeat neurological examination revealed no focal deficits except for a new right homonymous hemianopsia. The ICH score was 0 with hemorrhage volume < 30 cc. Blood pressure goal of SBP <160 was maintained with intravenous nicardipine infusion; headache was managed with acetaminophen 500 mg q 12 h and seizure prophylaxis with levetiracetam 500 mg q 12 h. Euvolemia and euglycemia were maintained (target glucose 100–180 mg/dL). Patient underwent conventional cerebral angiogram

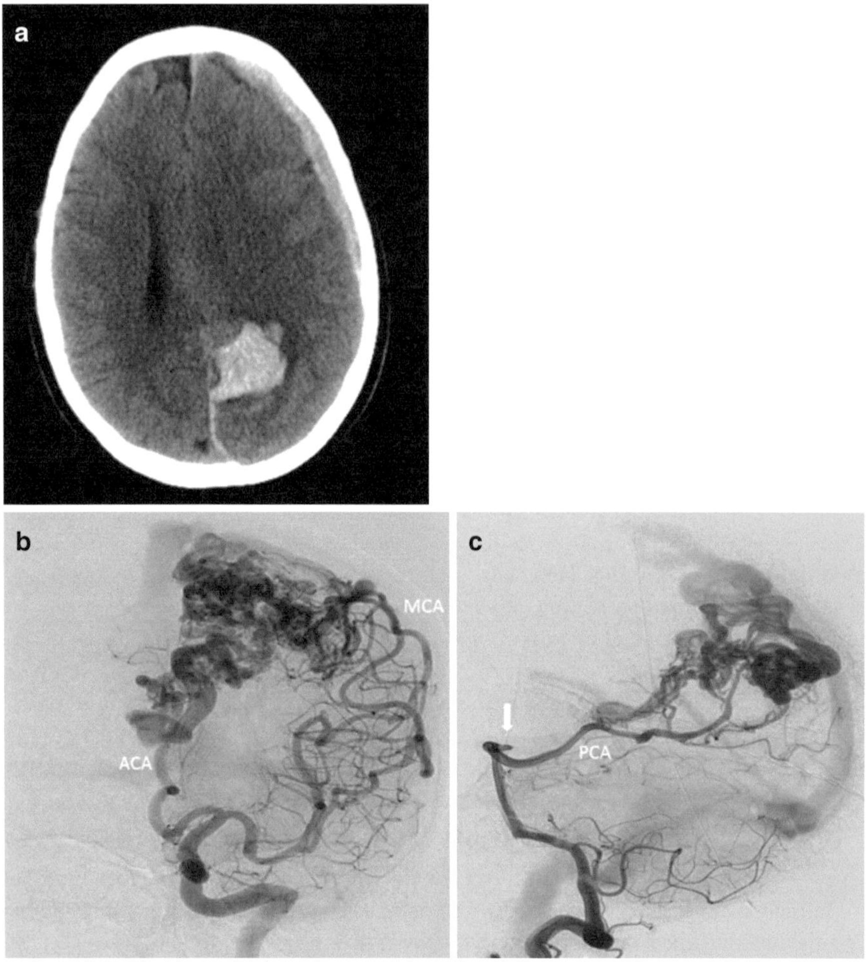

Fig. 9.2 (**a**) CT head without contrast showing intraparenchymal (left parieto-occipital) and left subdural hematoma (left frontal convexity). (**b**, **c**) Angiographic image of the arteriovenous malformation with anterior, middle, and posterior cerebral arteries (ACA, MCA, PCA). A small aneurysm (white arrow) from proximal segment of the PCA. (**d**, **e**) Angiographic image showing arterial feeders from the left PCA before (**d**) and after (**e**) embolization and aneurysm coiling (white arrow). (**f**) An image showing a large flow-related aneurysm (white arrow) of left posterior inferior cerebellar artery supplying the arteriovenous malformation

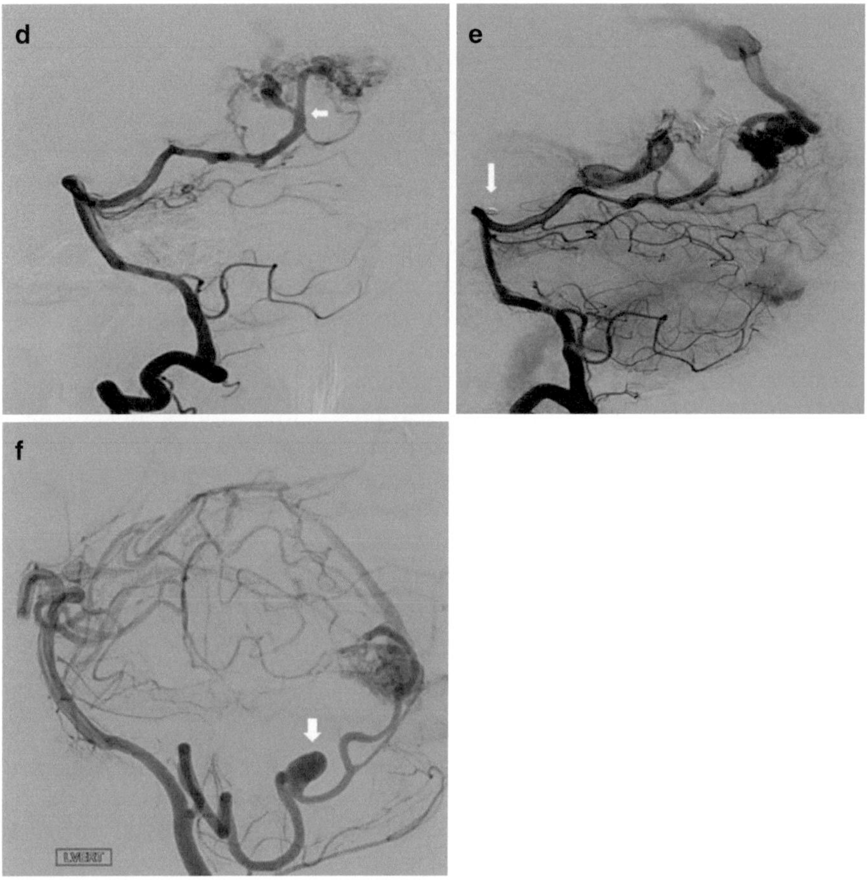

Fig. 9.2 (continued)

which demonstrated a Spetzler-Martin grade IV AVM (Fig. 9.2b, c). The size of the nidus measured 5.9 cm anterioposteriorly, 3.9 cm horizontally, and 4.7 cm cranio-caudally. The left PCA had a small aneurysm measuring 2.5 mm (Fig. 9.2c) in the proximal segment at the basilar tip and a dysplastic segment distally. There was evidence of azygos ACA with large pedicle feeding the superior aspect of the AVM. Venous drainage involved cortical veins draining into the superior sagittal sinus and deep drainage into the vein of Galen and straight sinus. Also evident were small feeding arteries from the left MCA feeders. Patient underwent left-sided burr hole craniotomy and evacuation of subdural hematoma. After a stable hospital course, the patient was discharged with a treatment plan of staged embolization followed by surgical resection and/or stereotactic radiosurgery (SRS). She underwent initial primary coiling of the feeding artery aneurysm of the left PCA and embolization to occlude the two feeders of the left PCA (Fig. 9.2d, e) using Onyx® liquid embolic agent (ev3, Irvine, CA).

Discussion

Brain AVMs represent an abnormal connection between the arterial and venous system in the brain without a well-defined intermediate capillary network. The term *nidus* is used to describe the entangled blood vessel of the AVM, and the size of which has significant treatment and prognostic implications. Incidence of bAVMs ranges from 0.7 to 1.3 per 100,000 population [21–23]. Although uncertain, the etiology of bAVMs is considered congenital, and these lesions may remain asymptomatic for decades (similar to case presented). Brain AVMs account for 2–4% of all hemorrhagic strokes [24]. Spontaneous intracranial hemorrhage, intraparenchymal and/or subarachnoid, accounts for as high as 40% of the clinical presentations in patients with bAVMs [25]. Apart from intracranial hemorrhage and chronic headaches (similar to case presented), patients may present with seizures, stroke, or transient ischemic attack and non-focal neurological symptoms. In unruptured bAVMs, the risk of hemorrhage is estimated to range approximately from 2% to 5% per year, and the risk is higher in bAMV patients with Spetzler-Martin grade IV or V and is associated with poor outcomes [26]. Mortality associated with ruptured AVMs ranges from 10% to 29% with initial hemorrhage and could reach 50% with posterior fossa involvement, particularly if involved with ruptured intranidal or flow-related arterial aneurysms [27]. In ruptured AVMs, risk of subsequent hemorrhage is high in the first year after hemorrhage (6–17%) [28].

Diagnostic evaluation starts in most cases after an incidental finding of hyperdense lesions on non-contrast CT head with focal areas of calcification or presence of “flow voids” on MRI brain T2-weighted sequence. Scientific evidence on management of bAVMs recommends tailored treatment of these unique vascular lesions based on patient’s age, clinical presentation, characteristics associated with high risk of hemorrhage and/or mortality such as large intranidal or flow-related aneurysms (Fig. 9.2f), deep venous drainage, venous outflow stenosis, single draining vein, involvement of vertebrobasilar system, periventricular or ventricular area of AVM location, etc. [29, 30]. While there is relative clarity on the role of intervention in ruptured bAVMs, there are no widely accepted guidelines for unruptured AVMs. A randomized trial of unruptured bAVMs comparing medical management to medical and intervention with embolization, radiosurgery, and/or surgery showed significantly more adverse events of stroke or death in the interventional arm [31]. Concerns raised about this clinical trial include underrepresentation of surgical treatment (4% surgery, 26% embolization, 27% radiosurgery), majority of Spetzler-Martin grade I–II lesions undergoing embolization, incomplete treatment with non-obliteration of AVM, and inadequate follow-up posttreatment. Treatment of bAVMs has inherent risks and may result in permanent neurological deficits [32]. The risk associated with surgical treatment in patients with Spetzler-Martin grades I–III is reported as low [33] and utilizing this grading system for estimating the morbidity and mortality associated with surgical intervention of bAVMs is recommended [34]. Brain AVM is a dynamic vascular condition, and in cases with partial embolization, neuroangiogenesis and growth of the bAVM after embolization are reported [35].

Therefore, it is conceivable that partial treatment with incomplete embolization of the nidus does not eliminate the risk of hemorrhage.

Endovascular treatment of AVMs frequently involves use of liquid embolic agents such as nBCA (n-butylcyanoacrylate) labelled as Trufill (Codman Neurovascular, Rayman, MA), an ethylene-vinyl alcohol polymer labelled as Onyx (ev3, Irvine, CA) and administered with dimethyl-sulfoxide (DMSO), or less frequently coils to decrease the flow in the feeding arteries followed by use of liquid embolic material for controlled and effective treatment. Embolization of arterial feeders and/or aneurysms of the AVM is frequently done prior to surgical resection to decrease intraoperative bleeding. Alternatively, embolization can be followed by stereotactic radiosurgery (SRS) or used independently to achieve angiographic cure in select cases. For acute ruptured AVMs, embolization procedure should be delayed by 1–2 weeks to allow for resolution of any edema or mass effect. Post-embolization, blood pressure management in the ICU is critical, particularly in situations such as early venous penetration and/or occlusion of venous drainage during embolization or after embolization of large nidus which may incite autoregulatory failure and breakthrough hemorrhage. Stereotactic radiosurgery (SRS) is considered a potential option in the management of Spetzler-Martin grade I–III AVMs that are small in size (< 3 cm of nidus) and deep seated and involve eloquent areas of the brain [36–38]. Treatment response is expected several years after the SRS (approximately 3–5 years), and the risk of hemorrhage during the early period may match the expected natural history of AVMs and is reduced overtime [31, 39, 40].

Conclusion

Brain AVMs frequently present with intracranial hemorrhage and carry a significant mortality and morbidity. Management of bAVMs is complex due to the dynamic nature of the disease. Conclusive evidence or consensus on the best management strategy for bAVMs is currently not available. As there is an inherent risk of lifetime hemorrhage in patients with bAVMs, a thorough diagnostic workup and therapeutic evaluation are recommended. A multimodality treatment approach with a goal of complete elimination of the AVM and balanced by a clinical benefit overtime is most preferred. Long-term angiographic follow-up may be essential to confirm stability of these vascular lesions.

Dural Arteriovenous Fistulas (DAVF)

Case A 62-year-old male presented with mild headache and visual disturbance. He had left homonymous hemianopsia and no other focal neurological deficits on exam. Initial non-contrast CT revealed a small right occipital intraparenchymal hemorrhage (Fig. 9.3a). Further investigations included a MRI brain with and

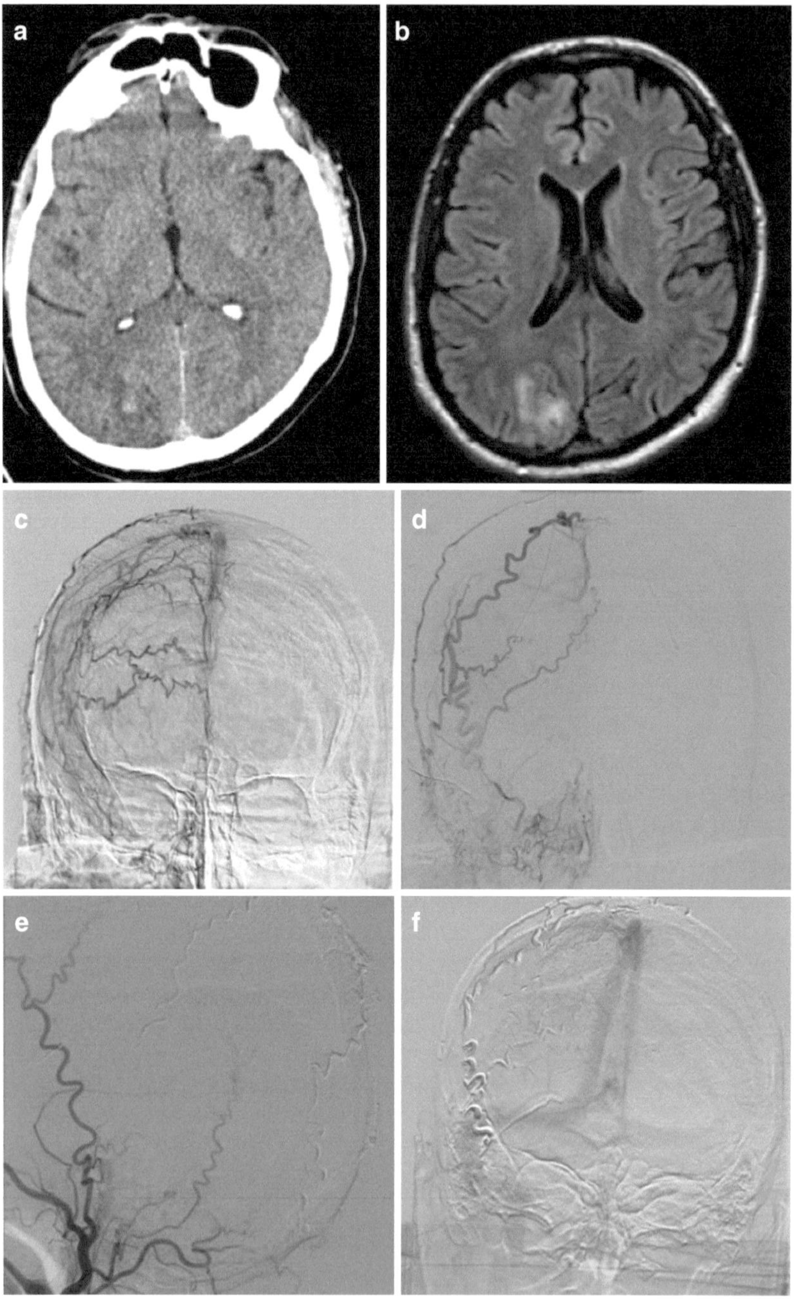

Fig. 9.3 (**a**, **b**) Non-contrast CT and MR imaging (FLAIR sequence) of head showing small right occipital hemorrhage with surrounding edema. (**c**, **d**) Angiography in anterior-posterior projection showing fistulous drainage from right external carotid artery branches to superior sagittal sinus and venous reflux. (**e**, **f**) Arterial and venous phases of angiography done post-embolization of occipital and superficial temporal artery branches connecting to the fistula

without contrast and MRA head. Again, occipital hemorrhage with surrounding edema and mild regional mass effect was noted (Fig. 9.3b). No clear abnormal vasculature was seen on MR angiography, but there was overabundance of flow voids within the region of hemorrhage on T2-weighted imaging suspicious for an underlying arteriovenous malformation. A conventional cerebral angiogram was performed which revealed evidence of Borden type III dural arteriovenous fistula (dAVF) with venous drainage directly into cortical veins and then into anterior and middle third of the superior sagittal sinus. Arterial connections of the dAVF were from bilateral external carotid arteries, mainly the right occipital artery (OA), middle meningeal artery (MMA), superficial temporal artery (STA), and the left MMA (Fig. 9.3c). Evidence of leptomeningeal venous drainage was noted, and patient underwent embolization of the OA, STA, and MMA feeders to shut down a significant number of fistulous connections (Fig. 9.3d–f). On follow-up cerebral angiography, previously noted meningeal venous reflux was no longer seen.

Discussion

Abnormal communications within the dura between dural arteries and, less frequently, the pial arteries and the dural venous sinuses are termed as dural arteriovenous fistulas (dAVFs). These vascular lesions in adults are frequently acquired unlike the other arteriovenous malformations. Different etiologies such as sinus thrombosis or surgery have been implicated in this phenomenon [41, 42]. In the pediatric population, the abnormal dural arteriovenous connections are associated with structural venous abnormalities and represent a distinct clinical group of vascular anomalies. Traumatic lesions involving the skull base and leading to intracranial arteriovenous shunts in previously normal vascular substrate, such as carotid-cavernous fistula, represents a distinct clinical subset and not discussed in this chapter. Clinical presentation of the dAVFs is commonly based on the location of fistulous connection and type of venous drainage. The widely used classifications of dAVFs are also based on the venous drainage in relationship to clinical presentation [43–45]. The two commonly involved venous sinuses are the transverse-sigmoid sinus and the cavernous sinus. Symptoms such as pulsatile tinnitus and/or headache are associated with transverse-sigmoid sinus and cranial nerve deficits and ocular symptoms with cavernous sinus. DAVFs may also present with many different signs and symptoms such as exophthalmos, papilledema from raised intracranial pressure, and focal neurological deficits. The most feared clinical presentation of DAVFs is spontaneous intracranial hemorrhage. The major determinant of hemorrhagic risk is the venous drainage pattern and severity of cortical venous reflux if present. In patients with dAVF, the incidence of ICH is reported as high as 42%, and commonly the hemorrhage is intraparenchymal [43, 46]. The annual risk of hemorrhage is reported as 8% and non-hemorrhagic neurological deficits as 7% [46, 47]. Patients with dAVF and initial presentation of ICH have a 35% risk of re-hemorrhage within the first few weeks [48]. Therefore, treatment is recommended in patients with leptomeningeal or cortical venous reflux, and conservative management is proposed for dAVFs without such drainage pattern.

Diagnostic evaluation of patients with neurological complaints frequently starts with non-contrast CT head, and presence of hemorrhage may warrant further evaluation with MRI of the brain. Prominent vasculature in the vicinity of the hemorrhage or along the cerebral or cerebellar convexities may be evident raising the possibility of AVM or dural-based AVF. Cerebral catheter angiography is essential to confirm the presence or absence of underlying dAVF and associated pattern of venous drainage with or without dangerous features such as venous ectasia or aneurysms [49].

Management of dAVFs depends on the type of venous drainage and lesions draining directly into the venous sinuses with antegrade flow, and no evidence of cortical venous reflux can be managed conservatively [41, 50, 51]. In cases with a high flow across the shunt affecting normal venous drainage of the brain or presence of clinical symptoms such as bruits, tinnitus, vision abnormalities, etc., intervention may be reasonable after weighing the benefits with the risks involved with treatment. Treatment of dAVFs could be performed in several stages if the lesions are multifocal or extensive [51]. If there is involvement of cavernous sinus with progressive visual impairment, then intervention would be needed urgently. Treatment may involve arterial approach to the AVF or retrograde venous approach after excluding venous obstruction, stenosis, or thrombosis [52]. Goal of treatment in cases with leptomeningeal or cortical venous reflux should be curative due to the aggressive nature of the disease and in select cases may require surgical disconnection of the shunting lesion post-endovascular therapy. Arterial embolization for treatment of dAVFs is beneficial in majority of the cases and cure achieved with endovascular approach in up to 88% of the cases [46, 47, 52]. Embolic materials regularly used for arterial approaches include nBCA and Onyx. Transvenous approach to shut off the cortical venous reflux by maintaining a patent venous sinus may be occasionally needed to cure the dAVFs. Surgical approaches such as intraoperative embolization, dural resection, etc. are reserved for failed endovascular treatments.

Conclusion

Dural arteriovenous fistulas in adults are acquired lesions involving the dural arteries, and their clinical presentation is often based on the venous drainage patterns. Lesions with cortical or leptomeningeal venous reflux have a relatively higher risk of hemorrhage or neurological deficits, and curative treatment of these lesions is recommended. Management of dAVFs mainly involves endovascular embolization via transarterial approach and in select cases transvenously using embolic materials with or without coils to obliterate the fistulous connections.

Acknowledgments Authors would like to thank Dr. Reid Gooch from the Department of Neurosurgery, Thomas Jefferson University for sharing a case of brain arteriovenous malformation for presentation in this chapter.

References

1. Bhattathiri PS, Gregson B, Prasad KS, Mendelow AD, STICH Investigators. Intraventricular hemorrhage and hydrocephalus after spontaneous intracerebral hemorrhage: results from the STICH trial. Acta Neurochir Suppl. 2006;96:65–8.
2. Witsch J, Bruce E, Meyers E, Velazquez A, Schmidt JM, Suwatcharangkoon S, et al. Intraventricular hemorrhage expansion in patients with spontaneous intracerebral hemorrhage. Neurology. 2015;84(10):989–94.
3. Passero S, Ulivelli M, Reale F. Primary intraventricular haemorrhage in adults. Acta Neurol Scand. 2002;105:115–9.
4. Zhu XL, Chan MS, Poon WS. Spontaneous intracranial hemorrhage: which patients need diagnostic cerebral angiography? A prospective study of 206 cases and review of the literature. Stroke. 1997;28:1406–9.
5. Hemphill JC 3rd, Greenberg SM, Anderson CS, Becker K, Bendok BR, Cushman M, et al. Guidelines for the management of spontaneous intracerebral hemorrhage: a guideline for healthcare professionals from the American Heart Association/American Stroke Association. Stroke. 2015;46:2032–60.
6. Wang YC, Lin CW, Shen CC, Lai SC, Kuo JS. Tissue plasminogen activator for the treatment of intraventricular hematoma: the dose-effect relationship. J Neurol Sci. 2002;202(1–2):35–41.
7. Ávila C, Lozano C, De La Cueva VA, Moliner J, López M, San Miguel F, et al. Intraventricular hemorrhage treated with intraventricular fibrinolysis: a 10-year experience. Med Intensiva. 2013;37:61–6.
8. Dunatov S, Antoncic I, Bralic M, Jurjevic A. Intraventricular thrombolysis with rt-PA in patients with intraventricular hemorrhage. Acta Neurol Scand. 2011;124:343–8.
9. Fountas KN, Kapsalaki EZ, Parish DC, Smith B, Smisson HF, Johnston KW, et al. Intraventricular administration of rt-PA in patients with intraventricular hemorrhage. South Med J. 2005;98:767–73.
10. Naff N, Williams MA, Keyl PM, Tuhrim S, Bullock MR, Mayer SA, et al. Low-dose recombinant tissue-type plasminogen activator enhances clot resolution in brain hemorrhage: the intraventricular hemorrhage thrombolysis trial. Stroke. 2011;42:3009–16.
11. Lapointe M, Haines S. Fibrinolytic therapy for intraventricular hemorrhage in adults. Cochrane Database Syst Rev. 2002:CD003692.
12. Khan NR, Tsivgoulis G, Lee SL, Jones GM, Green CS, Katsanos AH, et al. Fibrinolysis for intraventricular hemorrhage: an updated meta-analysis and systematic review of the literature. Stroke. 2014;45:2662–9.
13. Hanley DF, Lane K, McBee N, Ziai W, Tuhrim S, Lees KR, et al. Thrombolytic removal of intraventricular haemorrhage in treatment of severe stroke: results of the randomised, multicentre, multiregion, placebo-controlled clear iii trial. Lancet. 2017;389(10069):603–11.
14. Wang D, Liu J, Norton C, Liu M, Selim M. Local fibrinolytic therapy for intraventricular hemorrhage: a meta-analysis of randomized controlled trials. 6th World Intracranial Hemorrhage Conference, Baltimore, May 2017 (abstract).
15. Dowlatshahi D, Demchuk AM, Flaherty ML, Ali M, Lyden PL, Smith EE, et al. Defining hematoma expansion in intracerebral hemorrhage: relationship with patient outcomes. Neurology. 2011;76(14):1238–44.
16. Brott T, Broderick J, Kothari R, Barsan W, Tomsick T, Sauerbeck L, et al. Early hemorrhage growth in patients with intracerebral hemorrhage. Stroke. 1997;28:1–5.

17. Diringer MN, Skolnick BE, Mayer SA, Steiner T, Davis SM, Brun NC, et al. Thromboembolic events with recombinant activated factor VII in spontaneous intracerebral hemorrhage: results from the Factor Seven for Acute Hemorrhagic Stroke (FAST) trial. Stroke. 2010;41:48–53.
18. Mayer SA, Brun NC, Begtrup K, Broderick J, Davis S, Diringer MN, et al. Efficacy and safety of recombinant activated factor VII for acute intracerebral hemorrhage. N Engl J Med. 2008;358(20):2127–37.
19. Mayer SA, Davis SM, Skolnick BE, Brun NC, Begtrup K, Broderick JP, et al. Can a subset of intracerebral hemorrhage patients benefit from hemostatic therapy with recombinant activated factor VII? Stroke. 2009;40:833–40.
20. Gladstone D, Aviv R, Demchuk A, Hill MD, Thorpe K, Khoury J, Sucharew H, De Masi S, Ka L, Mamdani M, Al-Ajlan F, Carrozzella J, Jauch E, Broderick JP, Flaherty M; for the SPOTLIGHT and STOP-IT Study Steering Committee and Investigators. Randomized trial of hemostatic therapy for 'Spot Sign' positive intracerebral hemorrhage: primary results from the SPOTLIGHT/STOP-IT Collaboration. AHA International Stroke Conference, Houston, February 2017 (abstract).
21. Brown RD Jr, Wiebers DO, Torner JC, O'Fallon WM. Incidence and prevalence of intracranial vascular malformations in Olmsted County, Minnesota, 1965 to 1992. Neurology. 1996;46(4):949–52.
22. Berman MF, Sciacca RR, Pile-Spellman J, Stapf C, Connolly ES Jr, Mohr JP, et al. The epidemiology of brain arteriovenous malformations. Neurosurgery. 2000;47(2):389–96; discussion 397.
23. ApSimon HT, Reef H, Phadke RV, Popovic EA. A population-based study of brain arteriovenous malformation: long-term treatment outcomes. Stroke. 33(12):2794–800.
24. Choi JH, Mohr JP. Brain arteriovenous malformations in adults. Lancet Neurol. 2005;4(5):299–308.
25. Brown RD Jr, Wiebers DO, Forbes G, O'Fallon WM, Piepgras DG, Marsh WR, et al. The natural history of unruptured intracranial arteriovenous malformations. J Neurosurg. 1998;68(3):352–7.
26. Mast H, Young WL, Koennecke HC, Sciacca RR, Osipov A, Pile-Spellman J, et al. Risk of spontaneous haemorrhage after diagnosis of cerebral arteriovenous malformation. Lancet. 1997;350(9084):1065–8.
27. Wilkins RH. Natural history of intracranial vascular malformations: a review. Neurosurgery. 1985;16(3):421–30.
28. Ondra SL, Troupp H, George ED, Schwab K. The natural history of symptomatic arteriovenous malformations of the brain: a 24-year follow-up assessment. J Neurosurg. 1990;73(3):387–91.
29. Stapf C, Mast H, Sciacca RR, Choi JH, Khaw AV, Connolly ES, et al. Predictors of hemorrhage in patients with untreated brain arteriovenous malformation. Neurology. 2006;66(9):1350–5.
30. Hetts SW, Cooke DL, Nelson J, Gupta N, Fullerton H, Amans MR, et al. Influence of patient age on angioarchitecture of brain arteriovenous malformations. AJNR Am J Neuroradiol. 2014;35(7):1376–80.
31. Mohr JP, Parides MK, Stapf C, Moquete E, Moy CS, Overbey JR, et al. Medical management with or without interventional therapy for unruptured brain arteriovenous malformations (ARUBA): a multicentre, non-blinded, randomised trial. Lancet. 2014;383(9917):614–21.
32. Hartmann A, Mast H, Mohr JP, Pile-Spellman J, Connolly ES, Sciacca RR, et al. Determinants of staged endovascular and surgical treatment outcome of brain arteriovenous malformations. Stroke. 2005;36(11):2431–5.
33. Cunha e Sa MJ, Stein BM, Solomon RA, McCormick PC. The treatment of associated intracranial aneurysms and arteriovenous malformations. J Neurosurg. 1992;77(6):853–9.
34. Hamilton MG, Spetzler RF. The prospective application of a grading system for arteriovenous malformations. Neurosurgery. 1994;34(1):2–6.
35. Sure U, Butz N, Siegel AM, Mennel HD, Bien S, Bertalanffy H. Treatment-induced neoangiogenesis in cerebral arteriovenous malformations. Clin Neurol Neurosurg. 2001;103(1):29–32.

36. Ding D, Starke RM, Kano H, Mathieu D, Huang PP, Kondziolka D, et al. Stereotactic radiosurgery for ARUBA (a randomized trial of unruptured brain arteriovenous malformations)-eligible Spetzler-Martin grade I and II arteriovenous malformations: a multicenter study. World Neurosurg. 2017;102:507–17.
37. Morgan MK, Hermann Wiedmann MK, Stoodley MA, Heller GZ. Microsurgery for Spetzler-Ponce class A and B arteriovenous malformations utilizing an outcome score adopted from gamma knife radiosurgery: a prospective cohort study. J Neurosurg. 2016;23:1–12.
38. Ding D, Yen CP, Starke RM, Xu Z, Sun X, Sheehan JP. Radiosurgery for Spetzler-Martin grade III arteriovenous malformations. J Neurosurg. 2014;120(4):959–69.
39. Ding D, Yen CP, Xu Z, Starke RM, Sheehan JP. Radiosurgery for patients with unruptured intracranial arteriovenous malformations. J Neurosurg. 2013;118(5):958–66.
40. Maruyama K, Kawahara N, Shin M, Tago M, Kishimoto J, Kurita H, et al. The risk of hemorrhage after radiosurgery for cerebral arteriovenous malformations. N Engl J Med. 2005;352(2):146–53.
41. Chaudhary MY, Sachdev VP, Cho SH, Weitzner I Jr, Puljic S, Huang YP. Dural arteriovenous malformation of the major venous sinuses: an acquired lesion. AJNR Am J Neuroradiol. 1982;3(1):13–9.
42. Watanabe A, Takahara Y, Ibuchi Y, Mizukami K. Two cases of dural arteriovenous malformation occurring after intracranial surgery. Neuroradiology. 1984;26(5):375–80.
43. Cognard C, Gobin YP, Pierot L, Bailly AL, Houdart E, Casasco A, et al. Cerebral dural arteriovenous fistulas: clinical and angiographic correlation with a revised classification of venous drainage. Radiology. 1995;194(3):671–80.
44. Borden JA, Wu JK, Shucart WA. A proposed classification for spinal and cranial dural arteriovenous fistulous malformations and implications for treatment. J Neurosurg. 1995;82(2):166–79. Erratum in: J Neurosurg. 1995 Apr;82(4):705–6.
45. Davies MA, TerBrugge K, Willinsky R, Coyne T, Saleh J, Wallace MC. The validity of classification for the clinical presentation of intracranial dural arteriovenous fistulas. J Neurosurg. 1996;85(5):830–7.
46. Davies MA, Saleh J, Ter Brugge K, Willinsky R, Wallace MC. The natural history and management of intracranial dural arteriovenous fistulae. Part 1: benig lesions. Interv Neuroradiol. 1997;3(4):295–302.
47. Davies MA, Ter Brugge K, Willinsky R, Wallace MC. The natural history and management of intracranial dural arteriovenous fistulae. Part 2: aggressive lesions. Interv Neuroradiol. 1997;3(4):303–11.
48. Duffau H, Lopes M, Janosevic V, Sichez JP, Faillot T, Capelle L, et al. Early rebleeding from intracranial dural arteriovenous fistulas: report of 20 cases and review of the literature. J Neurosurg. 1999;90(1):78–84.
49. Willinsky R, Terbrugge K, Montanera W, Mikulis D, Wallace MC. Venous congestion: an MR finding in dural arteriovenous malformations with cortical venous drainage. AJNR Am J Neuroradiol. 1994;15(8):1501–7.
50. van Dijk JM, terBrugge KG, Willinsky RA, Wallace MC. Clinical course of cranial dural arteriovenous fistulas with long-term persistent cortical venous reflux. Stroke. 2002;33(5):1233–6.
51. van Dijk JM, TerBrugge KG, Willinsky RA, Wallace MC. Multiplicity of dural arteriovenous fistulas. J Neurosurg. 2002;96(1):76–8.
52. Roy D, Raymond J. The role of transvenous embolization in the treatment of intracranial dural arteriovenous fistulas. Neurosurgery. 1997;40(6):1133–41.

Chapter 10
Special Systems of Care Considerations in Intracerebral Haemorrhage

Aravind Ganesh and Michael D. Hill

Case Example

Mrs. Retiree was a 65-year-old smoker with a history of hypertension, living independently at home. She presented to the emergency department of a regional hospital with a new moderate-intensity headache accompanied by mild right arm numbness and weakness that had begun fairly suddenly 5 h ago. Her presentation was triaged as a "headache", and consequently she waited for an hour before being examined by an emergency physician, by which point her weakness had worsened and she had developed word-finding difficulties. A CT head was obtained within the next hour, which demonstrated a left frontal lobar haemorrhage with an estimated volume of 10 mL but no mass effect. A telephone referral was made to the neurosurgery team at the nearest tertiary hospital (7 h after onset), who reviewed the images remotely and declined the request to transfer the patient as there was no apparent indication for neurosurgical intervention. In the meantime, the patient was admitted to a busy general medical ward, where hourly blood pressure readings remained

A. Ganesh (✉)
Calgary Stroke Program, Department of Clinical Neurosciences, Cumming School of Medicine, University of Calgary, Calgary, Canada

Centre for Prevention of Stroke and Dementia, Nuffield Department of Clinical Neurosciences, University of Oxford, Oxford, UK

M. D. Hill
Calgary Stroke Program, Department of Clinical Neurosciences, Cumming School of Medicine, University of Calgary, Calgary, Canada

Department of Radiology, Department of Community Health Sciences, Department of Medicine, and Hotchkiss Brain Institute, Cumming School of Medicine, University of Calgary, Calgary, Canada

B. Ovbiagele, A. I. Qureshi (eds.), *Intracerebral Hemorrhage Therapeutics*,
https://doi.org/10.1007/978-3-319-77063-5_10

elevated (170–180 systolic). The ward did not have a protocol for neurological monitoring. She continued to complain about her headache. Fourteen hours after symptom onset, the nurse noticed that the patient was no longer responding to questions. The on-call medical resident found her to have dense right hemiparesis and global aphasia, and repeated the CT head which showed marked hematoma expansion with 1.5 cm midline shift and intraventricular extension. The neurosurgical team was contacted again, and arrangements were made to transfer her to the tertiary hospital. She suffered from severe generalized tonic-clonic seizures in the ambulance, which did not settle with intravenous lorazepam. She was unable to protect her airway, could not be intubated en route, and was pronounced dead upon her arrival to the tertiary hospital.

The Case for Integrated Stroke Systems of Care

As Mrs. Retiree's unfortunate case demonstrates, the management of intracerebral haemorrhage (ICH) presents a variety of complex challenges all along the continuum of care and is profoundly impacted by the availability and utilization of specialized healthcare resources. Given the specialized resources required to deliver high-quality stroke care, the Canadian Stroke Best Practice Recommendations, the American Stroke Association (ASA), and the World Stroke Organization's Global Stroke Services Guidelines have recommended the implementation of organized systems of stroke care delivery [1–3].

To have a stroke system of care means that care is coordinated and optimized along the entire stroke care continuum, from primary prevention to rehabilitation [2]. These include the designation of comprehensive stroke centres [4], development of regional strategies to guarantee appropriate interventions like emergency medical services (EMS) routing policies, pre- and in-hospital care protocols, stroke unit care, as well as inter-provider collaboration, the use of telemedicine to aid patient care in remote facilities, access to post-stroke rehabilitation, and the integration of quality of improvement programs [1]. Mrs. Retiree's case demonstrates several examples of mishaps along the stroke continuum of care that can be addressed by specific strategies; these are summarized in Table 10.1, with references to the relevant chapter section where such strategies are discussed.

Stroke systems of care apply to all stroke types, haemorrhagic and ischemic, though the largest effect of such systems will apply to ischemic stroke, simply because it is more prevalent. However, ICH is currently orphaned as a stroke type with a distinct lack of clearly proven acute interventions. Stroke unit care is the only intervention applicable to all stroke types including haemorrhage that is proven to result in reduced morbidity and mortality. Evidence for stroke systems of care arises from consideration of stroke as a whole, and this overview will assume that this evidence applies well to both ischemic and haemorrhagic stroke types.

Table 10.1 Potential issues along the stroke care continuum highlighted by Mrs. Retiree's[a] case and the relevant system-of-care strategy discussed in this chapter

Continuum of care issue	System-of-care strategy	Relevant chapter section
Smoking Hypertension	Smoking cessation campaigns Early identification and control of hypertension	*Prevention and Public Awareness*: Modifiable Risk Factors for ICH
5 h from onset to seeking help	Public education about stroke symptoms and urgency of treatment (e.g. FAST campaign)	Public Awareness of Stroke Symptoms
Triaged as "headache" owing to this being the main complaint	Acute onset of focal neurological symptoms should trigger a stroke code and rapid assessment	*Hyper-acute and Acute ICH Management*
Admitted to a regional centre without stroke expertise	Stroke code should trigger pre-hospital protocols like EMS routing to comprehensive stroke centres	*Pre-hospital Protocols*: EMS Routing Protocols
CT head obtained 2 h after presentation. No follow-up CT obtained until severe deterioration, despite clinical signs of potential hematoma expansion	Stroke code should trigger emergent neuroimaging (<25 min). Protocols for early follow-up imaging in high-risk or clinically deteriorating patients should be in place	In-hospital Care Protocols
Admitted to general medical ward and not stroke unit; neurological monitoring not performed. ICU admission not considered, given potential for airway compromise	ICH patients should be cared for on a stroke/neurocritical unit with multidisciplinary team input and specialized nursing care	Care on Stroke Units or Neurologic Intensive Care Units ICH-Specific Intensity of Care Quality Metrics
BPs elevations not adequately treated	Pre-hospital and in-hospital care protocols should aim for early BP control	ICH-Specific Intensity of Care Quality Metrics
Inter-hospital transfer refused owing to no neurosurgical indication; transfer undertaken without adequate stabilization of the patient	ICH patients should be redirected to appropriate centres to ensure complex care needs are met; inter-hospital transfer protocols should be in place to ensure safe transfers	Inter-hospital transfers

[a]Mock patient based on an aggregation of real cases

Stroke Systems of Care as an Intervention

The systematic organization of stroke care is a population-level intervention that applies to all stroke types. A recent ASA policy statement estimated that a 2–3% reduction in annual stroke mortality by such a system could translate into 20,000 fewer deaths in the United States and roughly 400,000 fewer deaths worldwide [5]. Although it is challenging to objectively demonstrate a causal benefit of such large-scale, multi-faceted interventions, there is compelling evidence favouring the implementation of integrated systems of stroke care.

A 2013 study demonstrated that implementation of the Ontario Stroke System in Ontario, Canada, in 2005 was associated with improved processes of care – in particular, a higher rate of care at designated stroke centres (from 40.0% to 46.5%) – as well as in stroke outcomes, including lower rates of discharge to long-term care facilities (from 16.9% to 14.8%) and decreased 30-day mortality, including for haemorrhagic stroke (from 38.3% to 34.4%) [6]. This study used piecewise regression analyses to distinguish the effect of the provincial stroke system from underlying temporal trends in care and outcomes between 2001 and 2010. Evidence on a national scale was provided by a 2016 study which found a 15% relative reduction in 30-day in-hospital mortality in Canadian provinces with integrated systems of stroke care, which was not observed in those without such systems, starting in the 2009/2010 fiscal year and sustained through to the 2013/2014 fiscal year [7]. The establishment of stroke systems was also associated with an increased availability of resources including stroke units, stroke prevention clinics, and telestroke services. Although these findings are most generalizable to the Canadian healthcare system, this general observation of decreased mortality in association with a multifactorial stroke system intervention can help inform policy decisions in other healthcare jurisdictions. Optimizing stroke care is likely to be cost-effective; it has been estimated that optimal stroke care in Canada would result in a cost avoidance of $682 million annually in direct and indirect healthcare costs [8].

Stroke systems of care are likely to evolve differently in different healthcare systems and geographies, particularly in single- versus multi-payer settings. The contrast between the American and Canadian healthcare systems is illustrative. The Canadian healthcare system is a collection of similar systems organized and funded by each province or territory [9]. Because of this centralization (essentially a single payer which is the province/territory), each province/territory can choose to regionalize stroke services to curtail cost and promote efficiency. These might include restricting the number of hospitals providing stroke care by geographical need and directing EMS to triage stroke patients preferentially to designated regional stroke centres. The multi-payer American system is decentralized, with much less federal or state-level coordination, meaning that allocation of resources is not directed necessarily at efficiency of population-level services but instead at maximizing efficiency at the level of the hospital or the hospital network; this may affect quality and raise stroke-specific costs at the population level [10]. This absence of a centralized structure can create barriers to monitoring and addressing regional issues to ensure that stroke systems act in the best interest of the all patients in a given region [11]. Stroke systems of care can also be expected to follow different development trajectories in lower- and middle-income countries, where a lack of adequate funds and expertise may mean a greater focus on certain aspects of stroke systems – like telestroke for rapid remote access to expert advice/evaluation, or rapid land/air patient transport protocols – to compensate for a dearth of resource-intensive stroke facilities.

Allowing for such inevitable heterogeneity, there are some core features and operating principles along the continuum of stroke care that can frame the organization of systems of care for ICH, each of which we will examine in turn: (a) prevention and public awareness, (b) hyper-acute and acute management, and (c) rehabilitation and community reintegration.

Prevention and Public Awareness

Modifiable Risk Factors for ICH

Globally, over 90% of the stroke burden is attributable to modifiable risk factors, with nearly three quarters related to behavioural factors [12]. Stroke systems of care can play a key upstream role in the prevention of ICH. Hypertension is the single most important risk factor for ICH [13]; while most hypertension-related ICH occurs in deep brain parenchymal nuclei, hypertension is also a risk factor for lobar ICH [14]. Meta-analyses have reported a 3.5-fold increased risk of ICH with hypertension [15], and more than a ninefold increase with blood pressures over 160/90 [16]. A recent report from the Trials of Hypertension Prevention (TOHP) found a direct linear association between average sodium intake, a modifiable risk factor, and mortality. Diabetes mellitus is associated with a 1.6-fold risk increase in ICH [17], but it remains unclear if treatment of diabetes mellitus reduces ICH risk. Smoking has been consistently shown to be a risk factor for ICH, with studies demonstrating a dose-response relationship with the number of cigarettes smoked and the risk of ICH [18, 19]. The relative risk for current versus non-smokers has been reported to be around 1.5 [15, 16]. Excessive alcohol consumption, including binge drinking, is a risk factor for ICH. Addressing these risk factors is both the function of the stroke prevention clinic, within a stroke system of care, and general public education with mass media campaigns [20–22].

The Role of Stroke Prevention Clinics

Following ICH, as with care following transient ischaemic attack (TIA) or ischaemic stroke (given shared risk factors), identifying the likely mechanism or cause of ICH is important to secondary prevention strategies. While hypertension is the most important risk factor for ICH, it can be well treated with currently available medication. Anticoagulant use may need review, and individual level decision-making may be required to decide if antithrombotic therapy continues to be indicated. Venous sinus thrombosis associated with ICH will require long-term anticoagulation, which appears to be safe in this setting [23]. In contrast, anticoagulants may be contraindicated after lobar haemorrhage with associated microbleeds in the brain suggestive of amyloid angiopathy [24]. Identification of structural arterial or venous lesions (arteriovenous malformations, arteriovenous fistulas, or aneurysms) has potential implications for subsequent neurosurgical, endovascular, or radiotherapy interventions.

Public Awareness of Stroke Symptoms

Early recognition of stroke symptoms and early medical attention is critical for maximizing the chance of a favourable outcome after stroke [25]. Because stroke is typically painless and therefore does not uniformly engender a sense of urgency [26] and many people do not know how to recognize stroke in another person and to seek help [27], stroke systems of care should take an active role in promoting public education about rapid recognition of stroke symptoms to optimize the hyper-acute presentation of stroke cases to medical attention. The Face-Arm-Speech-Time (FAST) campaign is an example of a highly successful international public awareness campaign that has been shown to have a sustained reduction on the time to first seeking medical attention after stroke [28]. In particular, the campaign appears to have promoted a shift towards directly contacting EMS (versus other sources of medical help like a general practitioner); increase in use of emergency services has repeatedly been cited as a critical factor in facilitating rapid assessment following stroke [29]. Importantly, such campaigns play a role not only in improving symptom recognition in patients at risk but also in improving stroke awareness in relatives, acquaintances, or other bystanders who are responsible for the actual call for medical assistance in almost 90% of major stroke cases [28]. Surveys of the general population in the United Kingdom have shown an increased ability to name stroke warning signs following the FAST campaign, suggesting that such improved initial diagnostic impressions in bystanders has likely contributed to the positive effects of the campaign on response times [30].

Hyper-acute and Acute ICH Management

The concept of "time is brain" that has permeated the care of hyper-acute ischaemic stroke applies equally to ICH, where different mechanisms of secondary brain damage also occur within the first few hours of symptom onset [25]. Hematoma growth >33% has been observed in one quarter of patients within the first hour and in roughly 40% within the first 20 h [31], with more than 70% of patients having some degree of hematoma expansion in the first day [32]. Hematoma expansion is associated with worse functional outcomes and increased mortality from ICH [32]. Perihaematomal oedema and intraventricular haemorrhage (IVH) are additional mechanisms of secondary damage; oedema grows rapidly in the first day but continues at a slower pace for 2 weeks [33], whereas IVH develops within the first few hours and is clearly associated with worse short- and long-term outcomes [34, 35].

Pre-hospital Protocols

EMS Routing Protocols

A recent analysis of pre-hospital delay times in patients with major stroke from the Oxford Vascular Study found that two-thirds of pre-hospital delay in those who sought emergency medical attention consisted of paramedic assessment and ambulance transport time [28]. This highlights the importance of pre-hospital protocols to rapidly identify and transport stroke patients to the correct emergency centre, which involves coordinated efforts among emergency departments as well as ground and air emergency transportation.

Pre-hospital identification of potential stroke cases is improved by adopting standardized tools like FAST, the Los Angeles Prehospital Stroke Screen, the Cincinnati Prehospital Stroke Scale, or the Hospital Evaluation Criteria [36] to rapidly identify and initiate a "code stroke" pathway. Protocols to allow EMS bypass to the most appropriate centre without pressures or incentives to stop at a less optimal hospital has been demonstrated to increase access to stroke centre care [1, 37]. Encouraging progress has been made in this area; in 2010, 49% of stroke hospitalizations in the United States occurred in jurisdictions with established EMS regional systems of acute stroke care, versus just 1% in 2004 [38].

Designation of Primary and Comprehensive Stroke Centres

Selection of appropriate centres for stroke care is facilitated by the designation of specific hospitals as comprehensive stroke centres (CSCs) and primary stroke centres (PSCs), as recommended by the Brain Attack Coalition (criteria summarized in Table 10.2) [4, 39]. It remains unclear if preferential routing of suspected ICH patients to CSCs improves outcomes. Clinical grading scales to identify ICH (e.g. the Siriraj score [40]) have been proposed but are simply not discriminative enough to identify ICH accurately. Pre-hospital clinical screening tools to identify ICH with a high degree of accuracy are still needed. Mobile Stroke CT ambulances may provide the best immediate option for early diagnosis and testing of field-based therapies; these are only available in selected cities around the world [41–44].

Development and certification of CSCs and PSCs must occur in parallel to the development of pre-hospital protocols; lack of access to such facilities, particularly in scarcely populated regions, can be a barrier to instituting acute stroke routing protocols [45]. However, adoption of EMS routing policies may itself provide incentive for more centres to achieve PSC accreditation, improving access to stroke

Table 10.2 Characteristics of comprehensive and primary stroke centres, with features compared or contrasted where appropriate [4, 39]

Comprehensive stroke centre (CSC)	Primary stroke centre (PSC)
Neurosurgical and endovascular capability, including clipping and coiling of intracranial aneurysms	
Advanced thrombolytic capability, including endovascular treatment	Capability to provide acute medical thrombolysis
Stroke unit care as well as intensive care unit	Stroke unit care (with telemetry monitoring)
Inter-disciplinary stroke team	Inter-disciplinary stroke team but may not be as complete or available as in a CSC
Advanced neurovascular imaging capability, such as MRI and various types of cerebral angiography	Computed tomography on site
Responsibility for stroke service coordination across a region and maintenance of a stroke registry	Responsibility for stroke service within a site

care: the yearly rate of eligible hospital conversion to PSC designation accelerated from 3.8% to 16.2% during the implementation of EMS routing policies in California [46]. From the healthcare system's perspective, this raises the question of how to optimize the number of stroke centres in a given region. Directing high case volume to a smaller number of institutions can help hone stroke-specific competencies among staff improving outcomes but may also result in the loss of skills at non-designated centres. Stroke patients may also be forced to deal with increased transport times to designated centres owing to restricted access. Alternately, if more hospitals gain CSC designation and increase their stroke admission volume, this can mean faster access to care for patients. The cost of CSC designation is a stretching of hospital resources such as neuroimaging and critical care nursing [47]. This situation poses a challenge for stakeholders charged with PSC/CSC designation criteria, who must strike an optimal balance between the healthcare establishment's need to sustainably invest limited resources and the public or consumer's need for timely access to certified stroke centres.

Evolving Pre-hospital Treatment Protocols

The additional availability of point-of-care laboratory testing for clotting parameters in mobile stroke CT ambulances means that ICH patients can have platelet or coagulation deficits treated even before they arrive in hospital. This can be especially valuable in cases of warfarin-related ICH, where rapid reversal (within 2 h of onset) has been advocated but significant delays are common [48]. The Cleveland mobile stroke unit reported rapid reversal of international normalized ratio (INR) with four-factor prothrombin complex concentrate in a case of warfarin-related ICH within 57 min of EMS dispatch [49], compared to the median onset-to-therapy time of 15 h in a recent haemorrhage registry [50].

Another emerging pre-hospital treatment consideration for ICH is blood pressure lowering in the field. While data from the ICH-ADAPT, INTERACT, and

INTERACT-2 RCTs have shown the safety of rapid BP lowering in ICH to a systolic target of 140 mmHg [51–53], the ATACH-2 study failed to show benefit of rapid lowering of BP in hospital using intravenous nicardipine [54]. Still, there is a physiological reason to believe that if blood pressure lowering is to work, it will have to be done extremely early after stroke onset. The feasibility of a definitive pre-hospital BP-lowering RCT in acute stroke has recently been demonstrated by the PIL-FAST pilot study of paramedic-initiated lisinopril [55]. The FAST-MAG trial, while negative for its primary outcome, has also demonstrated the feasibility of large-scale pre-hospital administration of a potentially neuroprotective agent in acute stroke [56]. By making their EMS provision amenable to large-scale trials or imminent in-the-field treatment options, stroke systems of care can stand to gain much from the advancement of pre-hospital stroke care.

In-Hospital Care Protocols

Once the patient with suspected stroke has arrived in the hospital, an in-hospital "code stroke" or "STAT stroke" pathway should kick into effect, with the immediate priority being to definitively establish the diagnosis of ischaemic or haemorrhagic stroke, if not already done. Once the patient has been definitively identified as having ICH, then their care should proceed along an ICH-specific pathway. Protocol-based care is associated with decreased length of stay and hospitalization costs [57].

Neurosurgical intervention is relevant for only a small minority of ICH patients; most patients with ICH should be admitted to a medical stroke unit. There is simply no evidence for benefit of early (emergency) craniotomy and haematoma evacuation. Stroke systems should facilitate relevant neurosurgical consultation in ICH patients where ventriculostomy for obstructive hydrocephalus and surgical evacuation of a cerebellar haemorrhage could be life-saving [5]. Early management priorities for in-hospital protocols should include emergency reversal of coagulopathies for which there is some modest evidence of benefit [58, 59], administration of anti-epileptic medications when seizures have complicated the patient's early clinical course, measures to control elevated intracranial pressure, deep venous thrombosis prophylaxis, and early mobilization and rehabilitation therapy [60–62].

ICH-Specific Intensity of Care Quality Metrics

A valuable framework for the organization of in-hospital protocols has recently been provided by the ICH-specific intensity of care quality metrics. These metrics were developed through a review of the available scientific evidence on quality indicators in ICH, or stroke in general or other directly relevant disease processes (like hyperglycemia) where ICH-specific data were lacking; 26 quality indicators related to 18 facets of care with thresholds for quality response for identified (summarized in Table 10.3) [63].

Table 10.3 ICH-specific quality of care metrics and proposed performance thresholds (Adapted from Qureshi et al. 2011 and 2013). To calculate intensity of care quality score, 1 point is assigned to each threshold met [64]

Variable	Definition	Proposed threshold(s) for performance
Emergency department (ED) evaluation time	Time to physician contact and hemodynamic monitoring	Performed within 10 min of ED arrival
Rapid acquisition of neuroimaging	Time interval between ED arrival and CT scan or MRI	Acquired within 25 min of ED arrival
ICU-type monitoring	Neurological and hemodynamic monitoring within 30-min intervals	Initiated within 10 min of ED arrival
Avoidance of DNR (do-not-resuscitate) or withdrawal of care status in first 24 h and DNR without cause within first 7 days	Appropriate causes include severe stroke, life-threatening brain damage, and significant comorbidities	No DNR/withdrawal of care status within 24 days of ED arrival, or *not applicable*
		No DNR/withdrawal of care status between 24 days and 7 days of ED arrival, unless there is a documented change in patient status
Treatment of acute hypertensive response	Systolic blood pressure (SBP) $\geq$180 mmHg per initial definition; following recent trials, SBP >140 may be more appropriate	Achieved target range within 2.5 h of the second of two consecutive measurements, or *not applicable*
Early intubation and mechanical ventilation	Indications: decreased level of consciousness (GCS < 10); hypoventilation or apnoea or decreased or ineffective respiratory effort; hypoxemia or hypercarbia; impaired airway protection; airway obstruction; recurrent aspiration; seizures >5 min; or craniotomy.	Intubation initiated within 30 min of identification of risk, or *not applicable*
Treatment of clinically significant intracranial mass effect or trans-tentorial herniation	Unilateral or bilateral pupillary enlargement or two spontaneous ICP readings >20 mmHg persisting for >5 min (if ICP monitoring is available)	Clinical reversal of herniation or attainment of ICP <20 mmHg within 60 min of detection, or *not applicable*
		No brain death status within 7 days of herniation or ICP elevation
Treatment of repetitive seizures and status epilepticus (clinical)	Continuous or repetitive seizure activity >5 min without recovery of consciousness	All motor seizure activity ceased within 20 min after the first recorded seizure and no return of seizure activity during next 40 min, or *not applicable*
Treatment of repetitive seizures and status epilepticus (subclinical)	Seizures seen only on electroencephalography or subtle signs at the bedside	All motor and electroencephalographic seizure activity ceased within 20 min after the first recorded seizure and no return of seizure activity during the next 40 min, or *not applicable*
		No recurrence of overt or subtle seizure within 12 h after first seizure or not applicable

Table 10.3 (continued)

Variable	Definition	Proposed threshold(s) for performance
Rapid reversal of elevated INR	INR >1.4 at admission	INR reversal (INR <1.4) within 2 h of first elevated INR >1.4, or *not applicable*
		At least two reversal agents administered within 2 h of first elevated INR >1.4, or *not applicable*
Treatment of elevated serum glucose concentration	Serum glucose >200 mg/dL within 72 h	Target glucose achieved within 4 h of detection of elevated glucose or *not applicable*
		No recurrent hyperglycemia within 72 h of admission
Treatment of hyperpyrexia	Temperature ≥ 38.3 °C on two consecutive measurements 1 h apart within 72 h	Time to normothermia (first T < 37.2 °C) <4 h, or *not applicable*
		No recurrent hyperpyrexia within 72 h of admission
Deep vein thrombosis prophylaxis	Low-molecular-weight heparin, heparin, or intermittent pneumatic compression	Administered in the first 48 h of arrival, or *not applicable*
Dysphagia screening	Bedside evaluations, videofluoroscopic assessment, or fiber-optic endoscopy	Performed within 72 h of arrival, or *not applicable*
Nutrition initiation	Enteric route preferred	Enteral feeding started within 72 h of arrival, or *not applicable*
Gastric ulcer prophylaxis	H2 blockers, proton blockers, or sucralfate	Administered within 48 h of symptom onset, or *not applicable*
Treatment of persistently elevated blood pressure	SBP ≥160 mmHg within 7 days; following recent trials, SBP >140 may be more appropriate	Initiated within 7 days of arrival, or *not applicable* or contraindication documented
Tracheostomy for persistent intubation or poor airway protection	Early percutaneous or surgical tracheostomy	Performed within 7 days of arrival, or *not applicable* or contraindication documented
Treatment of hospital-acquired or ventilator-associated pneumonia	New or progressive radiographic infiltrate and at least two of fever, leucocytosis, or purulent tracheal secretions, during ICU stay	Institution of intravenous antibiotics within 24 h of first persistent fever (≥38.3 °C on consecutive measurements 1 h apart)
		No new antibiotic substituted or added within 10 days of initiating first antibiotic

When a pilot study using these indicators was performed in 25 patients, the lowest performance scores were observed for early intubation and mechanical ventilation, treatment of significant mass effect or trans-tentorial herniation, and timely acquisition of neuroimaging, whereas the highest scores were seen for the treatment of status epilepticus or any seizure within 2 weeks of admission and prevention of gastric ulcers [63]. A validation study was then undertaken in 50 consecutive patients with ICH admitted within 24 h of symptom onset, with each patient's care scored from 0 to 26 based on the attainment of the threshold for appropriate performance for each parameter [64]. Higher scores correlated with lower in-hospital mortality, and the receiver operating characteristic curve demonstrated a high discriminating ability of these metrics for that outcome (*c*-statistic of 0.91); the association was evident even after adjusting for known prognostic variables like initial GCS score, haematoma volume, and intraventricular haemorrhage [64]. These findings support the broader use of these metrics for standardizing in-hospital care for ICH. Ultimately, these metrics provide a template that is amenable to modification based on new evidence; for example, the originally proposed BP targets can be modified based on recent RCT studies in ICH (Table 10.3).

Care on Stroke Units or Neurologic Intensive Care Units

Organized stroke unit care provided by specialized multidisciplinary teams on a discrete ward dedicated to stroke patients has been found to have a robust, demonstrably stable effect in reducing stroke mortality, when compared to alternative forms of care delivery [65, 66].

A review of 31 trials, involving 6936 participants, compared stroke unit care with alternative service provision and found that stroke unit care was consistently associated with improved outcomes; such patients are more likely to be alive and independently living at home at 1 year post-stroke [65]. Centralization of acute stroke care into hyper-acute stroke units increases the likelihood that patients will receive evidence-based clinical interventions [67].

Similar benefits have been observed in ICH patients. A Spanish study of ICH patients at a facility before and after the introduction of integrated care on a stroke unit observed a significant reduction in average stay, with improved scores on the Rankin scale at discharge, more patients discharged to rehabilitation centres, and fewer sent to long-term care facilities [68]. There were also fewer complications like hydrocephalus, re-bleeding, sepsis, and renal failure. Evidence of a mortality benefit in ICH was provided by a Norwegian prospective controlled study of 56 ICH patients admitted to an acute stroke unit, versus 65 ICH patients treated on general medical wards, and found that the 30-day mortality was 39% in the acute stroke unit compared to 63% in the general medical ward, while 1-year mortality rates were 52% and 69%, respectively (both statistically significant) [69]. This difference in 1-year mortality was driven by the large difference in 30-day survival, as there was no difference in survival between 30 and 365 days.

For ICH patients in particular, admission to a dedicated neurologic intensive care unit (ICU) with stroke expertise – versus just a stroke unit – for at least 24 h after the clinic event may be a reasonable protocol. The AHA/ASA Stroke Council have recommended that monitoring and management of ICH patients should take place in an ICU setting, given the high risk of neurological deterioration, frequent elevations in intracranial pressure, cardiovascular instability (including frequent BP elevations), the frequent need for intubation and ventilation, and multiple complicating medical issues within the first 24 h [70–72]. Investing in such neuro-specific critical care resources can have a meaningful impact on care. For instance, the introduction of a neurocritical team, including a full-time neuro-intensivist, and implementation of intensive-care protocol for key aspects of care like mechanical ventilation, deep vein thrombosis treatment, gastrointestinal prophylaxis, infection control, sedation, glucose control, core body temperature, and BP control were associated with significantly lower in-hospital mortality and length of stay but without changes in readmission rates or long-term mortality in one ICU-based study [73]. In addition, a multivariable analysis of prospectively collected data over 3 years by Project Impact from 52 participating ICUs and two neurocritical ICUs (around 40,000 patient records) found that not being on a neuro-ICU was associated with an increase in hospital mortality (OR 3.4) after adjustment for patient demographics, ICH severity, and ICU/institutional characteristics [74]. The added benefits of neurocritical care may be related to different approaches to BP management, withdrawal of care, coagulopathy correction, caregiver experience, comorbidity or complication management, and general supportive care [63].

Ultimately, whether ICH patients are housed on a stroke unit or neurologic ICU, they should receive close and specialized nursing care that involves careful monitoring for the possibility of clinical worsening from various complications.

Inter-hospital Protocols

Inter-hospital Transfers

Getting patients with suspected stroke to the right facility the first time must be a priority in a stroke system, given that time delays may exclude ischemic stroke patients from some acute therapies once they finally arrive at a PSC/CSC [75–77]. The secondary transfer of such patients to a PSC/CSC to initiate treatment can greatly worsen the delay from symptom onset to acute therapy [78]. With ICH, the urgency of transfer is dampened by the absence of proven acute interventions; however, transfers may help facilitate appropriate care in a stroke unit or neurologic ICU. To navigate such situations, it is important for stroke systems to have transfer protocols in place.

Inter-hospital transfer of ICH patients to receive neuro-ICU care may improve the quality of care but may also be associated with complications, particularly if transfer times are not optimized. A New York-based prospective single-centre study of patients with haemorrhagic stroke (including ICH) found that while complications generally did not differ between patients who were transferred to the neuro-ICU versus those directly admitted, longer transfer time among transferred patients was associated with a significantly greater risk of aneurysm re-bleed and tracheostomy [79]. Transferred patients had worse cognitive outcome at 3 months but there were no differences in death, disability, or length of stay.

The adequacy of the ICH patient's vital signs – airway, breathing, and circulation status – must be rapidly assessed and stabilized before inter-hospital transfer occurs

[80–82]. During the initial management and transport, aforementioned measures to prevent or minimize mechanisms of secondary injury should still be undertaken. A single-centre prospective study in Taiwan found that inter-hospital transfer neurological deterioration – defined as a GCS score drop of two or more points from last measure at the first facility to first measure at the second facility – occurred in 36/217 patients (16.6%) and was predicted by arrival SBP ≥180 mmHg, in addition to the known prognostic factors of infratentorial ICH, presence of intraventricular haemorrhage, and larger ICH [83]. This further highlights the need for pre-transfer treatment of critical parameters like BP.

One question that remains is whether observed potential benefits of inter-hospital transfer simply reflect the favourable baseline characteristics of those patients selected for transfer. For example, a study of 760 consecutive ICH admissions to a designated stroke centre in Connecticut, of which 321 (42.2%) were inter-hospital transfers, found that transferred patients were younger, had lower ICH scores, higher GCS, and lower SBP than direct admissions [84]. A retrospective cohort study of 1364 consecutive ICH patients admitted to 14 acute and specialist hospitals in Salford (United Kingdom), of whom 140 were transferred, also found that the decision to transfer was more likely with younger patients but also in women, brainstem or cerebellar bleeds, and larger haematomas [85]. However, independent of other prognostic factors, transferred patients had a significantly lower risk of death versus those remaining at the referring centre, whether they or not they ended up having a surgical intervention. This suggests that aggressive supportive care at specialized centres (i.e. CSCs) can improve survival in ICH. If observed estimates of neuro-ICU-based functional outcome distributions are proven accurate, then there is a strong cost-effectiveness argument for stroke systems to invest in the transfer of ICH patients to specialized neuro-ICUs according to a recently published decision analytic model [86].

For selected patients, early neurosurgical consultation is warranted, and inter-hospital transfers may be undertaken to ensure this. Patients with large cerebellar ICH or evidence of hydrocephalus will benefit from consideration of surgical intervention. Inter-hospital transfer should include the establishment of written protocols identifying criteria for such transfers, individuals responsible for coordinating the transfer, patient monitoring during the transfer, and communication of transfer outcome [5].

The Role of Telestroke Services

Telestroke – the use of voice and video telecommunications technology in stroke care – offers further opportunities for both pre-hospital and collaborative inter-hospital diagnosis and management in acute stroke. Pilot studies have explored the concept of ambulance-based telemedicine to facilitate rapid and accurate pre-hospital stroke triage; whereas older studies were limited by earlier-generation broadband [87–89], more recent studies using modern cellular connectivity have shown greater reliability [90, 91]. A recent study using standardized patients has also demonstrated the reliability of a low-cost, tablet-based platform and commercial cellular networks to perform pre-hospital neurological assessments in rural and urban settings [92]. Such remote assessments can also be valuable when considering inter-hospital transfers to ensure appropriate preparation and pre-transfer stabilization of the patients. Telestroke services can also be used by allied health professionals. Speech therapists recently reported use of remote videofluoroscopy to direct their examination of dysphagia with the aid of on-site clinicians, finding moderate agreement with on-site assessors and good agreement in treatment recommendations [93].

A systematic review of 18 telestroke studies found that such services can lead to better functional health outcomes including reduced mortality, compared with conventional care [94]. Telestroke services also appear to be cost-effective. For example, in the Telemedical Project for Integrative Stroke Care (TEMPiS) network, 30-month costs were calculated for patients treated in hospitals with telestroke units versus those without specialized care; whereas inpatient costs were higher in TEMPiS hospitals, costs of aftercare were lower compared with conventional hospitals, resulting in equal absolute costs by 30 months [95]. Costs of aftercare per year survived were lower in TEMPiS patients, making long-term cost savings very likely. Two other studies using decision-analytic models based on data from hospitals in the United States calculated the effects of increased numbers of ischaemic stroke patients treated with intravenous thrombolysis and estimated relevant cost savings in the long term as a result of decreased disability [96, 97]. ICH-specific models have not been published.

Rehabilitation and Community Reintegration

Successful rehabilitation after stroke consists of six main areas of focus: (1) training for maximum recovery, (2) prevention and treatment of co-morbid conditions, (3) enhancement of psychosocial coping, (4) promotion of integration into the community, (5) prevention of recurrent strokes or other vascular events, and (6) enhancement of quality of life [98]. Rehabilitation of stroke survivors should begin early but should not be started overly aggressively; the AVERT trial recently found that a higher-dose, very early (<24 h) mobilization protocol was associated with a lower odds of favourable outcome at 3 months [99]. Several studies have demonstrated that organized multidisciplinary stroke rehabilitation reduces death, disability, and institutionalization [98]. Such services should be directed by a physiatrist or neurologist experienced in stroke rehabilitation, and CSCs should have physical, occupational, and speech therapists readily available for patient assessment and therapy during the acute hospitalization [4]. Post-stroke care should also include assessment and support for cognitive decline, depression, and social consequences of stroke [100].

There have been a few different organized approaches to post-stroke rehabilitation following acute care: (1) acute stroke units that discharge patients early, usually within 7 days, for further inpatient or outpatient rehabilitation; (2) rehabilitation stroke units that accept such patients after 7 days and focus on rehabilitation; and (3) comprehensive stroke units that accept patients acutely and also provide rehabilitation for many weeks if needed [101]. Comprehensive units have demonstrated the greatest overall benefit, achieving both a significant reduction in length of stay and the greatest reduction in combined death/disability outcomes [101]. Cross-sectional, "before-and-after" comparisons, and randomized controlled studies have indicated that co-located acute/rehabilitation stroke care promotes better length-of-stay and/or functional outcome when compared to the acute or rehabilitation stroke unit models [102–104]. Outpatient rehabilitation programs can also improve outcomes and prevent deterioration in stroke survivors [105].

Integrated models of community reintegration and secondary prevention, such as the ICARUSS (Integrated Care for the Reduction of Secondary Stroke) model in Australia, can reduce recurrent events. ICARUSS is a multimodal program involving collaboration between a specialist stroke service, a hospital coordinator, and the patient's general practitioner to promote the management of vascular risk factors through ongoing patient contact and education. This model has been shown to be associated with a successful reduction in systolic blood pressure, modification of body mass index, greater exercise engagement, and reduced disability in the 12 months post-stroke versus usual care in an RCT; 10% of these patients had ICH [106].

Conclusion

Stroke systems of care play an essential role in good ICH patient care. They have a central role in education, infrastructure and protocol development, institutional accreditation, and continuous quality improvement across the continuum of stroke care. An integrated approach to stroke care, with carefully designed policies that address the complex challenges and care needs along each step of the continuum from prevention and public awareness to hyper-acute/acute management and ultimately rehabilitation and community reintegration, can help ensure that patients with ICH have the best chance at disability-free survival.

References

1. Schwamm L, Pancioli A, Acker JE, et al. Recommendations for the establishment of stroke systems of care: recommendations from the American Stroke Association's Task Force on the Development of Stroke Systems. Stroke. 2005;36(3):690–703.
2. Lindsay P, Bayley M, McDonald A, Graham I, Warner G, Phillips S. Toward a more effective approach to stroke: Canadian Best Practice Recommendations for Stroke Care. Can Med Assoc J. 2008;178(11):1418–25.

3. Lindsay P, Furie KL, Davis SM, Donnan GA, Norrving B. World Stroke Organization global stroke services guidelines and action plan. Int J Stroke. 2014;9 Suppl A100:4–13.
4. Alberts M, Latchaw R, Selman W, et al. Recommendations for comprehensive stroke centers: a consensus statement from the Brain Attack Coalition. Stroke. 2005;36(7):1597–616.
5. Higashida R, Alberts MJ, Alexander DN, et al. Interactions within stroke systems of care: a policy statement from the American Heart Association/American Stroke Association. Stroke. 2013;44(10):2961–84.
6. Kapral M, Fang J, Silver F, et al. Effect of a provincial system of stroke care delivery on stroke care and outcomes. Can Med Assoc J. 2013;185(10):E483–91.
7. Ganesh A, Lindsay P, Fang J, et al. Integrated systems of stroke care and reduction in 30-day mortality: a retrospective analysis. Neurology. 2016;86(10):898–904.
8. Krueger H, Lindsay P, Cote R, Kapral MK, Kaczorowski J, Hill MD. Cost avoidance associated with optimal stroke care in Canada. Stroke. 2012;43(8):2198–206.
9. Lewis S. A system in name only--access, variation, and reform in Canada's provinces. N Engl J Med. 2015;372(6):497–500.
10. Fuchs VR. How and why US health care differs from that in other OECD countries. JAMA. 2013;309(1):33–4.
11. Fletcher JJ, Majersik JJ. Stroke systems of care: The sum is greater than the parts. Neurology. 2016;86(10):886–7.
12. Feigin VL, Roth GA, Naghavi M, et al. Global burden of stroke and risk factors in 188 countries, during 1990-2013: a systematic analysis for the Global Burden of Disease Study 2013. Lancet Neurol. 2016;15(9):913–24.
13. Ikram MA, Wieberdink RG, Koudstaal PJ. International epidemiology of intracerebral hemorrhage. Curr Atheroscler Rep. 2012;14(4):300–6.
14. Zia E, Hedblad B, Pessah-Rasmussen H, Berglund G, Janzon L, Engstrom G. Blood pressure in relation to the incidence of cerebral infarction and intracerebral hemorrhage. Hypertensive hemorrhage: debated nomenclature is still relevant. Stroke. 2007;38(10):2681–5.
15. Ariesen MJ, Claus SP, Rinkel GJ, Algra A. Risk factors for intracerebral hemorrhage in the general population: a systematic review. Stroke. 2003;34(8):2060–5.
16. O'Donnell MJ, Xavier D, Liu L, et al. Risk factors for ischaemic and intracerebral haemorrhagic stroke in 22 countries (the INTERSTROKE study): a case-control study. Lancet. 2010;376(9735):112–23.
17. Emerging Risk Factors C, Sarwar N, Gao P, et al. Diabetes mellitus, fasting blood glucose concentration, and risk of vascular disease: a collaborative meta-analysis of 102 prospective studies. Lancet. 2010;375(9733):2215–22.
18. Zhang Y, Tuomilehto J, Jousilahti P, Wang Y, Antikainen R, Hu G. Lifestyle factors on the risks of ischemic and hemorrhagic stroke. Arch Intern Med. 2011;171(20):1811–8.
19. Andersen KK, Olsen TS, Dehlendorff C, Kammersgaard LP. Hemorrhagic and ischemic strokes compared: stroke severity, mortality, and risk factors. Stroke. 2009;40(6):2068–72.
20. Xu X, Alexander RL Jr, Simpson SA, et al. A cost-effectiveness analysis of the first federally funded antismoking campaign. Am J Prev Med. 2015;48(3):318–25.
21. Wakefield MA, Loken B, Hornik RC. Use of mass media campaigns to change health behaviour. Lancet. 2010;376(9748):1261–71.
22. Mouradian MS, Hussain MS, Lari H, et al. The impact of a stroke prevention clinic in diagnosing modifiable risk factors for stroke. Can J Neurol Sci. 2005;32(4):496–500.
23. Coutinho J, de Bruijn SF, Deveber G, Stam J. Anticoagulation for cerebral venous sinus thrombosis. Cochrane Database Syst Rev. 2011(8):CD002005.
24. Viswanathan A, Greenberg SM. Cerebral amyloid angiopathy in the elderly. Ann Neurol. 2011;70(6):871–80.
25. Rabinstein AA, Anderson CD. Time is brain also counts for ICH. Neurology. 2015;84(10):970–1.
26. Langdorf MI, Bearie BJ, Kazzi AA, Blasko B, Kohl A. Patients' vs. Physicians' assessments of emergencies: the Prudent Layperson Standard. Cal J Emerg Med. 2003;4(4):75–81.

27. Greenlund KJ, Neff LJ, Zheng ZJ, et al. Low public recognition of major stroke symptoms. Am J Prev Med. 2003;25(4):315–9.
28. Wolters FJ, Paul NL, Li L, Rothwell PM, Oxford VS. Sustained impact of UK FAST-test public education on response to stroke: a population-based time-series study. Int J Stroke. 2015;10(7):1108–14.
29. Fassbender K, Balucani C, Walter S, Levine SR, Haass A, Grotta J. Streamlining of prehospital stroke management: the golden hour. Lancet Neurol. 2013;12(6):585–96.
30. Robinson TG, Reid A, Haunton VJ, Wilson A, Naylor AR. The face arm speech test: does it encourage rapid recognition of important stroke warning symptoms? Emerg Med J. 2013;30(6):467–71.
31. Brott T, Broderick J, Kothari R, et al. Early hemorrhage growth in patients with intracerebral hemorrhage. Stroke. 1997;28(1):1–5.
32. Davis SM, Broderick J, Hennerici M, et al. Hematoma growth is a determinant of mortality and poor outcome after intracerebral hemorrhage. Neurology. 2006;66(8):1175–81.
33. Balami JS, Buchan AM. Complications of intracerebral haemorrhage. Lancet Neurol. 2012;11(1):101–18.
34. Witsch J, Bruce E, Meyers E, et al. Intraventricular hemorrhage expansion in patients with spontaneous intracerebral hemorrhage. Neurology. 2015;84(10):989–94.
35. Maas MB, Nemeth AJ, Rosenberg NF, Kosteva AR, Prabhakaran S, Naidech AM. Delayed intraventricular hemorrhage is common and worsens outcomes in intracerebral hemorrhage. Neurology. 2013;80(14):1295–9.
36. Goldstein LB, Simel DL. Is this patient having a stroke? JAMA. 2005;293(19):2391–402.
37. Sanossian N, Liebeskind DS, Eckstein M, et al. Routing ambulances to designated centers increases access to stroke center care and enrollment in prehospital research. Stroke. 2015;46(10):2886–90.
38. Hanks N, Wen G, He S, et al. Expansion of U.S. emergency medical service routing for stroke care: 2000-2010. West J Emerg Med. 2014;15(4):499–503.
39. Alberts MJ, Latchaw RE, Jagoda A, et al. Revised and updated recommendations for the establishment of primary stroke centers: a summary statement from the brain attack coalition. Stroke. 2011;42(9):2651–65.
40. Mwita CC, Kajia D, Gwer S, Etyang A, Newton CR. Accuracy of clinical stroke scores for distinguishing stroke subtypes in resource poor settings: a systematic review of diagnostic test accuracy. J Neurosci Rural Pract. 2014;5(4):330–9.
41. John S, Stock S, Cerejo R, et al. Brain imaging using mobile CT: current status and future prospects. J Neuroimaging. 2016;26(1):5–15.
42. Ebinger M, Winter B, Wendt M, et al. Effect of the use of ambulance-based thrombolysis on time to thrombolysis in acute ischemic stroke: a randomized clinical trial. JAMA. 2014;311(16):1622–31.
43. Walter S, Kostopoulos P, Haass A, et al. Diagnosis and treatment of patients with stroke in a mobile stroke unit versus in hospital: a randomised controlled trial. Lancet Neurol. 2012;11(5):397–404.
44. Kunz A, Ebinger M, Geisler F, et al. Functional outcomes of pre-hospital thrombolysis in a mobile stroke treatment unit compared with conventional care: an observational registry study. Lancet Neurol. 2016;15(10):1035–43.
45. Dimitrov N, Koenig W, Bosson N, et al. Variability in criteria for emergency medical services routing of acute stroke patients to designated stroke center hospitals. West J Emerg Med. 2015;16(5):743–6.
46. Schuberg S, Song S, Saver JL, Mack WJ, Cen SY, Sanossian N. Impact of emergency medical services stroke routing protocols on Primary Stroke Center certification in California. Stroke. 2013;44(12):3584–6.
47. Janjua N, Qureshi AI, Zaidat OO. Systemization of advanced stroke care: the dollars and sense of comprehensive stroke centers. J Neurointerv Surg. 2014;6(3):162–5.
48. Goldstein JN, Thomas SH, Frontiero V, et al. Timing of fresh frozen plasma administration and rapid correction of coagulopathy in warfarin-related intracerebral hemorrhage. Stroke. 2006;37(1):151–5.

49. Gomes JA, Ahrens CL, Hussain MS, et al. Prehospital reversal of warfarin-related coagulopathy in intracerebral hemorrhage in a mobile stroke treatment unit. Stroke. 2015;46(5):e118–20.
50. Frontera JA, Gordon E, Zach V, et al. Reversal of coagulopathy using prothrombin complex concentrates is associated with improved outcome compared to fresh frozen plasma in warfarin-associated intracranial hemorrhage. Neurocrit Care. 2014;21(3):397–406.
51. Anderson CS, Heeley E, Huang Y, et al. Rapid blood-pressure lowering in patients with acute intracerebral hemorrhage. N Engl J Med. 2013;368(25):2355–65.
52. Anderson CS, Huang Y, Wang JG, et al. Intensive blood pressure reduction in acute cerebral haemorrhage trial (INTERACT): a randomised pilot trial. Lancet Neurol. 2008;7(5):391–9.
53. Butcher KS, Jeerakathil T, Hill M, et al. The intracerebral hemorrhage acutely decreasing arterial pressure trial. Stroke. 2013;44(3):620–6.
54. Qureshi AI, Palesch YY, Barsan WG, et al. Intensive blood-pressure lowering in patients with acute cerebral hemorrhage. N Engl J Med. 2016;375(11):1033–43.
55. Shaw L, Price C, McLure S, et al. Paramedic Initiated Lisinopril For Acute Stroke Treatment (PIL-FAST): results from the pilot randomised controlled trial. Emerg Med J. 2014;31(12):994–9.
56. Saver JL, Starkman S, Eckstein M, et al. Prehospital use of magnesium sulfate as neuroprotection in acute stroke. N Engl J Med. 2015;372(6):528–36.
57. Wentworth DA, Atkinson RP. Implementation of an acute stroke program decreases hospitalization costs and length of stay. Stroke. 1996;27(6):1040–3.
58. Kuramatsu JB, Gerner ST, Schellinger PD, et al. Anticoagulant reversal, blood pressure levels, and anticoagulant resumption in patients with anticoagulation-related intracerebral hemorrhage. JAMA. 2015;313(8):824–36.
59. Parry-Jones AR, Di Napoli M, Goldstein JN, et al. Reversal strategies for vitamin K antagonists in acute intracerebral hemorrhage. Ann Neurol. 2015;78(1):54–62.
60. Flower O, Smith M. The acute management of intracerebral hemorrhage. Curr Opin Crit Care. 2011;17(2):106–14.
61. Latorre JG, Greer DM. Management of acute intracranial hypertension: a review. Neurologist. 2009;15(4):193–207.
62. Elliott J, Smith M. The acute management of intracerebral hemorrhage: a clinical review. Anesth Analg. 2010;110(5):1419–27.
63. Qureshi AI. Intracerebral hemorrhage specific intensity of care quality metrics. Neurocrit Care. 2011;14(2):291–317.
64. Qureshi AI, Majidi S, Chaudhry SA, Qureshi MH, Suri MF. Validation of intracerebral hemorrhage-specific intensity of care quality metrics. J Stroke Cerebrovasc Dis. 2013;22(5):661–7.
65. Stroke Unit Trialists' Collaboration. Organized inpatient (stroke unit) care for stroke. Cochrane Database Syst Rev. 2013;9:CD000197. https://doi.org/10.1002/14651858.CD000197.pub3
66. Candelise L, Gattinoni M, Bersano A, et al. Stroke-unit care for acute stroke patients: an observational follow-up study. Lancet. 2007;369(9558):299–305.
67. Ramsay AI, Morris S, Hoffman A, et al. Effects of centralizing acute stroke services on stroke care provision in two large metropolitan areas in England. Stroke. 2015;46(8):2244–51.
68. Fuentes B, Diez-Tejedor E. The advantages of a stroke unit in the treatment of intracerebral hemorrhage. Rev Neurol. 2000;31(2):171–4.
69. Ronning OM, Guldvog B, Stavem K. The benefit of an acute stroke unit in patients with intracranial haemorrhage: a controlled trial. J Neurol Neurosurg Psychiatry. 2001;70(5):631–4.
70. Broderick J, Connolly S, Feldmann E, et al. Guidelines for the management of spontaneous intracerebral hemorrhage in adults: 2007 update: a guideline from the American Heart Association/American Stroke Association Stroke Council, High Blood Pressure Research Council, and the Quality of Care and Outcomes in Research Interdisciplinary Working Group. Stroke. 2007;38(6):2001–23.
71. Qureshi AI, Mendelow AD, Hanley DF. Intracerebral haemorrhage. Lancet. 2009;373(9675):1632–44.
72. Qureshi AI, Tuhrim S, Broderick JP, Batjer HH, Hondo H, Hanley DF. Spontaneous intracerebral hemorrhage. N Engl J Med. 2001;344(19):1450–60.

73. Suarez JI, Zaidat OO, Suri MF, et al. Length of stay and mortality in neurocritically ill patients: impact of a specialized neurocritical care team. Crit Care Med. 2004;32(11):2311–7.
74. Diringer MN, Edwards DF. Admission to a neurologic/neurosurgical intensive care unit is associated with reduced mortality rate after intracerebral hemorrhage. Crit Care Med. 2001;29(3):635–40.
75. Fogelholm R, Murros K, Rissanen A, Ilmavirta M. Factors delaying hospital admission after acute stroke. Stroke. 1996;27(3):398–400.
76. Yu RF, San Jose MC, Manzanilla BM, Oris MY, Gan R. Sources and reasons for delays in the care of acute stroke patients. J Neurol Sci. 2002;199(1–2):49–54.
77. Wester P, Radberg J, Lundgren B, Peltonen M. Factors associated with delayed admission to hospital and in-hospital delays in acute stroke and TIA: a prospective, multicenter study. Seek-Medical-Attention-in-Time Study Group. Stroke. 1999;30(1):40–8.
78. Crocco TJ, Grotta JC, Jauch EC, et al. EMS management of acute stroke--prehospital triage (resource document to NAEMSP position statement). Prehosp Emerg Care. 2007;11(3):313–7.
79. Catalano AR, Winn HR, Gordon E, Frontera JA. Impact of interhospital transfer on complications and outcome after intracranial hemorrhage. Neurocrit Care. 2012;17(3):324–33.
80. Jauch EC, Saver JL, Adams HP Jr, et al. Guidelines for the early management of patients with acute ischemic stroke: a guideline for healthcare professionals from the American Heart Association/American Stroke Association. Stroke. 2013;44(3):870–947.
81. Morgenstern LB, Hemphill JC 3rd, Anderson C, et al. Guidelines for the management of spontaneous intracerebral hemorrhage: a guideline for healthcare professionals from the American Heart Association/American Stroke Association. Stroke. 2010;41(9):2108–29.
82. Adams R, Acker J, Alberts M, et al. Recommendations for improving the quality of care through stroke centers and systems: an examination of stroke center identification options: multidisciplinary consensus recommendations from the Advisory Working Group on Stroke Center Identification Options of the American Stroke Association. Stroke. 2002;33(1):e1–7.
83. Fan JS, Chen YC, Huang HH, Yen DH, How CK, Huang MS. Interhospital transfer neurological deterioration in patients with spontaneous intracerebral haemorrhage: incidence and risk factors. Postgrad Med J. 2017;93(1100):349–53.
84. Kilbourn KJ, Killory BD, Fortunato G, et al. Clinical characteristics and outcomes of patients with intracerebral hemorrhage after Interhospital transfer to a designated stroke center. Conn Med. 2015;79(6):335–41.
85. Abid KA, Vail A, Patel HC, King AT, Tyrrell PJ, Parry-Jones AR. Which factors influence decisions to transfer and treat patients with acute intracerebral haemorrhage and which are associated with prognosis? A retrospective cohort study. BMJ Open. 2013;3(12):e003684.
86. Fletcher JJ, Kotagal V, Mammoser A, Peterson M, Morgenstern LB, Burke JF. Cost-effectiveness of transfers to centers with neurological intensive care units after intracerebral hemorrhage. Stroke. 2015;46(1):58–64.
87. LaMonte MP, Xiao Y, Hu PF, et al. Shortening time to stroke treatment using ambulance telemedicine: TeleBAT. J Stroke Cerebrovasc Dis. 2004;13(4):148–54.
88. Liman TG, Winter B, Waldschmidt C, et al. Telestroke ambulances in prehospital stroke management: concept and pilot feasibility study. Stroke. 2012;43(8):2086–90.
89. Bergrath S, Reich A, Rossaint R, et al. Feasibility of prehospital teleconsultation in acute stroke – a pilot study in clinical routine. PLoS One. 2012;7(5):e36796.
90. Van Hooff RJ, Cambron M, Van Dyck R, et al. Prehospital unassisted assessment of stroke severity using telemedicine: a feasibility study. Stroke. 2013;44(10):2907–9.
91. Wu TC, Nguyen C, Ankrom C, et al. Prehospital utility of rapid stroke evaluation using in-ambulance telemedicine: a pilot feasibility study. Stroke. 2014;45(8):2342–7.
92. Chapman Smith SN, Govindarajan P, Padrick MM, et al. A low-cost, tablet-based option for prehospital neurologic assessment: The iTREAT Study. Neurology. 2016;87(1):19–26.
93. Malandraki GA, McCullough G, He X, McWeeny E, Perlman AL. Teledynamic evaluation of oropharyngeal swallowing. J Speech Lang Hear Res. 2011;54(6):1497–505.
94. Johansson T, Wild C. Telemedicine in acute stroke management: systematic review. Int J Technol Assess Health Care. 2010;26(2):149–55.

95. Schenkel J, Reitmeir P, Von Reden S, et al. Cost analysis of telemedical treatment of stroke. Gesundheitswesen. 2013;75(7):405–12.
96. Nelson RE, Saltzman GM, Skalabrin EJ, Demaerschalk BM, Majersik JJ. The cost-effectiveness of telestroke in the treatment of acute ischemic stroke. Neurology. 2011;77(17):1590–8.
97. Switzer JA, Demaerschalk BM, Xie J, Fan L, Villa KF, Wu EQ. Cost-effectiveness of hub-and-spoke telestroke networks for the management of acute ischemic stroke from the hospitals' perspectives. Circ Cardiovasc Qual Outcomes. 2013;6(1):18–26.
98. Gresham GE, Alexander D, Bishop DS, et al. American Heart Association Prevention Conference. IV. Prevention and rehabilitation of stroke. Rehabilitation. Stroke. 1997;28(7):1522–6.
99. Group ATC, Bernhardt J, Langhorne P, et al. Efficacy and safety of very early mobilisation within 24 h of stroke onset (AVERT): a randomised controlled trial. Lancet. 2015;386(9988):46–55.
100. McGuire JR, Harvey RL. The prevention and management of complications after stroke. Phys Med Rehabil Clin N Am. 1999;10(4):857–74. ix
101. Foley N, Salter K, Teasell R. Specialized stroke services: a meta-analysis comparing three models of care. Cerebrovasc Dis. 2007;23(2–3):194–202.
102. Ang YH, Chan DK, Heng DM, Shen Q. Patient outcomes and length of stay in a stroke unit offering both acute and rehabilitation services. Med J Aust. 2003;178(7):333–6.
103. Chiu A, Shen Q, Cheuk G, Cordato D, Chan DK. Establishment of a stroke unit in a district hospital: review of experience. Intern Med J. 2007;37(2):73–8.
104. Chan DK, Levi C, Cordato D, et al. Health service management study for stroke: a randomized controlled trial to evaluate two models of stroke care. Int J Stroke. 2014;9(4):400–5.
105. Helgason CM, Wolf PA. American Heart Association Prevention Conference IV: prevention and rehabilitation of stroke: executive summary. Circulation. 1997;96(2):701–7.
106. Joubert J, Reid C, Barton D, et al. Integrated care improves risk-factor modification after stroke: initial results of the Integrated Care for the Reduction of Secondary Stroke model. J Neurol Neurosurg Psychiatry. 2009;80(3):279–84.

Chapter 11
ICH Rehabilitation and Recovery

Benjamin A. Abramoff, Nicole D. Mahdi, Maria Beran, and Samir R. Belagaje

Case

A 47-year-old African-American male with a past medical history of uncontrolled hypertension presented with new-onset dysarthria and decreased response time. Initial head CT showed a large right frontoparietal intraparenchymal hemorrhage with midline shift of 9 mm, as well as a thin right convexity subdural hematoma. His systolic blood pressure was greater than 200. The patient was taken urgently to the OR for surgical decompression. Follow-up CT showed improvement of mass effect. During the hospitalization, he had a witnessed seizure and was started on levetiracetam.

Eighteen days following admission, he was discharged from the acute hospital and transferred to a rehabilitation hospital. At that point, he was requiring moderate to maximal assistance. Deficits included left hemiplegia and development of spasticity. His rehabilitation stay was complicated by right common femoral vein deep vein thrombosis requiring inferior vena cava filter placement and a Klebsiella urinary tract infection leading to increased fatigue during therapy sessions which was ultimately treated with antibiotics.

Despite these setbacks, the patient made progress during his rehab course. His increased tone and spasticity was treated with baclofen and daily range of motion

B. A. Abramoff · M. Beran
Physical Medicine and Rehabilitation, Emory University Hospital, Atlanta, GA, USA

N. D. Mahdi
Stroke Program, Northwest Hospital, The Sandra and Malcolm Berman Brain and Spine Institute, Baltimore, MD, USA

S. R. Belagaje (✉)
Neurology and Rehabiliation Medicine, Emory University, Atlanta, GA, USA
e-mail: samir.r.belagaje@emory.edu; sbelaga@emory.edu

B. Ovbiagele, A. I. Qureshi (eds.), *Intracerebral Hemorrhage Therapeutics*,
https://doi.org/10.1007/978-3-319-77063-5_11

exercises. With physical and occupational therapy, he worked on mobility, upper and lower extremity dressing, transfers, self-care, toileting, bathing, as well as range of motion, strength, and gait. Speech language pathologists addressed his speech, swallowing, and cognitive deficits. Diet was ultimately progressed from nothing by mouth to regular consistency. His functional independence measure (FIM) score improved to a minimal assistance at time of discharge. He had no seizure-like events while in rehabilitation, and his family is wondering if the levetiracetam may be stopped.

The above case illustrates the typical rehabilitation course that a patient with hemorrhagic stroke goes through after their initial hospitalization. Despite receiving appropriate acute treatment in the hospital, the patient continued to have functional deficits preventing his return home. With a dedicated team of professionals, he was able to have significant recovery. This chapter will introduce the key statistics, concepts, issues, and techniques surrounding rehabilitation of the hemorrhagic stroke survivor with a focus on the evidence behind them.

The chapter begins by examining the statistics, factors, and trends in hemorrhage stroke rehabilitation followed by an overview of key principles underlying stroke rehabilitation. In addition, the chapter will focus on the issues and considerations more specifically associated with hemorrhagic stroke rehabilitation. It concludes with a discussion on future trends.

Outcomes and Prognosis

Mortality

There is a high rate of mortality following intracerebral hemorrhage (ICH) particularly within the first 2 days [1]. As seen in Table 11.1, the mortality rate following ICH is greatest in the first month and subsequently decreases.

Alternative survival figures place the 1-year survival rate at 46% and 5-year survival rate at 29% [3]. In a population-based cohort study consisting of 140 patients beginning 3 months following a spontaneous ICH, the 7-year mortality in ICH patients was 32.9% versus 19.4% in age- and sex-matched controls who had not suffered an ICH [4]. The mortality after recurrent ICH has been shown to be worse than after the initial ICH with in-hospital mortality reported to be between 32% and 56% [4]. A more detailed discussion on prognosis is found in a prior chapter.

Table 11.1 Mortality following ICH over time [1, 2]

Time since ICH onset	24 h	2 days	28 days	1 year
Mortality rate	16%	24%	50%	53%

Functional Outcomes in Ischemic Vs Hemorrhagic Strokes

There is conflicting evidence as to whether prognosis differs in ischemic compared to hemorrhagic strokes when controlling for other stroke factors. Barber et al. found that mortality rates were similar in ICH compared to ischemic strokes when both groups were matched on age, level of consciousness (as measured by GCS), and handicap (as measured by modified Rankin score (mRS)) [5]. In another study of patients who survived the first 2 days following ICH, patients were matched with those with ischemic strokes on age, level of consciousness (as measured by GCS), and handicap (as measured by mRS). There were not any differences between the two groups in terms of survival and handicap at 1 year which led the authors to conclude that the extent of the brain lesion, not the type of stroke, determined the outcome after a 2-day survival [1]. Andersen et al. found ICH was associated with an overall higher mortality risk compared to ischemic strokes as a result of both the higher severity level and the classification as hemorrhagic. The mortality risk gradually decreased, and after 3 months the stroke type did not correlate with mortality [6].

Paolucci et al. assessed the influence of stroke type on rehabilitation outcomes by matching hemorrhagic and ischemic patients for stroke severity, age, disability, sex, and time between onset and inpatient rehabilitation admission. At the time of discharge from inpatient rehabilitation, better functional recovery and mobility status was seen in the ICH patients compared to the ischemic stroke patients. The authors speculated the difference could potentially be due to better neurological recovery as hematomas resolve and brain compression improves in the ICH group. They also found a lower percentage of persistent urinary incontinence in the ICH stroke patients (4.7%) compared to ischemic stroke patients (12.4%). However the length of stay and percent of discharges to home were similar between the groups [7]. Other studies have shown ICH patients were more disabled on admission to rehabilitation compared to ischemic stroke patients, based on lower motor function scores and lower total, cognitive, and motor functional independence measure (FIM) scores [8, 9]. The ICH patients had a greater functional improvement after rehabilitation according to their functional independence measure (FIM) and motor function scores, even after adjustment for admission FIM, length of stay, age, and time from stroke onset to rehabilitation admission [8, 9].

General Stroke Rehabilitation Principles

Clinical Rehabilitation Principles and Pathways

The recovery team and rehabilitation pathways following an ICH are varied. The most recent guidelines for the management of a spontaneous ICH published jointly by the American Heart Association and American Stroke Association provide a Level IA recommendation that patients with ICH have access to interdisciplinary rehabilitation and a Level IB recommendation that patients begin rehabilitation as early as possible and continue their rehabilitation into the community setting [10].

The Stroke Patient Care Continuum

A recent Cochrane review outlined the various patient pathways following a stroke with different levels of interdisciplinary team involvement (Table 11.2) [11].

Including patients with hemorrhagic strokes, patients who received organized stroke unit care have higher survival, independence, and return to home with continued benefits potentially sustained up to 10 years. Dedicated stroke wards have demonstrated improved outcomes compared to mobile stroke teams as well as a trend toward improved outcomes compared to mixed rehabilitation wards [11].

In a meta-analysis comparing the different types of stroke wards (acute stroke units, rehabilitation units, and comprehensive units), Chan et al. found that comprehensive units led to reduced lengths of stay, decreased death and dependency, and improved functional outcomes compared to acute stroke and rehabilitation units [12]. Langhorne et al. found in a review of eight clinical trials that stroke units prevent death and disability in those with hemorrhagic stroke at least as much as those with ischemic strokes [13].

Rehabilitation efforts are not limited to the inpatient setting. A review of 14 trials found that stroke survivors discharged from an inpatient setting and continuing home-based rehabilitation improved their ability to perform activities of daily living [14]. Other potential patient settings include outpatient clinics, transitional/long-term acute care hospitals, home-health-based care, day treatment programs, assisted living facilities, and skilled nursing facilities.

Table 11.2 Inpatient rehabilitation settings

Type	Admission	Discharge	Features
Acute, intensive	Acute (hours)	Days	High nurse staffing; life-support facilities
Acute, semi-intensive	Acute (hours)	Days	Close physiological monitoring
Comprehensive	Acute (hours)	Days to weeks	Acute care/rehabilitation; conventional staffing
Integrated TCM	Acute (hours)	Days	Comprehensive stroke unit with integrated TCM (e.g., acupuncture)
Rehabilitation	Delayed (days)	Weeks	Rehabilitation
Mobile team	Variable	Days to weeks	Medical/rehabilitation advice
Mixed rehabilitation	Variable	Weeks	Mixed patient group; rehabilitation

From John Wiley and Sons, Stroke Unit Trialists' Collaboration [11], Table 1
TCM traditional Chinese medicine

Members of the Rehabilitation Team

Comprehensive, organized, interdisciplinary, team-based care is a key component of rehabilitation, and evidence shows that it enhances recovery and independence while decreasing mortality [11, 15, 16]. The members of the rehabilitation team are varied and have different roles (Table 11.3).

The patient's family also becomes a critical part of the patient care team following an ICH as they are often responsible for the long-term care of the patient and can assist in functional recovery.

Table 11.3 Members of the Stroke Rehabilitation Team.

Discipline	World Wide Web site	Description
Certified rehabilitation counselors	www.crccertification.com	Assist individuals with disabilities to maximize their vocational and avocational living goals in the most integrated setting possible through the application of the counseling process, including vocational and counseling, case management, referral, and service coordination; identifying and addressing employment and attitudinal barriers; and job analysis, development, and placement services.
Neuropsychologists	www.apa.org	Specialize in brain-behavior relationships and have extensive training in anatomy, physiology, and neuropathology. They identify and treat cognitive and neurobehavioral dysfunction and through assessment also monitor recovery and thereby enhance community reintegration.
Occupational therapists	www.aota.org	Focus on the "skills of living" necessary for independent and satisfying living. OT services include customized treatment programs to perform daily activities, comprehensive home and job site evaluations and adaptation recommendation, performance skills assessment and interventions, adaptive equipment recommendations and training, and family and caregiver education.
Rehabilitation nurses (RNs)	www.rehabnurse.org	Manage complex medical issues, provide ongoing patient and caregiver education, and establish care plans to maintain optimal wellness. RNs use a holistic approach to fulfill patients' medical, environmental, spiritual, vocational, and educational needs via principles from other disciplines and their own unique medical expertise (bowel, bladder, and skin management). In all care settings, RNs function as coordinators/case managers, collaborators, and counselors. A registered nurse with at least 2 years of practice in rehabilitation who passes the Association of Rehabilitation Nurses examination can earn the Certified Rehabilitation Nurse distinction.

(continued)

Table 11.3 (continued)

Discipline	World Wide Web site	Description
Physical therapists	www.apta.org	Experts in examining and treating neuromuscular problems that affect the abilities of individuals to move. PTs practice in many settings and with all age groups.
Physicians	www.aapmr.org	Usually coordinate the rehabilitation team and manage medical conditions pertaining to stroke and comorbidities. A physician may be a physiatrist (i.e., specializing in physical medicine and rehabilitation and thus restoration of function in individuals with problems that range from simple physical mobility to more complex cognitive issues).
Recreational therapists	www.atra-online.com	Provide treatment services and recreation activities to individuals with disabilities to facilitate independent physical, cognitive, emotional, and social functioning by enhancing individuals' current skills and assisting new skill development for daily living and community function. Besides discharge planning for community reintegration, they help individuals develop or redevelop social, discretionary time, decision-making, coping, self-advocacy, and basic skills to enhance overall quality of life.
Social workers'	www.naswdc.org	Assist individuals, groups, or communities restore or enhance their capacity for social functioning, while creating societal conditions favorable to their goals. Requires knowledge of human development and behavior; social, economic, and cultural institutions; and interactions among these factors. Social workers help prevent crises; counsel individuals, families, and communities to facilitate coping with everyday stresses; and identify resources to allow individuals with disabilities to remain in the community.
SLPs	www.asha.org	Assess speech, language, and other cognitive functions, as well as swallowing, and provide interventions and counseling/education to address language and speech disorders (e.g., aphasia, apraxia of speech, dysarthria, and cognitive-communication impairment). SLPs also intervene when swallowing and cognitive disorders exist. They provide services to all age groups and in all care settings.

From Miller et al. [15], Table 3, http://stroke.ahajournals.org/content/41/10/2402.long, with permission of Wolters Kluwer Health, Inc

RN indicates rehabilitation nurse

Mechanisms of Recovery

Primary injury occurs in hemorrhagic stroke due to disruption of the brain's cellular architecture and mass effect. Secondary injuries include the adverse effects of thrombin, inflammation, complement activation, free radicals, and glutamate-induced excitotoxicity [17, 18]. These mechanisms can potentially continue to cause damage days to weeks after initial injury [19–21].

Less research in the field of the recovery has been done with respect to hemorrhagic injuries compared to ischemic injury [22]. Nonetheless, the limited research to date suggests that reduction in edema and neuroplasticity are the main recovery mechanisms from hemorrhagic injury: there is evidence in rodents that the time course of the formation and resolution of edema closely matches the neurological deficits [20]. Efforts to reduce the mass effect from clot and/or edema may thus help to improve recovery by reducing perihematomal ischemia and improving cerebral blood flow [23]. Neuroplasticity is the ability of the brain and its synaptic connections to change in response to internal or external stimuli. It is a widely accepted mechanism for recovery after stroke.

At the cellular level, following ICH, there is increased proliferation of neural stem cells in the perihematomal region within 1–3 days [24]. There is also evidence of possible increase in dendritic branching indicating the formation of new synapses [20, 21]. From rodent models, there is evidence that rehabilitation may enhance dendritic growth and reduce tissue loss following ICH [20].

Factors Impacting Functional Recovery

Numerous factors play a role in stroke recovery and subsequent improvement in function (Fig. 11.1).

From: [25]

Age: Older patients who have had ICH have been found to have worse disability at 90 days compared to younger patients. A patient over 75 was four times more likely to be dependent at 90 days compared to those less than 52 years old. Pain,

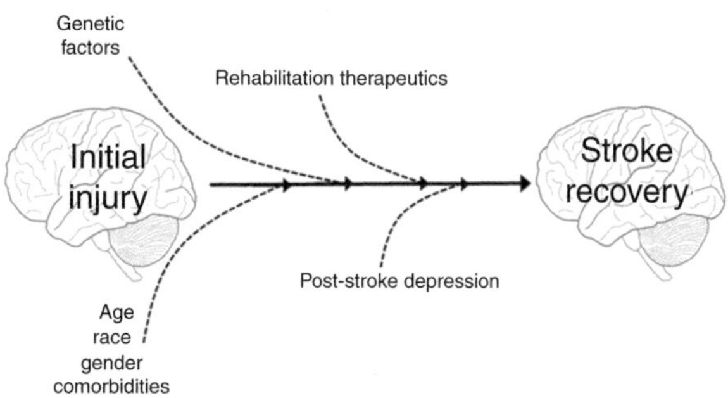

Fig. 11.1 The factors involved in stroke recovery. (From Feng and Belagaje [25], Fig. 1, © Georg Thieme Verlag KG)

mobility, self-care, participation in activities, and depression were all noted to increase with patient age [26].

Race: Racial disparities have been noted in some studies investigating rehabilitation therapies from stroke although the evidence is mixed. There is also evidence that black patients have worse functional outcomes compared to white patients [27].

Socioeconomic Status: Poor socioeconomic status has also been tied to impaired recovery outcomes [25, 27].

Gender: Women tend to have worse functional outcomes following strokes compared to men in multiple domains including physical impairments, limitations in ADLs, quality of life, and depression. They are also more likely to be institutionalized [28, 29]. In ICH, there is evidence that female sex may be an independent predictor of worse outcome, particularly in the early poststroke period [30, 31].

Stroke Location: Lobar intracerebral hemorrhages are more likely to lead to poor functional outcome compared to non-lobar ICH. There are no clear differences in functional outcome based on laterality. These studies have been limited by focus on motor outcomes and not precisely defining the neuroanatomical locations of the ICH. There is some evidence for poorer outcomes with thalamic bleeds [32]. Ventricular extension of blood is another poor sign of functional outcome [33].

Stroke Volume: Hemorrhage volume is one of the most important predictors of short- and long-term functional outcome in patients with ICH. A volume of hemorrhage greater than 30 ml is generally associated with worse functional outcomes, while a volume less than 20 ml is associated with better functional outcomes. A volume between 20 and 30 ml has less clear implication of functional recovery [33].

Outcome Scoring Systems: Numerous grading systems have been developed to evaluate the functional outcomes of patients with intracerebral hemorrhage. The ICH-GS (composed of age, initial GCS, ICH location, ICH volume (dichotomized by location of bleed)), and intraventricular extension have been used to predict functional outcome at 30 days [34]. The mEDICH has also been used to evaluate functional outcome at hospital discharge and is made up of initial GCS, ICH volume, INR, IVH, and location [35]. The FUNC score is comprised of ICH volume, age, ICH location, GCS, and pre-ICH cognitive impairment and is able to accurately predict functional independence at 90 days. Figure 11.2 demonstrates the percent of patients who became functionally independent at different time points following ICH according to their initial FUNC score. None (0%) of the patients with a FUNC score less than 4 had functional independence at 90 days. Eighty-two percent of patients with a FUNC score of 11 achieved functional independence [36]. A comparison of the different methods at hospital discharge found the mEDICH as the most reliable at predicting good functional outcome at hospital discharge [37].

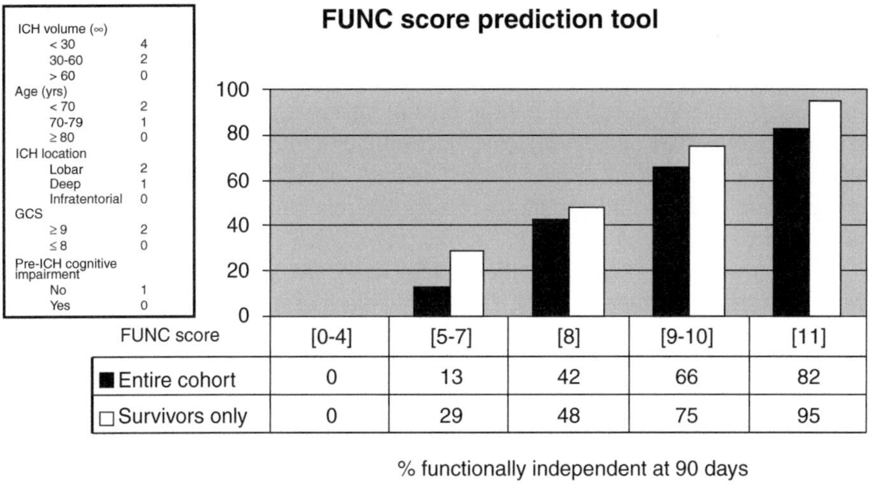

Fig. 11.2 Predictive ability of FUNC score. (From Rost et al. [36], Fig. 1, http://stroke.ahajournals.org/content/39/8/2304, with permission of Wolters Kluwer Health, Inc.)

Timing, Intensity, and Safety of Intracerebral Hemorrhage Rehabilitation

For all strokes, certain aspects of rehabilitation remain unknown. These questions include timing, intensity, and dosing of rehabilitation. These questions are even more apparent in the hemorrhagic stroke population as very few studies have investigated these questions specifically in this population.

As specific guidelines for early mobilization do not exist, one common concern is starting therapy very early may raise blood pressures which may lead to worsening hemorrhage and outcomes. To further complicate matters, there are not clear blood pressure parameters that are deemed safe to initiate therapy. In surveys of stroke care professionals, patients with hemorrhagic strokes were felt to start later mobilization than those with ischemic strokes [38, 39]. However, prolonged bedrest increases the risk of complications related to immobility including pressure sores, aspiration pneumonia, and deep vein thrombosis.

In the only dedicated large study specific to ICH to date, 243 subjects with ICH at multiple centers in China were randomized to very early rehabilitation compared to standard care. Survival and functional outcomes were measured. The intensity between the very early rehabilitation (starting rehabilitation within 48 h) and the standard of care group (rehabilitation starting on day 7) were comparable. At 6 months, patients receiving the standard of care were more likely to have died (adjusted hazard ratio, 4.44; 95% confidence interval [CI], 1.24–15.87) [40]. The generalizability of this study is uncertain given the standard of care group started therapy on day 7 which is usually later than therapy is started in the Western hemisphere, including US centers. Nevertheless, it suggests that patients may benefit from early rehabilitation. This is supported by other studies showing patients with hemorrhagic strokes undergoing early rehabilitation (starting within 24 h of their stroke) have been found to have better recovery of ADLs and motor functioning compared to patients undergoing more standard rehabilitation without an increase in mortality [41].

In contrast to these findings, the A Very Early Rehabilitation Trial (AVERT), 2104 hospitalized stroke subjects (258 of whom had intracerebral hemorrhages) were randomized to receive customary therapy or a very early intervention. In the intervention arm, first mobilization aimed to begin within 24 h following stroke onset with the additional goals of being upright and out of bed at least twice daily. This intervention was for the first 14 days poststroke or until discharge from the acute stroke unit and delivered by a physiotherapy team including a trained nurse. Those who were mobilized had worse outcomes defined as a modified Rankin Score <3 compared to standard care (46% vs 50%; adjusted odds ratio [OR] = 0·73, p = 0·004) [42]. In a prespecified dose response analysis of the trial, patients who were mobilized earlier and had more frequent sessions were more likely to have favorable outcomes compared to those who had increased length of out of bed activity, thereby suggesting more frequent, shorter out of bed activity is possibly the preferred dosing of rehabilitation [43].

In the ICARE trial, 361 subjects were given rehabilitation in one of three arms: Accelerated Skill Acquisition Program (ASAP), dose-equivalent occupational therapy (DEUCC), or monitoring-only occupational therapy (UCC). Motor outcomes were not significantly different between the three groups. Twelve percent (n = 43) of the subjects had intracerebral hemorrhage with equal numbers among the three interventions. There are no further subsequent analysis on this subgroup to date [44].

In the Locomotor Experience Applied Post-Stroke (LEAPS) trial, Duncan et al. tested the role of body-weight-supported treadmill against standard home physical therapy program and also attempted to provide further answers into the timing of rehabilitation. In this single-blinded trial, 408 subjects, 70 (17.2%) of which had hemorrhagic strokes, were randomly assigned to 1 of 3 arms lasting 12 to 16 weeks: a home-based exercise starting 2 months after the stroke or the body-weight-supported treadmill locomotor program, starting either at 2 or 6 months after the stroke.

The primary outcome of the study was the proportion of participants with improved walking function 1 year after the stroke. Most participants (52%) improved their walking function, but there were no significant differences between the three arms (change of 0.23 m/s in early locomotor group vs. 0.24 m/s in late locomotor group vs. 0.25 m/s for home exercise group). Serious adverse events were similar in all three arms, as were minor events, except that there was significantly more dizziness or faintness (p = 0.008) in the locomotor groups [45]. These results suggest that there is not a difference in poststroke walking improvement between body-weight-supported treadmill devices and a home-based physical therapy program.

Special Rehabilitation Considerations for ICH

For those patients who survive the acute phase of ICH, there are a variety of post-stroke complications that pose a significant impact on recovery and rehabilitation. This section will describe a variety of special considerations specific to ICH rehabilitation and how they impact long-term outcomes. As a summary, Table 11.4 consists of common post-ICH sequelae along with possible pharmacologic and non-pharmacologic treatments. These treatments have varying levels of evidence in stroke, and particularly post-ICH patients, and primary sources should be reviewed prior to prescribing.

Table 11.4 Common post-ICH sequelae and proposed treatment options

Common post-ICH sequelae	Proposed and accepted treatment options
Hemiparesis	*Pharmacologic*: Selective serotonin reuptake inhibitors Amphetamines *Non-pharmacologic*: Physical and occupational therapy (constraint therapy, mirror therapy) Functional electrical stimulation Specialized equipment
Spasticity	*Pharmacologic*: Botulinum toxin Phenol/alcohol neurolysis Intrathecal therapy (Baclofen) Baclofen Tizanidine Dantrolene Benzodiazpines *Non-Pharmacologic*: Daily stretching Physical therapy Splinting [77]
Seizures	Prophylactic seizure medications are not recommended if no prior history of seizures [72]
Dysphagia/aspiration	*Pharmacologic*: Cilostazol Angiotensin-converting enzyme inhibitors Amantadine *Non-pharmacologic*: Exercises/swallowing rehabilitation Postural and behavioral compensatory strategies Texture/consistency of food Nutrition consult Nasogastric/orogastric feeding tubes, gastrostomy, jejunostomy [78]

(continued)

Table 11.4 (continued)

Common post-ICH sequelae	Proposed and accepted treatment options
Neurogenic bladder	*Pharmacologic*: Anticholinergics (oxybutynin) and botulinum toxin for detrusor overactivity Cholinergics (Bethanechol) for urinary retention Adrenergic antagonists (Tamsulosin) for sphincter dyssynergy/urinary outlet obstruction *Non-pharmacologic*: Behavioral techniques: timed voiding, manual maneuvers, fluid restriction, physical therapy External, indwelling, and intermittent catheterizations Surgical procedures Consider urodynamic testing for further evaluation of bladder function [79]
Neurogenic bowel	*Pharmacologic*: Fiber Laxatives Rectal stimulants *Non-pharmacologic*: Abdominal massage Manual evacuation Toilet transfer training Bathroom equipment (bedside commode) Timed toileting [80]
Falls	*Pharmacologic*: Avoid polypharmacy, sedating alcohol, and medications *Non-pharmacologic*: Exercise, balance, cognitive and safety training, supervision Assistive devices (visual aids) Environmental hazard removal Prevention and treatment of osteopenia/osteoporosis to prevent fractures [81]
Psychiatric issues: depression, anxiety, emotionalism, relationship difficulties	*Pharmacologic*: Selective serotonin reuptake inhibitors Tricyclic antidepressants Monoamine oxidase inhibitors Buspirone *Non-pharmacologic*: Electroconvulsive therapy Peer support Recreational therapy Psychotherapy (counseling, cognitive behavioral therapy, motivational interviewing) Family counseling [82, 83]

Table 11.4 (continued)

Common post-ICH sequelae	Proposed and accepted treatment options
Sexual dysfunction	*Pharmacologic*: Phosphodiesterase-5 inhibitors Intracavernosal Intraurethral suppositories Hormonal therapy Avoid medications that can worsen sexual function: antidepressants, SSRIs, anticholinergics, opioids *Non-pharmacologic*: Physical therapy Mechanical devices, Counseling/psychotherapy [84]
Hemiplegic shoulder pain	*Pharmacologic*: Corticosteroid injections Platelet-rich plasmin Stem cells Suprascapular nerve blocks Botulinum toxin *Non-pharmacologic*: Physical therapy Massaging Support devices (slings, arm board) Electrical stimulation [85]
Other causes of pain following stroke: complex regional pain syndrome, spasticity-related pain, poststroke pain, neuropathic pain	*Pharmacologic*: Topical Agents NSAIDs Opioids Antiepileptic Antidepressant Lidocaine Ketamine Systemic corticosteroids Intrathecal therapy: opioids, ziconotide, baclofen *Non-pharmacologic*: Neurostimulatory techniques Transcutaneous electrical stimulation Acupuncture Desensitization Contrast baths Ultrasound Sympathectomy Pain psychology [86]
Fatigue	*Pharmacologic*: Antidepressants Neurostimulants (methylphenidate, modafinil) *Non-pharmacologic*: Treatment of sleep apnea Psychosocial therapy (education, CBT) Physical therapy Aerobic exercise [87]

(continued)

Table 11.4 (continued)

Common post-ICH sequelae	Proposed and accepted treatment options
Visual and visuospatial issues	*Pharmacologic*: Dopamine agonists Neurostimulants *Non-pharmacologic*: Visual therapy Eye patching Mirror therapy Prisms [88]
Aphasia	*Pharmacologic*: Amantadine Amphetamines Acetylcholinesterase inhibitors (donepezil, galantamine) Memantine Piracetam Bromocriptine *Non-pharmacologic*: Speech and language therapy Transcranial magnetic/electrical stimulation [89]
Cognitive and attention impairment, vascular dementia	*Pharmacologic*: Acetylcholinesterase inhibitors NMDA receptor antagonists Calcium channel blockers *Non-pharmacologic:* Cognitive therapy Treatment of depression Control risk factors for vascular dementia

Seizures and ICH

It is well recognized that seizures commonly occur after stroke, with varying incidences reported from 2% to 33% depending on the type of study, time windows described, and stroke type analyzed [46–52]. This incidence may actually be underreported given subclinical electrographic seizures are not included in most studies. Predictive factors that have been found to be independently associated with poststroke seizures include hemorrhagic stroke, lobar or cortical location of stroke, and 10-point increase in stroke severity on the Scandinavian Stroke Scale [46, 48]. For hemorrhagic strokes, the local mass effect from edema, development of hydrocephalus, and presence of blood products can be a nidus for epileptogenic activity. Later onset seizures are suspected to be due to gliosis and scarring that may become an epileptogenic focus during the healing process after both ischemic and hemorrhagic stroke.

One controversial issue is the impact of seizures on early and long-term prognosis in ICH patients. De Herdt et al. explored the risk of early seizures in ICH and did not show any influence of their occurrence on hospital mortality or functional outcome at 6 months [49]. This finding contrasts results of a study by Szaflarski et al. who showed that early post-ICH seizures occurring within the first 24 h were associated with a higher incidence of 30-day mortality [47]. A more recent study by

Madzar et al. showed a trend favoring an association of post-ICH seizures with poorer outcomes, but this data did not reach statistical significance [52]. With respect to late-onset seizures, Rossi et al. found an association with worse functional outcome after 3 years of follow-up [50]. There remains limited definitive evidence of a direct correlation of post-ICH seizures with poor outcomes as the association may be related to the inherent increased mortality seen in ICH patients that may not be greatly altered by the development of seizures in either the acute or late phase of ICH recovery.

Hydrocephalus and ICH

Another complication associated with ICH is intraventricular hemorrhage (IVH) extension, which reportedly occurs in 30–50% of patients and has been shown to be an independent predictor of poor outcomes and carries an overall mortality rate of up to 75% [53]. Subsequently, the development of acute hydrocephalus is reported in up to 50–67% of patients with ICH and most often seen with thalamic hemorrhages due to the close proximity to the third ventricle [53–55]. Hydrocephalus management often involves placement of an external ventricular drainage (EVD) in up to 30–50% of patients which can lead to further complications due to prolonged hospital stays, increased infection risk, and immobility. The increased intracranial pressure (ICP) due to hydrocephalus leads to rapid clinical deterioration including death from brain herniation. Patients may require placement of a VP shunt for permanent diversion of CSF to reduce hydrocephalus recurrence if the EVD is unable to be removed.

Studies have suggested that the presence of hydrocephalus with ICH an independent predictor of poor outcomes [53, 54]. Diringer et al. showed that each 1 point increase in hydrocephalus severity, as measured using a 24-point score grading the degree of hydrocephalus within the various regions of the ventricular system, was associated with a 1.64-fold increase in mortality risk [56]. In the study, fewer patients with hydrocephalus were discharged to rehab or home, and over 60% of patients required admission to a nursing home or did not survive hospitalization [56]. Of those patients who survived, there was no difference in FIM scores at 3 months between patients with and without hydrocephalus. The study concluded that hydrocephalus is an independent predictor of mortality after ICH.

Spasticity in ICH

It is well recognized that surviving stroke patients suffer from residual upper motor neuron symptoms including muscle spasticity with prevalence ranging from 19% to 42% [57]. Spasticity can limit mobility and cause discomfort, all of which can impact poststroke recovery, efficacy of rehabilitation, and performance of activities of daily living. Hemorrhagic stroke is a predictor of poststroke spasticity [58]. One can hypothesize that given the degree of disability in ICH patients which is often higher than ischemic stroke patients, as well as tendency to sustain longer hospital stays and subsequent delays to early and aggressive poststroke therapy, these patients may have a higher prevalence of poststroke spasticity. Rehabilitation techniques for poststroke spasticity are currently generalized to help with functional outcomes for all stroke types. A variety of techniques used for poststroke spasticity include muscle strengthening exercises, treadmill training, use of orthotics, oral antispasmodics, nerve blockade, botulinum toxin injections, and intrathecal baclofen therapy.

Neuropsychiatric Complications of ICH

The proposed etiologies of poststroke mood disorders specifically in ICH may be attributed to the mass effect on various brain structures involved in emotion and behavior such as the amygdala and prefrontal cortex by the primary injury [59]. The subsequent inflammatory response on affected areas can therefore result in secondary injury [59]. An even simpler explanation would be a psychological reaction to one suffering a devastating neurological injury resulting in physical impairment affecting one's prior functional independence [59, 60]. Regardless, the profound complexity of ICH makes defining the exact mechanisms involved in poststroke mental illness difficult.

Poststroke depression (PSD) is a well-recognized complication of stroke, regardless of type, location, or severity. It has a prevalence ranging anywhere from 11% to 78% depending on study design [60, 61]. There are many confounders that affect PSD prevalence such as the incidence of pre-stroke depression, which is seen in up to 16% of the general elderly population. Pre-stroke depression likely influences the subsequent development of depression after stroke [60]. A recent systematic review showed that depression had a negative effect on functional outcomes after stroke, with associations of PSD with decreased quality of life, poor life satisfaction, less efficient use of rehab services, increased need for institutional services, and higher mortality. Individuals suffering from PSD are likely less motivated or physically able, especially in severely impaired patients, to participate and engage in rehabilitation, in both the acute and long-term stroke recovery period. Given the negative impact of depression on the ability to effectively rehabilitate from a stroke, it is important to identify those patients at risk for PSD and therefore initiate early interventions to aid in successful stroke recovery.

Dementia and ICH

Cognitive impairment following stroke is a contribution to the worldwide burden of new-onset dementia, which occurs in approximately 10% of patients after their first stroke and increases to 30% after recurrent stroke [62]. Although various studies exploring the prevalence of and risk factors for poststroke dementia, only a minority of them include ICH patients. A small cross-sectional study first reported a prevalence of post-ICH dementia of 23% after 3 years [63]. A larger prospective cohort study of ICH patients without preexisting dementia showed an incidence of dementia of 14% at 1-year follow-up and an incidence of 28% at 4-year follow-up. Risk factors associated with new-onset dementia included superficial siderosis, higher number of cerebral microbleeds, and increased cortical atrophy [64, 65]. In addition, the incidence of post-ICH dementia was two times higher in those with lobar hemorrhages, which may correlate with the known association of cortically located ICH with cerebral amyloid angiopathy (CAA) [65]. CAA has been reported in over 40% of patients with ICH and subsequent cognitive decline, although CAA has been independently associated with cognitive impairment, even in the absence of extensive Alzheimer's disease pathology [65, 66].

Thus, poststroke dementia poses a challenge to successful rehabilitation not only in the acute but in the long-term poststroke period. Cognitive impairment has been shown to be a powerful predictor for functional outcomes after stroke, with evidence suggesting that these individuals have reduced recovery potential due to reduced optimism, memory impairment, and deficiencies in performance of activities of daily living [66]. Further research on how dementia impacts stroke survivors is needed as well as more treatments to guide rehabilitation techniques in this patient population.

Medications in ICH Rehabilitation

Patients often suffer from depressed level of consciousness or impaired attention following ICH, both of which can limit effective poststroke rehabilitation. Thus, neurostimulants are often used to enhance arousal in order for patients to participate in more aggressive rehabilitation in both the short- and long-term recovery period and possibly even prevent extended care facility placement [67]. Despite the widespread use and potential of these medications, evidence of clear efficacy is lacking. In small studies, methylphenidate and dextroamphetamine, two commonly studied neurostimulants, improved function and speech [67]. Unfortunately, these agents carry the risk of hypertension; as blood pressure often needs to be strictly controlled in ICH patients, they may not be the ideal choices used in this patient population. Alternative neurostimulants include modafinil and amantadine, which are also used to aid in increased alertness in poststroke patients. More studies directly studying neurostimulant use in stroke patients are needed to make conclusive recommendations on which agents may in fact be beneficial and positively impact poststroke rehabilitation.

As mentioned earlier, depression is a well-recognized complication of stroke; consequently, antidepressants are commonly prescribed to patients after stroke to help during the rehabilitation process. There have been some studies specifically looking at selective serotonin reuptake inhibitors (SSRIs) and the risk of hemorrhagic stroke, and they demonstrate that SSRIs inhibit platelet aggregation [68, 69]. Other studies have not shown such a correlation, even with concomitant antiplatelet or anticoagulant use [69]. The controversy in SSRI risk needs to be weighed against evidence from multiple studies demonstrating benefit from SSRI. Both ischemic and hemorrhagic stroke patients have been found to have less dependency, improved motor recovery, and reduced depression with SSRIs [70]. Basic science research has demonstrated that SSRIs play a role in inhibiting pro-inflammatory cytokine production, thus positively impacting stroke recovery given its potential to augment neurogenesis and synaptic plasticity [71].

Given the increased incidence of seizures following ICH as compared to ischemic stroke, many patients are placed on antiepileptic drugs (AEDs) for seizure prophylaxis in the acute period. There is evidence showing that brief prophylaxis may reduce the risk of early seizures with lobar hemorrhage [72]. However, AEDs commonly have several side effects that may impact effective rehabilitation participation such as dizziness, drowsiness, and cognitive impairment [73]. In the Cerebral Hemorrhage and NXY-059 Trial (CHANT), early use of AEDs was strongly independently associated with severe disability and death in ICH; hypothesized mechanisms included both the sedative and cardiovascular effects of AEDs [74]. In particular, prophylactic use of phenytoin has been associated with fever and worse functional outcomes after ICH while not reducing the risk of seizures [75].

There are a variety of pharmacologic treatments available to manage poststroke spasticity including muscle relaxers and benzodiazepines, all of which have centrally acting side effects. Some of the common side effects of these agents share are dizziness, sedation, and cognitive slowing, which can negatively impact the efficacy of poststroke rehabilitation [76]. In addition, consistent use of these agents can be associated with withdrawal seizures if dependency is achieved, particularly with frequent baclofen and benzodiazepine use. Therefore, a need exists to find a balance between the benefits of lowering muscle tone with these medications while at the same time minimizing side effects. Alternatives, such as botulinum toxin, should also be considered in order to most benefit patients in the rehabilitation period.

Summary

Rehabilitation is an important component of care of hemorrhagic stroke patients. Despite the advances in prevention and acute treatment, stroke survivors will continue to need rehabilitation. Recovery begins as soon as the patient enters the healthcare system. Despite having worse deficits than ischemic stroke patients, hemorrhagic patients make larger gains in formal rehabilitation. Future recovery and rehabilitation studies need to focus specifically on the hemorrhagic stroke population to better understand their care. By understanding the general trends of hemorrhagic stroke recovery, incorporating and applying general rehabilitation principles, and recognizing and managing the special rehabilitation issues associated with hemorrhagic strokes, one can optimize outcomes.

References

1. Franke CL, van Swieten JC, Algra A, van Gijn J. Prognostic factors in patients with intracerebral haematoma. J Neurol Neurosurg Psychiatry. 1992;55(8):653–7.
2. Fogelholm R, Murros K, Rissanen A, Avikainen S. Long term survival after primary intracerebral haemorrhage: a retrospective population based study. J Neurol Neurosurg Psychiatry. 2005;76(11):1534–8.
3. Poon MT, Fonville AF, Al-Shahi Salman R. Long-term prognosis after intracerebral haemorrhage: systematic review and meta-analysis. J Neurol Neurosurg Psychiatry. 2014;85(6):660–7.
4. Saloheimo P, Lapp TM, Juvela S, Hillbom M. The impact of functional status at three months on long-term survival after spontaneous intracerebral hemorrhage. Stroke. 2006;37(2):487–91.
5. Barber M, Roditi G, Stott DJ, Langhorne P. Poor outcome in primary intracerebral haemorrhage: results of a matched comparison. Postgrad Med J. 2004;80(940):89–92.
6. Andersen KK, Olsen TS, Dehlendorff C, Kammersgaard LP. Hemorrhagic and ischemic strokes compared: stroke severity, mortality, and risk factors. Stroke. 2009;40(6):2068–72.
7. Paolucci S, Antonucci G, Grasso MG, Bragoni M, Coiro P, De Angelis D, et al. Functional outcome of ischemic and hemorrhagic stroke patients after inpatient rehabilitation: a matched comparison. Stroke. 2003;34(12):2861–5.
8. Katrak PH, Black D, Peeva V. Do stroke patients with intracerebral hemorrhage have a better functional outcome than patients with cerebral infarction? PM R. 2009;1(5):427–33.
9. Kelly PJ, Furie KL, Shafqat S, Rallis N, Chang Y, Stein J. Functional recovery following rehabilitation after hemorrhagic and ischemic stroke. Arch Phys Med Rehabil. 2003;84(7):968–72.
10. Hemphill JC 3rd, Greenberg SM, Anderson CS, Becker K, Bendok BR, Cushman M, et al. Guidelines for the Management of Spontaneous Intracerebral Hemorrhage: a guideline for healthcare professionals from the American Heart Association/American Stroke Association. Stroke. 2015;46(7):2032–60.
11. Stroke Unit Trialists' Collaboration. Organised inpatient (stroke unit) care for stroke. Cochrane Database Syst Rev. 2013;(9):Cd000197.
12. Chan DK, Cordato D, O'Rourke F, Chan DL, Pollack M, Middleton S, et al. Comprehensive stroke units: a review of comparative evidence and experience. Int J Stroke Off J Int Stroke Soc. 2013;8(4):260–4.
13. Langhorne P, Fearon P, Ronning OM, Kaste M, Palomaki H, Vemmos K, et al. Stroke unit care benefits patients with intracerebral hemorrhage: systematic review and meta-analysis. Stroke. 2013;44(11):3044–9.
14. Legg L, Langhorne P. Rehabilitation therapy services for stroke patients living at home: systematic review of randomised trials. Lancet. 2004;363(9406):352–6.
15. Miller EL, Murray L, Richards L, Zorowitz RD, Bakas T, Clark P, et al. Comprehensive overview of nursing and interdisciplinary rehabilitation care of the stroke patient: a scientific statement from the American Heart Association. Stroke. 2010;41(10):2402–48.
16. Keith RA. The comprehensive treatment team in rehabilitation. Arch Phys Med Rehabil. 1991;72(5):269–74.
17. Keep RF, Hua Y, Xi G. Intracerebral haemorrhage: mechanisms of injury and therapeutic targets. Lancet Neurol. 2012;11(8):720–31.
18. Xi G, Keep RF, Hoff JT. Mechanisms of brain injury after intracerebral haemorrhage. Lancet Neurol. 2006;5(1):53–63.
19. Mracsko E, Veltkamp R. Neuroinflammation after intracerebral hemorrhage. Front Cell Neurosci. 2014;8:388.
20. MacLellan CL, Silasi G, Auriat AM, Colbourne F. Rodent models of intracerebral hemorrhage. Stroke. 2010;41(10 Suppl):S95–8.
21. Nguyen AP, Huynh HD, Sjovold SB, Colbourne F. Progressive brain damage and alterations in dendritic arborization after collagenase-induced intracerebral hemorrhage in rats. Curr Neurovasc Res. 2008;5(3):171–7.

22. Jang SH. A review of motor recovery mechanisms in patients with stroke. NeuroRehabilitation. 2007;22(4):253–9.
23. NINDS ICH Workshop Participants. Priorities for clinical research in intracerebral hemorrhage: report from a National Institute of Neurological Disorders and Stroke workshop. Stroke. 2005;36(3):e23–41.
24. Shen J, Xie L, Mao X, Zhou Y, Zhan R, Greenberg DA, et al. Neurogenesis after primary intracerebral hemorrhage in adult human brain. J Cereb Blood Flow Metab. 2008;28(8):1460–8.
25. Feng W, Belagaje SR. Recent advances in stroke recovery and rehabilitation. Semin Neurol. 2013;33(5):498–506.
26. Radholm K, Arima H, Lindley RI, Wang J, Tzourio C, Robinson T, et al. Older age is a strong predictor for poor outcome in intracerebral haemorrhage: the INTERACT2 study. Age Ageing. 2015;44(3):422–7.
27. Stansbury JP, Jia H, Williams LS, Vogel WB, Duncan PW. Ethnic disparities in stroke: epidemiology, acute care, and postacute outcomes. Stroke. 2005;36(2):374–86.
28. Reeves MJ, Bushnell CD, Howard G, Gargano JW, Duncan PW, Lynch G, et al. Sex differences in stroke: epidemiology, clinical presentation, medical care, and outcomes. Lancet Neurol. 2008;7(10):915–26.
29. Petrea RE, Beiser AS, Seshadri S, Kelly-Hayes M, Kase CS, Wolf PA. Gender differences in stroke incidence and poststroke disability in the Framingham heart study. Stroke. 2009;40(4):1032–7.
30. Zhou J, Zhang Y, Arima H, Zhao Y, Zhao H, Zheng D, et al. Sex differences in clinical characteristics and outcomes after intracerebral haemorrhage: results from a 12-month prospective stroke registry in Nanjing, China. BMC Neurol. 2014;14:172.
31. Ganti L, Jain A, Yerragondu N, Jain M, Bellolio MF, Gilmore RM, et al. Female gender remains an independent risk factor for poor outcome after acute nontraumatic intracerebral hemorrhage. Neurol Res Int. 2013;2013:219097.
32. Sreekrishnan A, Dearborn JL, Greer DM, Shi FD, Hwang DY, Leasure AC, et al. Intracerebral hemorrhage location and functional outcomes of patients: a systematic literature review and meta-analysis. Neurocrit Care. 2016;25(3):384–91.
33. LoPresti MA, Bruce SS, Camacho E, Kunchala S, Dubois BG, Bruce E, et al. Hematoma volume as the major determinant of outcomes after intracerebral hemorrhage. J Neurol Sci. 2014;345(1–2):3–7.
34. Ruiz-Sandoval JL, Chiquete E, Romero-Vargas S, Padilla-Martinez JJ, Gonzalez-Cornejo S. Grading scale for prediction of outcome in primary intracerebral hemorrhages. Stroke. 2007;38(5):1641–4.
35. Masotti L, Di Napoli M, Godoy DA, Lorenzini G. Predictive ability of a modified version of emergency department intracerebral hemorrhage grading scale for short-term prognosis of intracerebral hemorrhage. J Stroke Cerebrovasc Dis Off J Natl Stroke Assoc. 2015;24(5):1100–4.
36. Rost NS, Smith EE, Chang Y, Snider RW, Chanderraj R, Schwab K, et al. Prediction of functional outcome in patients with primary intracerebral hemorrhage: the FUNC score. Stroke. 2008;39(8):2304–9.
37. Masotti L, Lorenzini G, Di Napoli M, Godoy DA. Prognostic ability of four clinical grading scores in spontaneous intracerebral hemorrhage. Acta Neurol Belg. 2017;117(1):325–7.
38. Sjoholm A, Skarin M, Linden T, Bernhardt J. Does evidence really matter? Professionals' opinions on the practice of early mobilization after stroke. J Multidiscip Healthc. 2011;4:367–76.
39. Skarin M, Bernhardt J, Sjoholm A, Nilsson M, Linden T. Better wear out sheets than shoes': a survey of 202 stroke professionals' early mobilisation practices and concerns. Int J Stroke Off J Int Stroke Soc. 2011;6(1):10–5.
40. Liu N, Cadilhac DA, Andrew NE, Zeng L, Li Z, Li J, et al. Randomized controlled trial of early rehabilitation after intracerebral hemorrhage stroke: difference in outcomes within 6 months of stroke. Stroke. 2014;45(12):3502–7.

41. Bai Y, Hu Y, Wu Y, Zhu Y, He Q, Jiang C, et al. A prospective, randomized, single-blinded trial on the effect of early rehabilitation on daily activities and motor function of patients with hemorrhagic stroke. J Clin Neurosci Off J Neurosurg Soc Australasia. 2012;19(10):1376–9.
42. AVERT Trial Collaboration Group. Efficacy and safety of very early mobilisation within 24 h of stroke onset (AVERT): a randomised controlled trial. Lancet. 2015;386(9988):46–55.
43. Bernhardt J, Churilov L, Ellery F, Collier J, Chamberlain J, Langhorne P, et al. Prespecified dose-response analysis for a very early rehabilitation trial (AVERT). Neurology. 2016;86(23):2138–45.
44. Winstein CJ, Wolf SL, Dromerick AW, Lane CJ, Nelsen MA, Lewthwaite R, et al. Effect of a task-oriented rehabilitation program on upper extremity recovery following motor stroke: the ICARE randomized clinical trial. JAMA. 2016;315(6):571–81.
45. Duncan PW, Sullivan KJ, Behrman AL, Azen SP, Wu SS, Nadeau SE, et al. Body-weight-supported treadmill rehabilitation after stroke. N Engl J Med. 2011;364(21):2026–36.
46. Bladin CF, Alexandrov AV, Bellavance A, Bornstein N, Chambers B, Cote R, et al. Seizures after stroke: a prospective multicenter study. Arch Neurol. 2000;57(11):1617–22.
47. Szaflarski JP, Rackley AY, Kleindorfer DO, Khoury J, Woo D, Miller R, et al. Incidence of seizures in the acute phase of stroke: a population-based study. Epilepsia. 2008;49(6):974–81.
48. Alberti A, Paciaroni M, Caso V, Venti M, Palmerini F, Agnelli G. Early seizures in patients with acute stroke: frequency, predictive factors, and effect on clinical outcome. Vasc Health Risk Manag. 2008;4(3):715–20.
49. De Herdt V, Dumont F, Henon H, Derambure P, Vonck K, Leys D, et al. Early seizures in intracerebral hemorrhage: incidence, associated factors, and outcome. Neurology. 2011;77(20):1794–800.
50. Rossi C, De Herdt V, Dequatre-Ponchelle N, Henon H, Leys D, Cordonnier C. Incidence and predictors of late seizures in intracerebral hemorrhages. Stroke. 2013;44(6):1723–5.
51. Haapaniemi E, Strbian D, Rossi C, Putaala J, Sipi T, Mustanoja S, et al. The CAVE score for predicting late seizures after intracerebral hemorrhage. Stroke. 2014;45(7):1971–6.
52. Madzar D, Kuramatsu JB, Gollwitzer S, Lucking H, Kloska SP, Hamer HM, et al. Seizures among long-term survivors of conservatively treated ICH patients: incidence, risk factors, and impact on functional outcome. Neurocrit Care. 2014;21(2):211–9.
53. Balami JS, Buchan AM. Complications of intracerebral haemorrhage. Lancet Neurol. 2012;11(1):101–18.
54. Zacharia BE, Vaughan KA, Hickman ZL, Bruce SS, Carpenter AM, Petersen NH, et al. Predictors of long-term shunt-dependent hydrocephalus in patients with intracerebral hemorrhage requiring emergency cerebrospinal fluid diversion. Neurosurg Focus. 2012;32(4):E5.
55. Bu Y, Chen M, Gao T, Wang X, Li X, Gao F. Mechanisms of hydrocephalus after intraventricular haemorrhage in adults. Stroke Vasc Neurol. 2016;1(1):23–7.
56. Diringer MN, Edwards DF, Zazulia AR. Hydrocephalus: a previously unrecognized predictor of poor outcome from supratentorial intracerebral hemorrhage. Stroke. 1998;29(7):1352–7.
57. Zorowitz RD, Gillard PJ, Brainin M. Poststroke spasticity: sequelae and burden on stroke survivors and caregivers. Neurology. 2013;80(3 Suppl 2):S45–52.
58. Lundstrom E, Terent A, Borg J. Prevalence of disabling spasticity 1 year after first-ever stroke. Eur J Neurol. 2008;15(6):533–9.
59. Snaphaan L, van der Werf S, Kanselaar K, de Leeuw FE. Post-stroke depressive symptoms are associated with post-stroke characteristics. Cerebrovasc Dis. 2009;28(6):551–7.
60. Hackett ML, Pickles K. Part I: frequency of depression after stroke: an updated systematic review and meta-analysis of observational studies. Int J Stroke Off J Int Stroke Soc. 2014;9(8):1017–25.
61. Kutlubaev MA, Hackett ML. Part II: predictors of depression after stroke and impact of depression on stroke outcome: an updated systematic review of observational studies. Int J Stroke Off J Int Stroke Soc. 2014;9(8):1026–36.
62. Moulin S, Labreuche J, Bombois S, Rossi C, Boulouis G, Henon H, et al. Dementia risk after spontaneous intracerebral haemorrhage: a prospective cohort study. Lancet Neurol. 2016;15(8):820–9.

63. Garcia PY, Roussel M, Bugnicourt JM, Lamy C, Canaple S, Peltier J, et al. Cognitive impairment and dementia after intracerebral hemorrhage: a cross-sectional study of a hospital-based series. J Stroke Cerebrovasc Dis Off J Natl Stroke Assoc. 2013;22(1):80–6.
64. Auriel E, Greenberg SM. The pathophysiology and clinical presentation of cerebral amyloid angiopathy. Curr Atheroscler Rep. 2012;14(4):343–50.
65. Greenberg SM, Gurol ME, Rosand J, Smith EE. Amyloid angiopathy-related vascular cognitive impairment. Stroke. 2004;35(11 Suppl 1):2616–9.
66. Gurr DB, Ibbitson J. How does cognitive ability affect stroke rehabilitation outcomes? Int J Ther Rehabil. 2012;19(8):458–62.
67. Napolitano E, Elovic EP, Qureshi AI. Pharmacological stimulant treatment of neurocognitive and functional deficits after traumatic and non-traumatic brain injury. Med Sci Monit. 2005;11(6):RA212–20.
68. Hackam DG, Mrkobrada M. Selective serotonin reuptake inhibitors and brain hemorrhage: a meta-analysis. Neurology. 2012;79(18):1862–5.
69. Kharofa J, Sekar P, Haverbusch M, Moomaw C, Flaherty M, Kissela B, et al. Selective serotonin reuptake inhibitors and risk of hemorrhagic stroke. Stroke. 2007;38(11):3049–51.
70. Mead GE, Hsieh CF, Lee R, Kutlubaev M, Claxton A, Hankey GJ, et al. Selective serotonin reuptake inhibitors for stroke recovery: a systematic review and meta-analysis. Stroke. 2013;44(3):844–50.
71. Mortensen JK, Larsson H, Johnsen SP, Andersen G. Impact of prestroke selective serotonin reuptake inhibitor treatment on stroke severity and mortality. Stroke. 2014;45(7):2121–3.
72. Broderick J, Connolly S, Feldmann E, Hanley D, Kase C, Krieger D, et al. Guidelines for the management of spontaneous intracerebral hemorrhage in adults: 2007 update: a guideline from the American Heart Association/American Stroke Association Stroke Council, High Blood Pressure Research Council, and the Quality of Care and Outcomes in Research Interdisciplinary Working Group. Stroke. 2007;38(6):2001–23.
73. Walia KS, Khan EA, Ko DH, Raza SS, Khan YN. Side effects of antiepileptics – a review. Pain Pract Off J World Inst Pain. 2004;4(3):194–203.
74. Messe SR, Sansing LH, Cucchiara BL, Herman ST, Lyden PD, Kasner SE. Prophylactic antiepileptic drug use is associated with poor outcome following ICH. Neurocrit Care. 2009;11(1):38–44.
75. Naidech AM, Garg RK, Liebling S, Levasseur K, Macken MP, Schuele SU, et al. Anticonvulsant use and outcomes after intracerebral hemorrhage. Stroke. 2009;40(12):3810–5.
76. Zorowitz RD. Road to recovery: drugs used in stroke rehabilitation. Expert Rev Neurother. 2004;4(2):219–31.
77. Francisco GE, McGuire JR. Poststroke spasticity management. Stroke. 2012;43(11):3132–6.
78. Vose A, Nonnenmacher J, Singer ML, Gonzalez-Fernandez M. Dysphagia Management in Acute and sub-acute Stroke. Curr Physi Med Rehabil Rep. 2014;2(4):197–206.
79. Linsenmeyer TA. Post-CVA voiding dysfunctions: clinical insights and literature review. NeuroRehabilitation. 2012;30(1):1–7.
80. Coggrave M, Norton C. Management of faecal incontinence and constipation in adults with central neurological diseases. Cochrane Database Syst Rev. 2013;(12):Cd002115.
81. Batchelor FA, Mackintosh SF, Said CM, Hill KD. Falls after stroke. Int J Stroke Off J Int Stroke Soc. 2012;7(6):482–90.
82. Hackett ML, Anderson CS, House A, Halteh C. Interventions for preventing depression after stroke. Cochrane Database Syst Rev. 2008;(3):Cd003689.
83. Campbell Burton CA, Holmes J, Murray J, Gillespie D, Lightbody CE, Watkins CL, et al. Interventions for treating anxiety after stroke. Cochrane Database Syst Rev. 2011;(12):Cd008860.
84. Nilsson MI, Fugl-Meyer K, von Koch L, Ytterberg C. Experiences of sexuality six years after stroke: a qualitative study. J Sex Med. 2017;14(6):797–803.

85. Viana R, Pereira S, Mehta S, Miller T, Teasell R. Evidence for therapeutic interventions for hemiplegic shoulder pain during the chronic stage of stroke: a review. Top Stroke Rehabil. 2012;19(6):514–22.
86. Harrison RA, Field TS. Post stroke pain: identification, assessment, and therapy. Cerebrovasc Dis. 2015;39(3–4):190–201.
87. Wu S, Kutlubaev MA, Chun HY, Cowey E, Pollock A, Macleod MR, et al. Interventions for post-stroke fatigue. Cochrane Database Syst Rev. 2015;(7):Cd007030.
88. Diamond PT. Rehabilitative management of post-stroke visuospatial inattention. Disabil Rehabil. 2001;23(10):407–12.
89. Greener J, Enderby P, Whurr R. Pharmacological treatment for aphasia following stroke. Cochrane Database Syst Rev. 2001;(4):CD000424.

Chapter 12
Clinical Trial Design in Subjects with Intracerebral Hemorrhage

Adeola Olowu and Nicole R. Gonzales

Introduction

Intracerebral hemorrhage imparts a high degree of disability and death. The greatest impact in decreasing the devastating nature of ICH is to prevent the disease altogether. Thus, screening, prevention, genetic, epidemiologic, and treatment trials are all equally important in decreasing the burden of this disease; however, the lack of effective treatment in the acute setting lends itself to a focus on clinical trials targeting acute treatment of ICH. Many aspects of clinical trial design in patients with ICH will draw from our successful experiences with ischemic stroke; however, the ICH patient population also offers unique considerations which will be discussed in this chapter. Lastly, the results of several large randomized controlled trials in patients with ICH have been reported over the last decade which provide important lessons that can be carried forward as we continue our efforts to develop treatment for this debilitating disease.

The last decade of clinical research in ICH has given us therapies which have achieved their physiologic goal, i.e., decreased hematoma expansion; however, this did not translate to improved clinical outcome based on the primary outcome measures [1–4]. While we have made considerable progress, definitive treatment which improves outcomes remains elusive. Heterogeneity of the patient population, patient recruitment and retention, finding the appropriate outcome measure, and timing at which to acquire this information all contribute to the challenges in finding efficacious treatment for ICH. In addition, there is a continued lack of understanding of the complex pathophysiology of disease which likely hampers our ability to detect treatment effect in our current clinical trial paradigm. In order to develop treatment, we need to more intimately understand the disease and recovery

A. Olowu · N. R. Gonzales (✉)
Department of Neurology, McGovern Medical School, Houston, TX, USA
e-mail: Nicole.R.Gonzales@uth.tmc.edu

B. Ovbiagele, A. I. Qureshi (eds.), *Intracerebral Hemorrhage Therapeutics*,
https://doi.org/10.1007/978-3-319-77063-5_12

process. In order to prove treatment efficacy, we need to adjust our clinical trial design to minimize known challenges and utilize our current technological and computational tools to develop new and efficient methods of evaluating investigational treatment.

General Concepts

Phase 1 trials are designed to establish a safe dose in humans and evaluate toxicity of a drug. Often, a specific aim is to estimate the maximum tolerated dose [5, 6]. Phase 2 studies examine feasibility, best dose, toxicity, and surrogate outcome markers of drug efficacy. In addition, phase 2 trials can be used to assess futility and can provide important information regarding the practical aspects of carrying out a larger clinical trial such as treatment administration and trial costs [5, 6]. In a phase 3 randomized controlled efficacy trial, participants are randomly assigned to an intervention or control group. The goal of the randomized controlled trial (RCT) evaluating therapy is to determine whether the treatment under evaluation is associated with an outcome. RCTs establish whether treatment is clinically efficacious [5, 7, 8].

With this framework in mind, there are several challenges in clinical trial design that are present in many conditions where patients present acutely with life-threatening illness. In these situations, rapid diagnostic evaluation and management decisions are made quickly with seemingly very little time for the additional processes that are necessary for clinical trial enrollment.

Ethical Considerations

Informed Consent

The challenges with informed consent in acute ICH treatment trials are similar to those in acute ischemic stroke (AIS) and other diseases in which patients present emergently with life-threatening conditions. Namely, can patients with this type of acute neurologic injury truly provide informed consent? When there is a time-sensitive aspect to treatment, can patients or their surrogate decision-makers really process the information needed to provide true informed consent [8]? What is the role of the clinician versus the clinical researcher and how does each influence informed consent [9]? On the other side of the coin, we also know that in acute stroke, the sooner treatment begins, the higher the chances for improved outcomes, in general. We know from our own work that when a surrogate is needed to provide informed consent it takes almost 20 min longer to obtain informed consent compared to cases where the patient can provide consent [10]. While there is no perfect scenario for the informed consent process in the emergent setting, clinical trial design can be sensitive to these issues with appropriate planning and training.

Patients with acute ICH may present with alteration in consciousness, aphasia, neglect, or other disabling deficit. In the acute setting of stroke, time is brain. Emergency responders aim to gather information necessary to initiate treatment as rapidly as possible. In most facilities, if the patient is not able to provide consent for participation in clinical research, a legally authorized representative (LAR) must be physically present to provide consent. Telephone consent is not typically allowed in most institutions. If there is no LAR at the bedside, then the patient will not be eligible for investigational studies; if the LAR subsequently arrives in the window for enrollment, then study-related procedures have been delayed [11]. Both scenarios can bias study results. In the best scenario, the LAR is at the bedside and, many times, discussion about clinical research begins in the hectic emergency department when the patient and family have just been delivered devastating news. Informed consent forms (ICFs) are lengthy and contain research, clinical, and legal information which can be overwhelming. The investigator must balance delivery of information and adjust discussion with each scenario and family dynamic. In this vulnerable state, patients may place all trust in their caregivers [9] or medical team for decision-making. There may be confusion in understanding what is standard of care and what is investigational when the clinician and researcher are the same person or part of the same team [9]. These are daunting responsibilities for patients, families, and investigators, and they must all be addressed in order for clinical research to be successful.

There is no single solution to the challenges of obtaining informed consent during emergent situations. Rather, it is important for investigators to be aware of these issues when designing clinical research trials so that the informed consent process happens correctly. Some potential approaches to these issues include ongoing discussion about consent even after enrollment and allowing the patient to provide consent once she has recovered well enough to do so [8]. To address the lengthy ICF, researchers can develop a short-form ICF [12] or a one-page summary of the trial [8] to accompany the complete ICF, with important points if the trial can be summarized succinctly and relevant institutional review board (IRB) is amenable to this process. Delay in obtaining consent for transferred or disabled patients requiring LAR consent or complete ineligibility of patients for clinical research without a LAR present can potentially be addressed with telemedicine and exemption from informed consent (EFIC).

Telemedicine provides the infrastructure to allow patients presenting to a hospital in a spoke/hub model to be offered participation in clinical research trials. Moreover, investigators can consent patients and their families for clinical trial enrollment remotely and begin study-related procedures either at the transferring facility [13, 14] or immediately upon arrival to the primary study site [15]. In addition, the FDA has provided guidance for exception from informed consent (EFIC) in emergency research when patients have a life-threatening medical condition necessitating urgent intervention and cannot provide consent due to their condition [16]. The circumstances under which EFIC is allowed are limited in scope but could be applicable to acute treatment trials evaluating therapy in patients with ICH in which the treatment is time-limited. EFIC also requires that available treatments are unsatisfactory; there must be the potential for direct benefit to the patient, and in order to provide benefit, treatment must be initiated before ICF can be obtained from the patient or the patient's LAR. The regulations also require community consultation and public disclosure in the communities where the research will take place. A summary of the regulations in the context of stroke-related research has been reported [17]. In addition, the American Heart Association Emergency Cardiovascular Care Committee and Council on Cardiopulmonary, Perioperative, and Critical Care have provided a template to assist with ensuring appropriate implementation of community consultation and public disclosure [18]. Lastly, researchers have reported on the views of patients and families enrolled in a RCT of an investigational agent for traumatic brain injury [19]. The majority of patients had positive attitudes toward the study inclusion and found their inclusion under EFIC acceptable [20].

The issue of obtaining true informed consent will always be a challenge in clinical trials for acute ICH therapy. Balancing the distribution of information for patients and families with rapid initiation of investigational treatment is an important responsibility of investigators. Continual reassessment and refinement of our informed consent processes will remain a focus of clinical trial design.

Clinical Trial Design Considerations

Patient Population

When developing inclusion and exclusion criteria for a clinical trial, the dilemma is whether to be inclusive or exclusive. If enrollment criteria are broad, then results will be generalizable and applicable to a larger number of patients. On the other hand, nonresponders may dampen treatment effect [9]. In contrast, if enrollment criteria are selective, this helps to minimize the heterogeneity of the patient population, may identify patients most likely to respond to treatment, and makes it more likely that a treatment effect will be seen if one truly exists. The trade-offs for selective inclusion/exclusion criteria are that the trial results may not be generalizable [5, 21], it may be difficult to enroll patients, and it may take longer to complete the trial. Development of new clinical, radiographic, and laboratory biomarkers can be incorporated into the patient selection algorithm to address the heterogeneity of this patient population [21, 22] (Fig. 12.1).

Clinical investigators are in search of treatment that will be applicable to all patients with a particular condition; however, the reality is that treatment may affect patients differently. Some patients may experience a large treatment benefit and others, a more modest effect, if any at all. Identification of the patient population which might respond to treatment may not be obvious in the initial phases of treatment

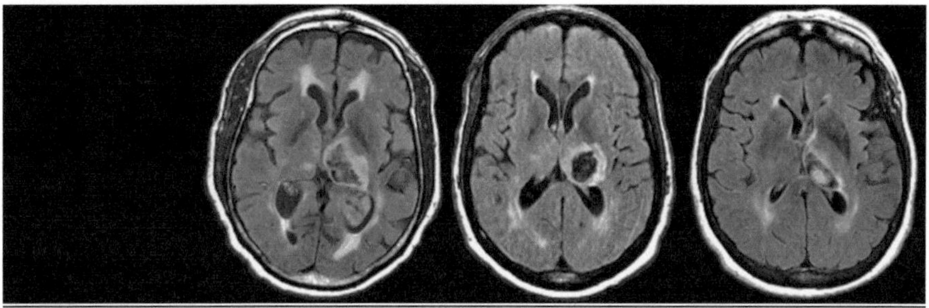

Age	46	59	57
ICH Volume	13.9	5.6	9.0
IVH?	Yes	Yes	No
GCS	14	14	14
NIHSS	16	10	7
Baseline mRS	0	0	0
180 Day mRS	3	2	1

Fig. 12.1 Clinical and Radiographic Heterogeneity in Patients with Intracerebral Hemorrhage. MRI images at presentation demonstrating the heterogeneity of patients with intracerebral hemorrhage even when the injury is in the same anatomic location. All three patients have a left thalamic hematoma; however, clinical and radiographic differences are apparent. ICH, intracerebral hemorrhage; IVH, intraventricular hemorrhage; GCS, Glasgow Coma Scale; NIHSS, National Institutes of Health Stroke Scale; mRS, modified Rankin Scale

development. We have seen this pattern in AIS where the treatment effect of IV tpa diminishes with time [23]. Thus, a larger treatment effect is present in patients who are treated with thrombolysis sooner after symptom onset. Similarly, if we consider recent endovascular trials in AIS as examples, after decades of not being able to demonstrate superiority of endovascular therapy over standard care, updated treatment devices, creation of a more homogeneous group of patients by limiting enrollment criteria by time, imaging, or lesion location, investigators were better able to accurately identify a group of responders to endovascular therapy [11, 24–27]. In the Factor Seven for Acute Hemorrhagic Stroke (FAST) trial, recombinant activated Factor VII (rFVIIa) demonstrated a dose-related decrease in hematoma expansion which did not translate to a clinical benefit [1]. Patient selection in this case may have played a role [3]. Since only about one third of patients are expected to have acute hematoma expansion [28], the treatment effects of rFVIIa may have been dampened by the enrollment of patients who were not likely to have hematoma enlargement and thus would not be expected to benefit from treatment. Identifying the subgroup of patients most likely to have hematoma expansion, e.g., with the spot sign, could identify the group of patients most likely to benefit from therapy trials targeting hematoma expansion [29]. While responder-based selection for enrollment criteria may limit generalizability [21], it may be a necessary step in demonstrating that acute treatment in ICH can affect outcomes.

Until recently, in-person or faxed consent was the only way to enroll a patient into a clinical trial. Depending on the time frame for enrollment, this limits the potential pool of study eligible patients to those presenting directly to the enrolling center. Patients who are transferred from an outside hospital may not be eligible for enrollment depending on the treatment window. Even if there is a prolonged time for enrollment, e.g., 24 h, transferred patients can potentially bias the study results if they are all enrolled and treated toward the end of the treatment window. As mentioned previously, telemedicine provides a mechanism by which study-related procedures can begin sooner when patients present to a facility with a spoke/hub model of telemedicine coverage. Clinical researchers have the opportunity to consent patients and/or their families for clinical trial enrollment remotely and begin study-related procedures, either at the transferring facility [13, 14] or immediately upon arrival to the primary study site [15]. The overall benefits of telemedicine are the following: (1) the investigational treatment is offered to patients who otherwise would not have been offered enrollment simply because of distance from an enrolling center, (2) increased enrollment helps to complete the trial faster, (3) there is increased generalizability as the geographic pool is enlarged, and (4) video consent avoids delay in treatment if family is not transported with the patient (e.g., air transport) who may not be able to provide consent. Incorporation of telemedicine into the clinical trial workflow will require additional resources and personnel for training, monitoring, in-servicing, and regulatory-related issues. In addition, depending on the intervention being evaluated, pharmacy and laboratory facilities may need to be involved [13]. The additional time and infrastructure development may be worth the investment if clinical trials are completed sooner and investigational studies are available to a greater number of patients.

Comparison Group

Single-arm studies can be completed quickly and require less resources than a clinical trial which includes a control group. Many phase 2 safety or dose-finding studies are single-arm studies. Even though we do not have a specific treatment approved for ICH, modernization of medicine is such that the development of stroke units and neurocritical care units may have an impact on outcomes and quality of care [30–32]. Thus, the use of historical estimates for outcomes could underestimate how well a control group actually does and overestimate the expected benefit of treatment [21, 33]. Since sample size estimation depends on the expected outcomes of a control group and anticipated benefit of the treatment [21], miscalculation can lead to an underpowered study. When possible, it is ideal to include a parallel control group in a randomized, controlled fashion.

Choice of Study Endpoint

Choosing the appropriate outcome at the right time is a critically important part of the clinical trial design. Outcomes measured in ICH typically include neurologic impairment, disability, and functional status. In addition, quality of life, resource utilization, and patient/caregiver feelings are also important outcome measures. Indirect measures of treatment effect such as biomarkers (e.g., radiographic or laboratory) can also be assessed [34, 35]. The choice of outcome measure depends on the phase of the investigation and the anticipated treatment effect. For example, in a phase 2 trial, safety, adverse events, or biomarkers might be primary outcome measures, and clinical or functional outcomes may be secondary outcome measures. Phase 3 clinical trials tend to use functional outcome as the primary outcome measure of drug efficacy. In addition, if treatment is expected to have a large impact on recovery, one might choose to dichotomize between good and bad outcome; for example, good outcome might be defined by modified Rankin scale score 0–1. On the other hand, if treatment is expected to have a more mild effect on outcomes, a researcher may choose to evaluate the entire range of the modified Rankin scale score (shift analyses) [36]. Clinical trials also evaluate quality of life and resource utilization outcomes. Incorporation of patient preferences and how outcomes are weighted in analyses is a current focus in cardiovascular disease and can be evaluated in the ICH population as well [37].

The most commonly used outcomes in clinical trials for ICH include mortality, functional outcome measured by the Barthel index (BI), modified Rankin scale score (mRS), Glasgow outcome scale (GOS), and the Stroke Impact Scale (SIS). The mRS and GOS are used to measure degree of disability. They are both ordered scales, and the main difference between the two measures is that the mRS has slightly more distinction between degree of "good" outcome [38]. The BI is a measure of ability to perform basic activities of daily living and mobility. The SIS measures patient or caregiver feelings and perspectives about residual deficits. Resource utilization and patient/caregiver perspectives will become a more common outcome measure in future trials. If a potential treatment is resource intensive but does not demonstrate improved outcomes compared with standard care, then cost utilization information and patient and family perspective can provide valuable information on whether the treatment should be pursued further. There may be other important outcomes which are valued by patients and families even if improved function is not demonstrated.

The best time point at which to measure outcome for ICH is unclear. The time point of 90 days after stroke onset is commonly used as the time at which to measure outcomes with the rationale that outcomes captured at a later time can be affected by late medical complications, rehabilitation therapy or other confounders which are not related to the investigational treatment [35]. Phase 3 clinical trials evaluating medical treatment for ICH have adopted a 3-month time point for assessment of clinical and functional outcomes, similar to clinical trials in AIS [1, 2, 39–41]. Phase 3 clinical trials evaluating surgical therapy measure functional outcomes at 6 months [42–44]. There is data which suggest that medically managed patients continue to have improvement measurable by the mRS score up to 6 months [45]. Thus, additional study is necessary to determine the ideal outcome measure(s) and timing at which to obtain this information in patients with ICH. Due to the complexity involved in anticipating treatment effect, choice of outcome measure, and method of evaluating the outcome measure, clinical researchers must work closely with an experienced statistical team who understands the patient population and disease.

ICH Therapy Trial Challenges and Unique Considerations

There are several challenges in patients with ICH which can directly impact clinical research trial design. ICH patients have clinical and radiographic features which contribute to a more severely affected patient population than AIS. These characteristics, e.g., IVH and coagulopathy-related ICH, introduce a higher in-hospital mortality and long-term disability rate which impacts sample size estimation, inclusion and exclusion criteria, and retention of patients in clinical trials. Given the high in-hospital mortality rate of ICH, predictors of early mortality would be useful to include in the randomization process. In contrast to AIS where standard care has been protocolized with standard metrics which are monitored [46], similar treatment standards are not as consistent for ICH. Routine care for patients with ICH is variable despite the guidelines [47], and it is unclear how variable treatment in a control group might affect outcomes. Clinical research protocols in patients with ICH must strictly define "standard care" for the control group or study designs which can accommodate the variability in clinical practice such as the use of hyperosmolar therapy, platelet transfusion, emergent surgery for herniating patients, and/or type of epileptic drugs for seizure prophylaxis should be explored (Table 12.1).

Combined Interventions

ICH causes both primary and secondary injuries. The primary insult is due to disruption of adjacent tissue with deposition of blood and subsequent mass effect [48]. Secondary injury occurs with development of edema, the inflammatory cascade, and direct cytotoxicity of red blood cell (RBC) breakdown products. The damage caused by ICH is multifactorial. It is intuitive that successful treatment might be multifaceted. Current treatment targets in ICH include prevention of hematoma expansion, removal of the toxic RBC breakdown products either surgically or pharmacologically, and cytoprotection [49]. Clinical trial designs which allow combined therapy should be explored. Evaluation of combined interventions reflects the real-world practice of medicine and could take into account the variability in our current "standard of care" for patients with ICH.

Table 12.1 Challenges in clinical trial design in acute intracerebral hemorrhage (ICH)

Challenges in ICH		Considerations
Severely affected patient population	Increased mortality and disability rates Inclusion of dying patients in clinical trials	Adaptive design, development of novel biomarkers for better risk stratification Novel endpoints including patient- and family-centered outcomes
Consent in the emergent setting	Not enough time for true informed consent in the acute setting	Short form or summary of important clinical trial points Ongoing discussion with family and patient even after initial consent
Consenting impaired patients	Ineligibility of patients for clinical trial enrollment without a surrogate present Delayed initiation of study-related procedures if surrogate shows up in a delayed fashion	Telemedicine consent Exemption from informed consent in the appropriate setting
Variable "standard care" in ICH	Unclear interpretation of control group outcomes if treatment is variable	Exploration of study designs which can incorporate common variable clinical practice (e.g., adaptive design, factorial design) Clearly define "standard care" in protocol
Enrollment inclusion/exclusion criteria	Nonresponders may dampen treatment effect Patient population heterogeneity	Responder-based selection for enrollment criteria
Single-arm studies, historical controls	Can overestimate treatment effect	Randomized, parallel control group
Retention in clinical trial	Transportation difficulty due to finances or disability Distance and time for travel Patient in a facility during short-term follow-up time point	Limit number of in-person follow-up visits Allow for transportation accommodations in the protocol and budget Study team can travel to the patient Telephone, telemedicine, or teleconferencing to obtain outcome data

ICH patients tend to be more severely disabled, and retention can be an issue. Due to new disability, patients sometimes have to move to be closer to family members who can participate in their care. Challenges for patients and families include transportation of a disabled patient, sometimes over long distances. At short-term follow-up (e.g., 30 days), some patients may still be in a facility (skilled nursing, long-term acute care, or rehabilitation). In order to improve data collection, long-term follow-up should accommodate this change in location by limiting the number of in-person follow-up visits or incorporating accommodations for this possibility in the protocol and budget. Some solutions include budgeting for transportation costs. In addition, patients can be transported to the primary study site. In such cases, sites may have to contract with a basic life support certified provider. Alternatively, the study team can travel to the patient. If the study team is following up with a patient in another facility, issues regarding credentialing may come into play. In order to improve retention, researchers should consider telemedicine or teleconferencing to obtain information [21, 50]. These "virtual visits" [22] can facilitate retention of patients who cannot travel due to financial hardship or disability. It is also reasonable to consider outcome measures that do not require in-person visits and can be obtained by telephone. Any accommodation that can minimize the need for travel or in-person visits is likely to improve data collection.

Novel Aspects in Clinical Trial Designs

Given the challenges in designing clinical research trials for patients with ICH, increasing limitations on funding, and the time it takes to complete trials, there is an urgent need to develop more efficient trial designs. It is difficult to do so within our traditional RCT framework, and it is imperative that clinical researchers explore ways to avoid the same pitfalls of prior trials. Ultimately, the way we carry out clinical trials in patients with ICH must adapt to the patient population, natural history of disease, and complexity of recovery. We have new computational power and new technology which make change possible. Efficiency can be incorporated in the pretrial planning phase as well as in the trial design. We have decades of clinical trials to learn from. Overestimating treatment effect or underestimating control group outcomes can lead to underpowered studies. Imbalances in baseline prognostic variables can make interpretation of results difficult. Inclusion of nonresponders dampens potential treatment effect. These are just some of the challenges which can be addressed with pretrial planning, adaptive methods of dose finding, randomization, and study monitoring. In addition, the incorporation of telemedicine into our workflow allows us to broaden our geographic reach and thus our patient population.

The US FDA Draft Guidance defines adaptive clinical trial as a study that modifies one or more aspects of the trial design based on prospectively planned evaluation of accumulating study data [51]. Adaptive design can be incorporated in dose escalation, randomization algorithms, study monitoring, determination of futility, and evaluation of outcome data. Indeed, some of these design aspects have already been utilized in stroke trials [52–57]. Adaptive design provides the ability to efficiently dose escalate, to adjust sample size estimates, and to make meaningful interpretations of available information in the absence of "statistical significance." It is important to understand the circumstances under which adaptive analyses are appropriate and their limitations [6, 58]; thus, an experienced statistical team is imperative.

Computer simulation utilizes mathematical models that mimic a real-world situation. Experiments can then be conducted to investigate or predict outcomes in this situation [59]. In clinical trials, simulation can be used at various points in trial design. Simulation can model disease progression and identify factors that contribute to variance in outcomes [22, 53]. In addition, simulation can be used to validate performance of randomization programming to ensure equal distribution of important prognostic variables among treatment groups [52].

Simulation is being utilized more in evaluation of neurologic treatment [22]. For example, the Stroke Hyperglycemia Insulin Network Effort (SHINE) trial utilized clinical trial simulation to better understand and address potential statistical limitations of their adaptive trial design [53]. The argatroban in combination with TPA Stroke Study used simulation to validate performance of the randomization program [52].

Regulatory and Financial Considerations

Keeping up with recruitment goals and adhering to a timeline for study completion within a fixed time is a herculean undertaking, especially in multicenter trials. When developing a timeline, keep in mind possible delays for IRB approval, developing and negotiating a budget and determination of "standard of care" costs vs. study-related costs. Investigators conducting a multicenter trial of surgical treatment for patients with ICH have reported delay in study initiation due to vastly different times in obtaining regulatory approval across institutions and countries [7]. As mentioned previously, because standard treatment for ICH can be variable, it can be difficult to adhere to one budget for each participating center. For example, if center A looks for a spot sign on all patients with ICH, then center A's standard of care is to perform a CT angiogram and post-contrast head CT on all their patients with ICH. Center B may only perform a non-contrast head CT and additional vascular imaging only when clinically indicated. Center B has a different "standard of care." One can imagine that in an ICH clinical trial where CTA is part of the study protocol, it may be more expensive to include center B because the budget would need to bear the financial burden of the CTA for each enrolled patient since it would not be considered standard of care for center B.

Conclusion

Thus far, identification of a treatment for ICH which improves outcomes has been elusive. In order to develop treatment, clinical researchers must continue to better understand the disease as well as adjust our clinical trial design to accommodate the complexities of the patient population and recovery process. Several well-designed clinical trials achieved the goal of limiting hematoma expansion, yet, this did not translate to improved outcomes. Our experience from these trials will inform our patient selection and stratification plans in future clinical trials. The smaller, sicker, and heterogeneous population of ICH patients warrants careful consideration of additional biomarkers which can help identify treatment responders. For future clinical trials in ICH, incorporation of adaptive design, computer simulation, and different types of outcome measures may be useful in identifying a meaningful effect of treatment.

A quick perusal of clinical trials in ICH listed on clinicaltrials.gov (accessed November 2016) demonstrated that almost 2/3 of registered clinical trials were focused on acute treatment. Less than 1/3 of listed studies reviewed were observational in nature and less than 1/10 targeted primary or secondary prevention of ICH. While there is an urgent need to develop acute treatment for ICH, the most dramatic impact for patients and families would be prevention of ICH altogether.

We continue to better understand the pathophysiology of ICH through our preclinical work and advancing technology. Technology also allows us to broaden the scope of clinical trials in ICH, figuratively and literally. As we apply these tools to our current practices, we remain hopeful that improved outcome in ICH is within reach.

References

1. Mayer SA, Brun NC, Begtrup K, Broderick J, Davis S, Diringer MN, et al. Efficacy and safety of recombinant activated factor VII for acute intracerebral hemorrhage. N Engl J Med. 2008;358(20):2127–37.
2. Anderson CS, Heeley E, Huang Y, Wang J, Stapf C, Delcourt C, et al. Rapid blood-pressure lowering in patients with acute intracerebral hemorrhage. N Engl J Med. 2013;368(25):2355–65.
3. Tuhrim S. Intracerebral hemorrhage – improving outcome by reducing volume? N Engl J Med. 2008;358(20):2174–6.
4. Anderson CS, Huang Y, Wang JG, Arima H, Neal B, Peng B, et al. Intensive blood pressure reduction in acute cerebral haemorrhage trial (INTERACT): a randomised pilot trial. Lancet Neurol. 2008;7(5):391–9.
5. Grotta JC, Albers G, Broderick JP, Kasner SE, Lo EH, Mendelow AD, et al. Stroke : pathophysiology, diagnosis, and management. 6th ed: Elsevier Inc; 2016. 1 online resource p.
6. Cheung K, Kaufmann P. Efficiency perspectives on adaptive designs in stroke clinical trials. Stroke. 2011;42(10):2990–4.
7. Kenyon GM, Mendelow AD, Gregson BA, Rowan E. Obtaining regulatory approval for multicentre randomised controlled trials: experiences in the STICH II trial. Br J Neurosurg. 2011;25(3):352–6.
8. Jadad AR, Enkin M, Jadad AR. Randomized controlled trials: questions, answers, and musings. Blackwell Publishing; Malden, Massachusetts. 2nd ed. xxiv, 136 p.
9. Slyter H. Ethical challenges in stroke research. Stroke. 1998;29(8):1725–9.
10. Masuca SR, Das DS, Delano D, Irani M, Pandurengan R, Barreto AD, et al. Abstract 3769: barriers to obtaining informed consent in acute stroke clinical trials. Stroke. 2012;43(Suppl 1):A3769-A.
11. Jovin TG, Chamorro A, Cobo E, de Miquel MA, Molina CA, Rovira A, et al. Thrombectomy within 8 hours after symptom onset in ischemic stroke. N Engl J Med. 2015;372(24):2296–306.
12. Stunkel L, Benson M, McLellan L, Sinaii N, Bedarida G, Emanuel E, et al. Comprehension and informed consent: assessing the effect of a short consent form. IRB. 2010;32(4):1–9.
13. Wu TC, Sarraj A, Jacobs A, Shen L, Indupuru H, Biscamp D, et al. Telemedicine-guided remote enrollment of patients into an acute stroke trial. Ann Clin Trans Neurol. 2015;2(1):38–42.
14. Alfredo Caceres J, Greer DM, Goldstein JN, Viswanathan A, Suarez JI, Brau L, et al. Enrollment of research subjects through telemedicine networks in a multicenter acute intracerebral hemorrhage clinical trial: design and methods. J Vasc Intervent Neurol. 2014;7(3):34–40.
15. Switzer JA, Hall CE, Close B, Nichols FT, Gross H, Bruno A, et al. A telestroke network enhances recruitment into acute stroke clinical trials. Stroke. 2010;41(3):566–9.

16. U.S. Department of Health and Human Services Food, Drug Administration Office of Good Clinical Practice Center for Drug Evaluation, Research Center for Biologics Evaluation, Research Center for Devices, Radiological Health. Guidance for institutional review boards. Clinical investigators, and sponsors; exception from informed consent requirements for emergency research. Washington, DC: U. S. Food and Drug Administration; 2013.
17. Bateman BT, Meyers PM, Schumacher HC, Mangla S, Pile-Spellman J. Conducting stroke research with an exception from the requirement for informed consent. Stroke. 2003;34(5):1317–23.
18. Halperin H, Paradis N, Mosesso V Jr, Nichol G, Sayre M, Ornato JP, et al. Recommendations for implementation of community consultation and public disclosure under the Food and Drug Administration's "Exception from informed consent requirements for emergency research": a special report from the American Heart Association Emergency Cardiovascular Care Committee and Council on Cardiopulmonary, Perioperative and Critical Care: endorsed by the American College of Emergency Physicians and the Society for Academic Emergency Medicine. Circulation. 2007;116(16):1855–63.
19. Wright DW, Yeatts SD, Silbergleit R, Palesch YY, Hertzberg VS, Frankel M, et al. Very early administration of progesterone for acute traumatic brain injury. N Engl J Med. 2014;371(26):2457–66.
20. Dickert NW, Scicluna VM, Baren JM, Biros MH, Fleischman RJ, Govindarajan PR, et al. Patients' perspectives of enrollment in research without consent: the patients' experiences in emergency research-progesterone for the treatment of traumatic brain injury study. Crit Care Med. 2015;43(3):603–12.
21. Zaidat OO, Liebeskind DS, Edgell RC, Amlie-Lefond CM, Kalia JS, Alexandrov AV. Clinical trial design for endovascular ischemic stroke intervention. Neurology. 2012;79(13 Suppl 1):S221–33.
22. Dorsey ER, Venuto C, Venkataraman V, Harris DA, Kieburtz K. Novel methods and technologies for 21st-century clinical trials: a review. JAMA Neurol. 2015;72(5):582–8.
23. Lees KR, Bluhmki E, von Kummer R, Brott TG, Toni D, Grotta JC, et al. Time to treatment with intravenous alteplase and outcome in stroke: an updated pooled analysis of ECASS, ATLANTIS, NINDS, and EPITHET trials. Lancet (London, England). 2010;375(9727):1695–703.
24. Berkhemer OA, Fransen PS, Beumer D, van den Berg LA, Lingsma HF, Yoo AJ, et al. A randomized trial of intraarterial treatment for acute ischemic stroke. N Engl J Med. 2015;372(1):11–20.
25. Goyal M, Demchuk AM, Menon BK, Eesa M, Rempel JL, Thornton J, et al. Randomized assessment of rapid endovascular treatment of ischemic stroke. N Engl J Med. 2015;372(11):1019–30.
26. Campbell BC, Mitchell PJ, Kleinig TJ, Dewey HM, Churilov L, Yassi N, et al. Endovascular therapy for ischemic stroke with perfusion-imaging selection. N Engl J Med. 2015;372(11):1009–18.
27. Saver JL, Goyal M, Bonafe A, Diener HC, Levy EI, Pereira VM, et al. Stent-retriever thrombectomy after intravenous t-PA vs. t-PA alone in stroke. N Engl J Med. 2015;372(24):2285–95.
28. Brott T, Broderick J, Kothari R, Barsan W, Tomsick T, Sauerbeck L, et al. Early hemorrhage growth in patients with intracerebral hemorrhage. Stroke. 1997;28(1):1.
29. Flaherty M, Jauch E. Spot sign for predicting and treating ICH growth study (STOP-IT) [updated 6/2011]. Available from: http://clinicaltrials.gov/ct2/show/NCT00810888; NLM Identifier: NCT00810888.
30. Diringer MN, Edwards DF. Admission to a neurologic/neurosurgical intensive care unit is associated with reduced mortality rate after intracerebral hemorrhage. Crit Care Med. 2001;29(3):635–40.
31. Varelas PN, Schultz L, Conti M, Spanaki M, Genarrelli T, Hacein-Bey L. The impact of a neuro-intensivist on patients with stroke admitted to a neurosciences intensive care unit. Neurocrit Care. 2008;9(3):293–9.
32. Burns JD, Green DM, Lau H, Winter M, Koyfman F, DeFusco CM, et al. The effect of a neurocritical care service without a dedicated neuro-ICU on quality of care in intracerebral hemorrhage. Neurocrit Care. 2013;18(3):305–12.

33. Jaffe J, AlKhawam L, Du H, Tobin K, O'Leary J, Pollock G, et al. Outcome predictors and spectrum of treatment eligibility with prospective protocolized management of intracerebral hemorrhage. Neurosurgery. 2009;64(3):436–45; discussion 45–6.
34. Fleming TR, Powers JH. Biomarkers and surrogate endpoints in clinical trials. Stat Med. 2012;31(25):2973–84.
35. Albers GW, Bogousslavsky J, Bozik MA, Brass LM, Broderick JP, Fisher M, Goldstein LB, Salazar-Grueso E, Zivin JA, Akitsuki S, Aranko K, Ashwood T, Atkinson RP, Bell RD, Brott TG, Cady WJ, Caplan LR, Coggins S, Cramer S, Cyrus P, Dayno J, Donald Easton J, Elliott PJ, Finklestein SP, Furlan AJ, Gamzu E, Glasky MS, Gordon K, Gorelick PB, Greenwood DT, Grotta JC, Gunn K, Hachinski V, Hacke W, Hall ED, Hsu CY, Michael Humphreys D, Ishikawa H, Jacobs AJ, Kaste M, Koroshetz WJ, Krams M, Lauritano AA, Leclerc J, Lees KR, Lesko L, Levine SR, Levy DE, Li F, Lyden PD, Masayasu H, McDermott J, Meibach RC, Meya U, Miyairi K, Niidome T, Oeda J, Michael Poole R, Ron ES, Sacco RL, Saltarelli MD, Shimizu K, Shook BJ, Soehngen M, Soehngen W, Stamler DA, Styren SD, Teal PA, Tilley BC, Traystman RJ, Walker MD, Wallin BA, Warach S, Ward DP, Wessel TC, Wettstein J, Stroke Therapy Academic Industry Roundtable II (STAIR-II), Writing Committee. Recommendations for clinical trial evaluation of acute stroke therapies. Stroke. 2001;32(7):1598.
36. Saver JL, Gornbein J. Treatment effects for which shift or binary analyses are advantageous in acute stroke trials. Neurology. 2009;72(15):1310–5.
37. Stafinski T, Menon D, Nardelli A, Bakal J, Ezekowitz J, Tymchak W, et al. Incorporating patient preferences into clinical trial design: results of the opinions of patients on treatment implications of new studies (OPTIONS) project. Am Heart J. 2015;169(1):122–31.e22.
38. Kasner SE. Clinical interpretation and use of stroke scales. Lancet Neurol. 2006;5(7):603–12.
39. Qureshi AI, Palesch YY, Barsan WG, Hanley DF, Hsu CY, Martin RL, et al. Intensive blood-pressure lowering in patients with acute cerebral hemorrhage. N Engl J Med. 2016;375(11):1033–43.
40. Lyden PD, Shuaib A, Lees KR, Davalos A, Davis SM, Diener H-C, et al. Safety and tolerability of NXY-059 for acute intracerebral hemorrhage. Stroke. 2007;38(8):2262.
41. Baharoglu MI, Cordonnier C, Salman RA-S, de Gans K, Koopman MM, Brand A, et al. Platelet transfusion versus standard care after acute stroke due to spontaneous cerebral haemorrhage associated with antiplatelet therapy (PATCH): a randomised, open-label, phase 3 trial. Lancet. 2016;387(10038):2605–13.
42. Mendelow AD, Gregson BA, Fernandes HM, Murray GD, Teasdale GM, Hope DT, et al. Early surgery versus initial conservative treatment in patients with spontaneous supratentorial intracerebral haematomas in the international surgical trial in intracerebral haemorrhage (STICH): a randomised trial. Lancet (London, England). 2005;365(9457):387–97.
43. Mendelow AD, Gregson BA, Rowan EN, Murray GD, Gholkar A, Mitchell PM. Early surgery versus initial conservative treatment in patients with spontaneous supratentorial lobar intracerebral haematomas (STICH II): a randomised trial. Lancet. 2013;382(9890):397–408.
44. Hanley DF, CLEAR III Investigators. Clot lysis: evaluating accelerated resolution of intraventricular hemorrhage (CLEAR III) results. International stroke conference, 2016; Los Angeles California; Oral Abstract LB12. 2016.
45. Sangha N, Irani M, Peng H, Rahbar MH, Martinez R, Barreto AD, Savitz SI, Wu T, Lopez G, Misra V, Ifejika N, Grotta JC, Gonzales NR. Longitudinal assessment of functional outcome in intracerebral hemorrhage. European stroke conference, Lisbon. 2012(Abstract #330).
46. The Specifications Manual for Joint Commission National Quality Measures (Version 2016A1) is periodically updated by The Joint Commission.
47. Hemphill JC 3rd, Greenberg SM, Anderson CS, Becker K, Bendok BR, Cushman M, et al. Guidelines for the management of spontaneous intracerebral hemorrhage: a guideline for healthcare professionals from the American Heart Association/American Stroke Association. Stroke. 2015;46(7):2032–60.
48. Xi G, Keep RF, Hoff JT. Mechanisms of brain injury after intracerebral haemorrhage. Lancet Neurol. 2006;5(1):53–63.

49. Gonzales NR. Ongoing clinical trials in intracerebral hemorrhage. Stroke. 2013;44(6 suppl 1):S70.
50. Augustine EF, Dorsey ER, Hauser RA, Elm JJ, Tilley BC, Kieburtz KK. Communicating with participants during the conduct of multi-center clinical trials. Clinl Trials (London, England). 2016;13:592.
51. U.S. Department of Health and Human Services, Food and Drug Administration, Center for Drug Evaluation and Research (CDER), Center for Biologics Evaluation and Research (CBER). Guidance for industry: adaptive design clinical trials for drugs and biologics. 2010. www.fda.gov/downloads/Drugs/.../Guidances/ucm201790.pdf on 11/20/16.
52. Rahbar MH, Dickerson AS, Cai C, Pedroza C, Hessabi M, Shen L, et al. Methodological issues for designing and conducting a multicenter, international clinical trial in acute stroke: experience from ARTSS-2 trial. Contemp Clin Trials. 2015;44:139.
53. Connor JT, Broglio KR, Durkalski V, Meurer WJ, Johnston KC. The stroke hyperglycemia insulin network effort (SHINE) trial: an adaptive trial design case study. Trials. 2015;16:72.
54. Elkind MS, Sacco RL, Macarthur RB, Peerschke E, Neils G, Andrews H, et al. High-dose lovastatin for acute ischemic stroke: results of the phase I dose escalation neuroprotection with statin therapy for acute recovery trial (NeuSTART). Cerebrovasc Dis (Basel, Switzerland). 2009;28(3):266–75.
55. Gonzales NR, Shah J, Sangha N, Sosa L, Martinez R, Shen L, et al. Design of a prospective, dose-escalation study evaluating the safety of pioglitazone for hematoma resolution in intracerebral hemorrhage (SHRINC). Int J Stroke Off J Int Stroke Soc. 2013;8(5):388–96.
56. Fagan SC, Waller JL, Nichols FT, Edwards DJ, Pettigrew LC, Clark WM, et al. Minocycline to improve neurologic outcome in stroke (MINOS): a dose-finding study. Stroke. 2010;41(10):2283–7.
57. Grieve AP, Krams M. ASTIN: a Bayesian adaptive dose-response trial in acute stroke. Clin Trials, (London, England). 2005;2(4):340–51; discussion 52–8, 64–78.
58. Howard G. Nonconventional clinical trial designs: approaches to provide more precise estimates of treatment effects with a smaller sample size, but at a cost. Stroke. 2007;38(2 Suppl):804–8.
59. Holford NH, Kimko HC, Monteleone JP, Peck CC. Simulation of clinical trials. Annu Rev Pharmacol Toxicol. 2000;40:209–34.

Index

B. Ovbiagele, A. I. Qureshi (eds.), *Intracerebral Hemorrhage Therapeutics*,
https://doi.org/10.1007/978-3-319-77063-5